Optimizing the Management of Fertility in Women over 40

Optimizing the Management of Fertility in Women over 40

Edited by

Dimitrios S. Nikolaou
Chelsea & Westminster Hospital

David B. Seifer
Yale School of Medicine

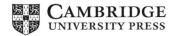

CAMBRIDGE
UNIVERSITY PRESS

CAMBRIDGE
UNIVERSITY PRESS

University Printing House, Cambridge CB2 8BS, United Kingdom

One Liberty Plaza, 20th Floor, New York, NY 10006, USA

477 Williamstown Road, Port Melbourne, VIC 3207, Australia

314–321, 3rd Floor, Plot 3, Splendor Forum, Jasola District Centre, New Delhi – 110025, India

103 Penang Road, #05–06/07, Visioncrest Commercial, Singapore 238467

Cambridge University Press is part of the University of Cambridge.

It furthers the University's mission by disseminating knowledge in the pursuit of education, learning, and research at the highest international levels of excellence.

www.cambridge.org
Information on this title: www.cambridge.org/9781316516829
DOI: 10.1017/9781009025270

First published 2022

Printed in the United Kingdom by TJ Books Limited, Padstow Cornwall

A catalogue record for this publication is available from the British Library.

ISBN 978-1-316-51682-9 Hardback

Dedication for **Dimitrios S. Nikolaou**:
To Egbert te Vede, Masoud Afnan and Nikos Kazantzakis
To my parents, Sotirios and Kyriaki, with infinite gratitude
for their sacrifices.
To my wife Dina, my companion and our 2 sons.
To my brother Vassilis.

Dedication for **David B. Seifer**
"May the love of my art inspire me at all times…" Maimonides

To the memory of my parents and to honor the members of my
family who have provided inspiration along my journey: my
mother, for her passion, intellectual curiosity and the pursuit of
knowledge; my father, for his mindset to challenge the norm
while being respectful of others; my brother for his quest of a
physical challenge and his embrace of the joy of life; my wife for
her commitment to excellence and her moral compass; and our
two wonderful sons for inspiring us to be the best versions of
ourselves and who are our legacy for the future.

Contents

Contributors

Paula Amato, MD

Division of Reproductive Endocrinology and Infertility, Department of Obstetrics and Gynecology Oregon Health & Science University, Portland, Oregon, USA

David H. Barad, MD, MS

The Center for Human Reproduction, New York, NY,USA The Foundation for Reproductive Medicine, New York, NY, USA

Éva Beaujouan

Wittgenstein Centre for Demography and Global Human Capital (IIASA, OeAW), University of Vienna, Vienna, Austria

Jennifer K. Blakemore, MD, MSc

Langone Fertility Center, New York University, New York, NY, USA

Pietro Bortoletto, MD

The Ronald O. Perelman and Claudia Cohen Center for Reproductive Medicine, Weill Cornell Medical College, New York, NY, USA

Timothy Bracewell-Milnes

Assisted Conception Unit, Chelsea and Westminster NHS Trust, London, UK

Beth Cartwright

Early Pregnancy Unit, Chelsea and Westminster Hospital, London, UK

Pritha Dasmahapatra, MBBS (Calcutta University), MRCOG

Chelsea & Westminster Hospital, London, UK

Shane Duffy, MB BS (Hons), DTM&H, DObst, DMEd, MSc, FRCOG

Chelsea & Westminster Hospital, London, UK

Norbert Gleicher, MD

The Center for Human Reproduction, New York, NY,USA The Foundation for Reproductive Medicine, New York, NY,USA Stem Cell Biology and Molecular Embryology Laboratory, The Rockefeller University, New York, NY,USA Department of Obstetrics and Gynecology, Medical University of Vienna, Austria

Tanya L. Glenn, MD

Division of Reproductive Endocrinology and Infertility, Department of Obstetrics, Gynecology, and Reproductive Sciences, Yale School of Medicine, New Haven, CT, USA

David L. Keefe, MD

Langone Fertility Center, New York University, New York, NY, USA

Alexandra Kermack

NIHR Clinical Lecturer/Registrar Obstetrics & Gynaecology School of Human Development and Health University of Southampton, UK

Winifred Mak, MD, PhD

Dell Medical School, University of Texas at Austin, TX, USA

Amir Mor, MD PhD

Division of Reproductive Endocrinology and Infertility, Department of Obstetrics, Gynecology, and Reproductive Sciences, Yale University School of Medicine, New Haven, CT, USA

Aditi Naik

Early Pregnancy Unit, Chelsea and Westminster Hospital, London, UK

Dimitrios S. Nikolaou, MD

Chelsea & Westminster Hospital, London, UK

Gwendolyn P. Quinn

Department of OB-GYN, Grossman School of Medicine, New York University, New York, NY, USA

Lauren Rouleau, MD, PhD

Department GynOb, Emory University, Atlanta, GA, USA

Vickie Schafer, PhD

Independent licensed psychologist

David B. Seifer, MD

Division of Reproductive Endocrinology and Infertility, Department of Obstetrics, Gynecology, and Reproductive Sciences, Yale School of Medicine, New Haven, CT, USA

Jacquelyn Shaw, MD

Langone Fertility Center, New York University, New York, NY, USA

Tomáš Sobotka

Wittgenstein Centre for Demography and Global Human Capital (IIASA, OeAW), University of Vienna, Vienna, Austria

Steven Spandorfer, MD

The Ronald O. Perelman and Claudia Cohen Center for Reproductive Medicine, Weill Cornell Medical College, New York, NY, USA

James P. Toner, MD, PhD

Emory Reproductive Center, Department GynOb, Emory University, Atlanta, GA, USA

Nicole Yoder, MD

Langone Fertility Center, New York University, New York, NY, USA

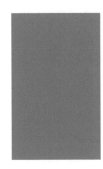

Introduction

Dimitrios S. Nikolaou and David B. Seifer

No one advises women to postpone childbearing until their 40s but a convergence of social, cultural, and economic factors over the last few decades has led to the expansion of this demographic of women who wish to conceive despite the odds. In most industrialized countries life expectancy continues to increase, in part due to advancing technology, better living conditions, and improved nutrition so many believe that the capacity to reproduce at a later age should follow. The topics in this book are in response to this growing population of women 40 plus seeking guidance and care from practitioners of reproductive medicine.

We have brought together a stellar group of international experts who diligently describe the best current evidence and their practice of treating women 40 and over who are trying to conceive. The table of contents includes chapters on demographic trends, contemporary insights from reproductive biology, optimal patient management, and support systems using patient experience architecture. Additional chapters include best practices in nutritional and preconceptional counseling, the most successful ART protocols and strategies as well as the most recent data on egg donation using fresh and frozen oocytes. Also included are chapters addressing optimal management of each stage of pregnancy, neonatal and long-term outcomes of children, ways to optimize these outcomes, and a discussion about the ethics of reproduction and fertility treatment in the 40 plus group. Rounding this off are sections on the discussion of emerging new reproductive technologies,

rethinking and redefining family planning, or "fertility planning" for the twenty-first century including the most recent data on ovarian reserve assessment.

This book is a call to arms for the medical and scientific community to fully collaborate to address unresolved clinical issues that will help this growing group of women. The maternal morbidity and mortality statistics in women over 40, especially over 45, are troubling. What can be done to improve the organized care of such women? The success rates of ART in the 40s have remained poor despite various advances in clinical and laboratory science. If the chance of success is low, what should the scope of management be and how can it be optimized? Infertility is a complex condition with physical, psychological, and social components. "Success" can have different meanings to different people in different contexts. For some it is a healthy baby. For others it may be the peace of mind that comes after "being heard" and having perhaps attempted some therapy. Even if it does not result in pregnancy, the therapeutic process may provide closure allowing one to move on with egg donation, child-free living, or the next meaningful chapter of their lives.

We want to thank our patients for their trust and love. They have been our inspiration. Also we thank our families, colleagues, teachers, and trainees for joining us on this journey. We are very grateful to Nick Dunton and Anna Whiting, of Cambridge University Press, who have been extremely supportive and a joy to work with.

Dimitrios S. Nikolaou, MD
David B. Seifer, MD

1

Is 40 the New 30? Increasing Reproductive Intentions and Fertility Rates beyond Age 40

Éva Beaujouan and Tomáš Sobotka

Introduction

Across the highly developed countries, reproduction trends of the last half a century are characterised by a continuous shift of parenthood towards more advanced reproductive ages [1–3]. The trend to later childbearing has been fuelled by a broad array of cultural and social changes such as higher education expansion, rise in gender equality and in women's employment, changes in partnership behaviour, rising economic uncertainty and shifts in family-related values and attitudes (e.g., [4]). Late reproduction has progressed hand in hand with a trend to a smaller family size, with two-child families becoming most prominent with respect to both fertility ideals and actual family size [5,6].

Initially, among women and men born in the 1950s and 1960s, later parenthood typically implied having children in their late 20s and early 30s rather than in their early- to mid-20s or in late teenage years. This trend was compatible with their desire to complete education and achieve relatively stable employment before starting a family, but also with their smaller family size preferences. Indeed, Habbema et al. [7] show that 90% of women intending to have two children and starting their pregnancy attempts around age 30 will eventually be able to reach their desired family size. Thus, for European women born between 1952 and 1972, later reproduction was not necessarily associated with lower fertility at a country level [8].

However, among the generations born in the 1970s and 1980s, many women were still childless in their mid-to-late 30s or even early 40s, and a substantial share still intended to have children [2,3]. This trend has potentially serious implications for women's and couples' fertility and well-being, and also for the future fertility rates across highly developed countries. Women planning pregnancies in later reproductive ages experience a rising risk of pregnancy complications, miscarriages and infer-

tility [9,10]. Therefore, many women postponing parenthood will not be able to realise their reproductive plans.

Highly educated women are at the forefront of delayed reproduction: level of education is closely related to later employment entry and parenthood postponement [11,12]. They also experience higher childlessness, although not everywhere: the Nordic countries saw the educational gradient in childlessness reverse, with lower-educated women now staying most often childless [13,14]. Highly educated women, who have invested in their career, face steeper opportunity costs of having children in terms of their potential loss of income and career interruption, especially in uncertain times or in countries where career is less compatible with parenthood. This may motivate them to postpone having children to minimise career disruption. On the other hand, findings from Finland and Sweden show that lower-educated women often have larger families, also because they are more likely to experience union disruption and 're-partnering' than the higher-educated women [15]. Union instability may thus motivate them to have another child at a more advanced age.

This chapter partly builds upon our earlier contributions on fertility and reproduction at more advanced reproductive ages, especially the study of Sobotka and Beaujouan (2018) [2]. We draw on vital statistics, register and survey data for European countries to outline the main trends in late reproduction, focussing on fertility plans and actual fertility rates among women past age 40. We pay special attention to education differences in late fertility and to trends in late reproduction among highly educated women. As data on late reproductive intentions and late fertility by education are not available for most countries, we illustrate the education stratification from survey and register data using examples from France, Norway and Great Britain. Given this limitation, our analysis of education differentials in late fertility may not be fully representative of other European countries.

Our chapter is structured as follows. First, we outline the key driving forces of the shift to delayed reproduction. Next, we highlight a rapid increase in late childbearing across Europe. We show that a rising share of women remaining childless or having only one child when reaching age 40 plan to have a child and, in turn, first and second birth rates past age 40 have been rising rapidly as well. We then discuss the role of medically assisted reproduction (MAR), which accounts for a rising share of late births. In conclusion, we argue that trends in childbearing past age 40 will become one of the critical factors determining the future of fertility and reproduction across the highly developed countries.

Background: How Do Current Social and Economic Trends Drive the Shift to Late Reproduction?

Historically, childbearing at late reproductive ages was widespread and associated with large families; many women continued having children until they became infertile [16,17]. An adoption of fertility-limiting behaviours in Europe, North America and Australia since the second half of the nineteenth century brought about a long-term decline in fertility rates among women aged 40 and older. In the 1980s, late fertility rates reached record low levels across the highly developed countries. As a result, late childbearing became relatively rare and irrelevant for the overall fertility levels [16].

The 'return' of late reproduction is linked to diverse social, economic, cultural and technological forces that made childbearing at more advanced reproductive ages both preferred and achievable (through widespread adoption of modern contraception and access to abortion) in most countries [4,18]. The 'gender revolution' – characterised by a broad rise in women's career aspirations, employment and non-family roles as well as the spread of gender egalitarian attitudes since the late 1960s (e.g., [19]) – was particularly important in that respect. In addition, major life course transitions closely linked to timing of parenthood, such as completion of education, residential

independence, transition to employment and union formation, shifted to later ages during the last half a century, contributing to delayed births (e.g., [20]). However, the key driver of delayed parenthood was the massive rise in higher education, which progressed fastest among women [21]. In contemporary societies participation in education is perceived as being incompatible with parenthood [22], with most people moving to live with a partner and having children only after completing education and establishing themselves in the labour market. Today, many young adults are enrolled in tertiary education into their late 20s; among the highly developed Organisation for Economic Co-operation and Development (OECD) countries, 16% of people aged 25–29 were still enrolled in education in 2018, and this share surpassed 25% in Denmark, Finland and Sweden [23].

Also, the interval between completing education and first birth has expanded considerably in the past decades [21]. This is partly explained by a changing labour market and, overall, a more precarious economic situation of young adults, especially since the global financial crisis around 2008–12. After completing their education, women and men often experience spells of unstable employment characterised by low pay, irregular work hours and time-limited contracts. Globalisation and skill-biased technological change have dampened wages and job opportunities, especially for male workers with middle and lower qualifications [24]. However, broader evidence suggests that young adults face economic headwinds across the board: in most economically developed countries, people in their 20s experienced deteriorating economic position and lower relative income in the 2000s and 2010s compared with previous generations [25]. Lower relative wages, student debts and skyrocketing housing prices, especially in bigger cities, contributed to this trend. Clark [26] demonstrated that age at first birth in the United States metropolitan areas is closely linked to housing costs for all education groups and race categories. In Europe, young adults face the most precarious economic situation in Southern Europe and in parts of Central and Eastern Europe: in these regions, many people aged 20–34 are 'NEETs', not in employment, education or training [27]. Prolonged education, unstable jobs and expensive housing translate into ever higher shares of young adults living with parents, a trend which also contributes to the ongoing delay in partnership formation and parenthood.

Later parenthood is also driven by long-term cultural and value changes typical of the 'second demographic transition' [28]. These include a decline in normative pressure related to having children, a stronger emphasis on individual autonomy and self-realisation, lower stability of partnerships and marriages, and higher standards and expectations placed on potential long-term partners. More women and men experience multiple partnerships before settling down and having children; women remaining childless at age 35 have often experienced relatively complex partnership trajectories [29]. Especially for the highly educated, parenthood becomes a carefully planned project and many experience difficulties in finding a partner when planning children. Having no partner clearly appears as a major obstacle in the realisation of fertility intentions later in life [29,30]. In East Asian societies, where marriage remains a precondition for childbearing, women increasingly postpone or avoid marriage due to the normative expectations about their parenthood and care responsibilities within marriage [31,32]. Delayed parenthood also results from subtle changes in the attitudes towards parenthood. Rotkirch [33], drawing from an example from Finland, argues that young adults have become more conflicted and ambiguous about parenthood, increasingly viewing it as a 'sacrifice' and stressing its potentially negative consequences, especially for climate change.

Although many explanations outlined above pertain especially to young adults, in combination they also explain why many women and men postpone childbearing into their late 30s or early 40s. Whether these presumably postponed births eventually take place or not is then closely related to the circumstances women encounter at these ages. Having a partner and feeling ready for parenthood play a central role [34]. The perception of the societal norms pertaining to childlessness and late childbearing also impacts the decision to have a child at a more advanced age [35,36]. Policies supporting combination of work and family life are of key importance for facilitating the decisions to have children at later ages, especially among higher-educated women [37,38]. Finally, cultural settings and norms influence availability of MAR and of alternative methods of conception as well as their actual use [39].

Increase in Childbearing Past Age 40 in All Countries and Across Education Groups

Fertility levels after age 40[1] have risen quickly across the highly developed countries during the last four decades [3]. In the 1980s, when late fertility rates were at record low levels across Europe, the share of the total fertility rate attributed to women aged 40+ ranged from 0.5% to 2% in most countries (Figure 1.1). The lowest values were reported in parts of Central and Eastern Europe (e.g., 0.4% in Czechia and 0.5% in Bulgaria) and the highest in Spain (3.2%) and Ireland (4.3%), where larger families were still common. Since then, late childbearing has become much more common: in 2018, births at age 40 and older accounted for 3% to 6% of the total fertility in most countries, with the highest values, around 7%, reported in Ireland, Italy and Spain. In the European Union as a whole, this share almost tripled from 1.6% in 1985 to 4.6% in 2018. Relative increase was fastest in countries with initially a very marginal share of late births, especially in Central and Eastern Europe. Increases in births taking place after age 45 were even faster, although starting from very low levels. For instance, the number of births in the European Union countries at extreme late reproductive ages of 50 and older jumped from 287 in 2002 to 1,554 in 2018 [40].

Generally, women with a degree are at the forefront of fertility postponement [41]. Late childbearing is also most common among them, as the example for Norway shows (Figure 1.2). Nonetheless, in Norway during the last 10 years, fertility at ages 40 and older has become more widespread among women across the whole education spectrum. In relative terms, late fertility in Norway increased fastest among lower-educated women, doubling from 2% to almost 4% from 2008 to 2018. This rise is likely linked to a rising selectivity of lower-educated women.

The profile of late fertility has transformed during the last half a century, from the dominance of larger families, where a majority of births at

---

[1] In this chapter, we refer to births and fertility rates among women aged 40 and older as 'late births', 'births at late reproductive ages', 'late childbearing' and 'late fertility'. These terms are used in a descriptive way, without implying normative judgement about preferred, optimal or appropriate age at motherhood.

5

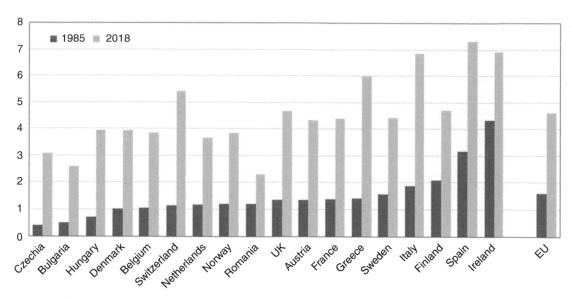

Figure 1.1 Share of fertility rates at ages 40+ on total fertility (in %) in selected European countries, 1985 and 2018 (countries ranked by late fertility rates in 1985).
Source: Own computations from Eurostat [40] database (Fertility rates by age [table demo_frate]).
Notes: EU data cover European Union in its 2018 boundaries, including the United Kingdom. Data for the EU in 1985 cover the EU in its boundary prior to 2005 and exclude Bulgaria, Croatia and Romania.

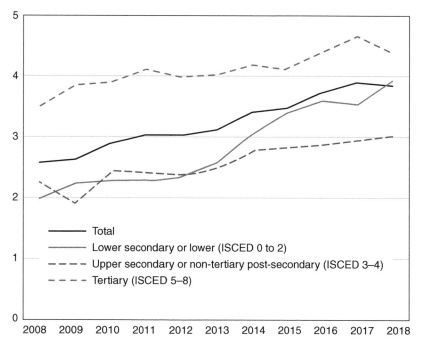

Figure 1.2 Share of fertility rates (%) at ages 40+ on total fertility rate by level of education in Norway, 2008–18.
Source: Own computation from Eurostat [40] database (live births by mother's age and educational attainment level [demo_faeduc] and population by age, sex and educational attainment [demo_pjanedu]).

ages 40+ were third or later births, to a dominance of first and second births among late mothers in most countries (Figure A1.1 in Appendix A). For instance, only 25% of births to mothers in the Netherlands aged 40 and older were first or second births in 1980, whereas fourth or later births accounted for 60% of all births. Almost four decades later the situation has reversed: in 2018, 62% of late births were first or second births and only 19% were fourth or higher-order births.

Fertility Intentions and Actual Fertility at Later Reproductive Ages: Sharpest Rise among Childless Women

In European countries, where most people favour having two children, trends in the share of women who do not have two children at age 40, in conjunction with their fertility intentions, give an important signal on the prospective 'demand' for late childbearing. The data reveal large cross-country diversity among European women in the evolution of childlessness and of having one child when reaching age 40 (Figure 1.3). Austria, the Netherlands and Sweden show only a modest rise in the share of women with fewer than two children, while Czechia and Spain depict a sharp and continuous increase in having no or one child among women born in the 1960s and 1970s. Southern European countries have high shares of childless women as well as of one-child mothers: for instance, in Spain, a majority (56%) of women born in 1978 had fewer than two children when reaching age 40, up from 38% among those born in 1960. The rise in the share of women with fewer than two children in late reproductive age is set to increase further among the women born past 1978: data for younger women aged 35 show a continuation of this trend, with 7 out of 10

Spanish women born in 1982 having fewer than two children by age 35. In most countries of Eastern and South-eastern Europe, including Romania, Russia and Ukraine, the share of women with fewer than two children at age 40 is also high, but in these countries one-child mothers clearly dominate this group and childlessness is less widespread.

As more women are having fewer than two children in their late 30s and early 40s, they often plan their first or second child later in life – often at ages when having children is becoming very uncertain or even unrealistic. Repeated surveys conducted in Great Britain show a sharp increase in reproductive intentions among women at more advanced reproductive ages: between 1979–84 and 2003–9, the share of childless women aged 35–39 intending to have a child jumped from 5% to 37% (Figure 1.4). A strong increase in parenthood intentions, although from a much lower level, is observed among women aged 40–42, many of whom are likely to experience infertility. A strong increase in fertility intentions is observed also among women with one child. Late fertility intentions have remained much less frequent among the mothers with two or more children. This pattern conforms to the widely shared two-child family norm across the highly developed countries [5]. Overall, planning children in late reproductive ages in Great Britain shifted from being a relatively

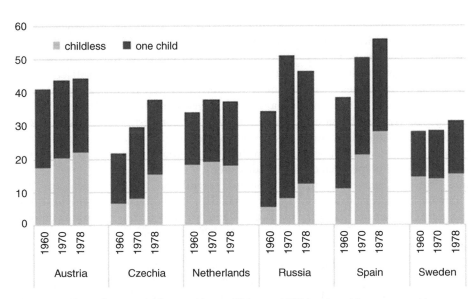

Figure 1.3 Share of women childless or with one child at age 40 (%) in selected European countries; women born in 1960, 1970 and 1978.
Source: Own computations from the Human Fertility Database (2021) [42].

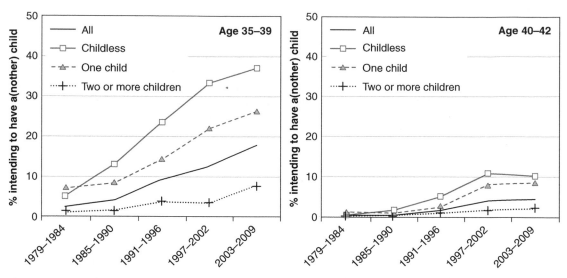

Figure 1.4 Share of women aged 35–39 and 40–42 who intend to have a child, by year and parity, Great Britain, 1979–2009.
Source: Own computations from the Centre for Population Change General Household Survey database [43].
Note: We use the question: 'Do you think that you will have any (more) children at all (after the one you are expecting)?'. Before 1991, possible answers were 'Yes', 'No' or 'Don't know'; from 1991, possible answers were 'Yes', 'Probably yes', 'Probably not', 'No', 'Don't know' (we group 'Yes' and 'Probably yes', which results in a series break in 1991). Proportions are calculated using survey weights [44]. Note that the total number of women observed over 30 surveys for this table is 12,729, and each proportion displayed is based on observations for more than 200 women.

marginal phenomenon to a rather common trend between the 1980s and 2000s.

The pattern observed in Great Britain is typical across the highly developed countries: reproductive plans at late childbearing ages have become strongly stratified by parity, with childless women planning to have a child most frequently, followed by those with one child, whereas a large majority of women with two or more children do not plan to have another child past age 40 [2]. However, considerable cross-country differences in the share of women planning a child after age 40 also illustrate many other factors influencing late fertility decisions: for instance, late childbearing intentions are most common among childless women in Western, Southern and Northern Europe, including Austria, Italy and France (Figure A1.2 in Appendix A). They remain less frequent across all parities in countries in Central and Eastern Europe, including Czechia and Poland, where the trend to delayed parenthood has started later than in other parts of Europe, during the 1990s [18,45].

Data for Great Britain illustrate the educational stratification in late childbearing intentions, which are most common among highly educated women (Table 1.1). Across all education groups few women aged 40–42 planned to have a(nother) child in the 1980s. However, their share increased steadily over time, and among highly educated women it reached almost 10% in 2003–9. This rising stratification was even more marked when selecting only women without a child or with one child (results not shown). More generally, in the late 2000s, highly educated women with no or one child were most likely to still wish a child at age 35–39 in Austria, France and Italy, countries where fertility postponement has been observed since the 1970s (Figure A1.3 in Appendix A). By contrast, there was no clear education differential in Czechia and Poland, where fertility postponement started about two decades later.

Because trends in fertility intentions are rarely available, it is difficult to generalise the upward trend in childbearing intentions among women with fewer than two children in late reproductive ages observed in Great Britain to other European countries. However, age-specific fertility trends by parity can be computed for a wider set of countries. They tend to mirror fertility intentions, although at a lower level, as many women who plan to have a child will not

Table 1.1 Share of women aged 40–42 who intend to have a(nother) child, by year and level of education, Great Britain, 1979–2009

	1979–84	1985–90	1991–6	1997–2002	2003–9
Low educated	0.5	0.5	1.5	2.9	3.3
Medium educated	0.8	0.4	2.1	3.8	4.0
High educated	–	2.8	2.8	8.5	9.5
All education levels	**0.5**	**0.6**	**1.7**	**4.1**	**4.6**

Source: see Figure 1.4.
Note: see Figure 1.4. The total number of women observed over 30 surveys for this table is 12,685, and each value in the table is based on observations for more than 200 women. Low education corresponds to ISCED 0–2, medium to ISCED 3–4 and high to ISCED 5–6 in the International Standard Classification of Education 1997.

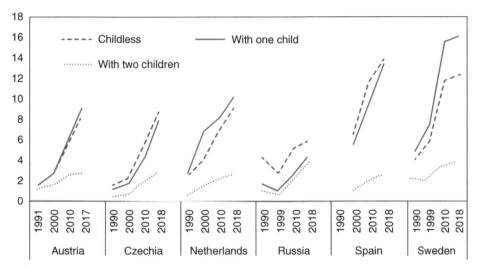

Figure 1.5 Share of women having a(nother) child past age 40 by parity status at age 40 (per 100 women of a given parity), selected European countries, 1990–2018.
Source: Own computations from the period fertility tables in the Human Fertility Database (2021).

realise their plans. Between 1990 and 2018, the likelihood of having (a)nother child past age 40 increased steeply among both childless women and women with one child (Figure 1.5). In both parity groups, late birth trends often moved in tandem, displaying almost identical levels in Austria, Czechia and Spain. Women with one child in the Netherlands and Sweden have a higher likelihood of having another child past age 40 compared with childless women, whereas the opposite pattern persists in Russia, where childlessness is less accepted, but women often have only one child. Except in Russia, there is a wide gap in the likelihood of having another child past age 40 between women with one and two children. In most countries, this gap has further widened over time, illustrating the continuing salience of a two-child family model and, generally, less frequent transition to a third birth across all ages.

Looking at late fertility by education gives additional insights on the mechanisms behind the rise in late first and second births. We use survey data for French women born in 1940–64, for whom we could reconstruct late birth trends by both parity and education (Table 1.2). Because the shift to delayed childbearing progressed relatively slowly in France, these women display only a gradual increase in childlessness at age 40. However, the data reveal a clear trend towards a higher share of women having their first or second child past age 40 and an emerging

9

Table 1.2 Share of women with no or one child at age 40, and share among them who have a child after age 40 (%), by level of education and year of birth, France (women born 1940–64)

	Education level	Share of women by number of children at age 40			Among them: share having a(nother) child past age 40		
		Year of birth			Year of birth		
		1940–4	1950–4	1960–4	1940–4	1950–4	1960–4
Childless	Lower	10.7	10.9	13.4	5.9	8.2	7.2
	Intermediate	11.9	12.9	13.4	4.5	7.4	8.3
	Higher	19.1	19.2	17.7	3.9	9.4	13.3
	All	**12.2**	**13.4**	**14.6**	**5.1**	**8.3**	**9.7**
With one child	Lower	17.4	18.6	17.4	2.7	3.8	7.4
	Intermediate	20.7	22.5	20.1	3.3	3.4	6.7
	Higher	19.6	19.1	17.7	7.2	7.7	11.9
	All	**18.7**	**20.2**	**18.7**	**3.5**	**4.4**	**8.2**

Source: Own computations from the French Survey on Family and Housing [46].
Notes: The total number of women observed for this table is 53,269, and each proportion displayed is based on observations for more than 300 women. Low education corresponds to ISCED 0–2, medium to ISCED 3–4 and high to ISCED 5–6 in the International Standard Classification of Education 1997.

education differentiation in this trend. Among women born in 1960–4, highly educated women with a degree stand out by displaying much higher likelihood of first birth past age 40 when compared with the women with both low and medium education.

Realising Fertility Intentions past Age 40: Impact of Infertility and of Age-Related Decline in Live Birth Rate Following IVF Treatments

As an ever higher number of women and couples are shifting their childbearing plans to late reproductive ages, the realisation of their fertility plans will increasingly rely on their access to MAR, its cost and on success rate of MAR at later ages. In vitro fertilisation using women's own fresh oocytes shows sharply declining success rates past age 40, with the majority of women not achieving live birth even after multiple treatment cycles [47,48]. In contrast to IVF with fresh oocytes, IVF using donor eggs or women's eggs cryopreserved at younger ages results in much higher live birth rates per treatment after age 40. However, many issues, including costs, legal regulations, ethical concerns, or – in the case of donor eggs – preference for own genetic offspring may limit the appeal of these methods for many women [49,50].

Despite these limitations, the use of MAR at later reproductive ages has been rising fast and MAR has contributed to a relatively high share of births and fertility rates above age 40 [51]. Many countries do not publish detailed and comparable data on MAR use and success rates by age. We therefore provide an illustration of the rising relevance of in vitro fertilisation for late fertility using detailed data for the United Kingdom, where the Human Fertilisation and Embryology Authority (HFEA) collects and publishes detailed data on assisted reproduction by age. Overall, the United Kingdom represents well broader European trends and has a similar share of IVF infants (2.7% in 2016) to the European average of 2.9% (table III in [52]).

In 2018 there were 13,617 IVF cycles in the UK among women aged 40 and older. This number compares with over 20,000 births among women aged 41 and older[2] and illustrates well the scope of unfulfilled 'demand' for children at later reproductive ages as well as the massive impact of infertility on limiting the realisation of late reproductive plans. Only one in six IVF cycles at ages 40+ resulted in live birth delivery. Despite this limited success rate, IVF contributed to a significant share of births and

---

[2] We relate IVF cycles at ages 40 and older to fertility rates lagged by 1 year, that is, among women aged 41 and older, to account crudely for the duration of pregnancy.

fertility rates at later reproductive ages. Our computations show that IVF accounted for 10.8% of live-born children among UK mothers at ages 41–43, 13.8% of children at ages 44–45 and over a quarter (25.3%) of children at ages 46 and older. This high share of IVF births at very late reproductive ages was achieved chiefly by use of donor oocytes. Our earlier analysis [53] showed that in the United States IVF – mostly using donor oocytes – contributed yet a higher share, 37.7%, of all live-born children among women aged 45 and older. As we illustrate in Figure A1.4 (Appendix A), the dominant role of IVF with donor eggs at very advanced reproductive ages is closely linked to the diverging trend with age in live birth rates between IVF treatments using women's own eggs and treatments using donor eggs. The former falls continuously to a low level of 6% at ages 43–44 and 4% thereafter, whereas live birth rates per IVF with donor eggs show a stable trend with age and remain at 30% even among women aged 45 and older.

Despite the rise in the number of IVF births at later reproductive ages and a gradual increase in the use of donor eggs and egg freezing, age remains a strong barrier to realising reproductive intentions. The analysis of reproductive intentions in Austria revealed that among women (but not among men) there was a steep decline in the share realising their fertility plans within 4 years past age 34 and a corresponding rise in the share of women giving up their fertility intentions: at ages 38–41, only 24% of women strongly intending a child realised their plans compared with 52% of men aged 38–45 and around 70% of women below age 35 [54]. The observed decline in the likelihood of realising fertility intentions with age among women follows the curve of declining physiological capacity to have a child (i.e., getting pregnant and carrying pregnancy to term) as estimated by Leridon [55]. However, the fall in the realisation of reproductive plans with age is steeper and the gap between the capacity to reproduce and the actual realisation of certain short-term fertility intentions widens among women past age 34, also on the new example of Austria (Figure 1.6). This might be due to a combination

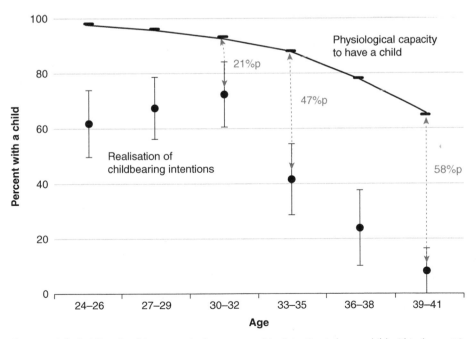

Figure 1.6 Probability of realising a certain short-term positive intention to have a child within the next 3 years among women in Austria and estimated curve of physiological capacity to have a child by age.
Sources and notes: Austrian Generations and Gender Survey [59] waves 2008–9 and follow-up 2012–13. Women were asked about their fertility intentions in the first wave and for the number of children they had between the waves in the second wave. See Beaujouan [60] for details on reconstructing the data on intentions realisation. The figure displays 95% confidence intervals, results are weighted with survey weights. The curve of physiological capacity to have a child is based on Leridon's estimates (table I, [61]).

of age-related biological and health factors (including longer waiting time to conception and more pregnancy complications), health limitations, less frequent sexual intercourse with union duration [56], but also personal circumstances (not having a partner, feeling too old for parenthood) that negatively impact the capacity realisation of fertility intentions at later reproductive ages [30,57,58].

Discussion: Is 40 the New 30? The Growing Importance of Late Fertility for the Realisation of Individual Reproductive Plans and for Future Fertility Rates

Age-related rise in infertility and the onset of menopause continue to impose a strong barrier to reproduction past age 40. In addition, as recently as in 2006–7 a majority of respondents in Europe perceived age 40 as a normative age deadline, after which women were considered too old for having children [61]. Our study of trends in late reproduction suggests that this barrier is being eroded by multiple forces. Reproduction is increasingly shifted to a 'grey zone', towards late 30s and early 40s, when most women can still achieve a pregnancy, but also face rising infertility, rising chance of miscarriage and pregnancy complications and overall declining chances of realising their reproductive plans [7].

Decades of a continuing trend to delayed parenthood have resulted in a growing share of women aged 35 and older who remain childless or have one child. In conjunction, surveys of reproductive intentions reveal that a rising number of these women plan to have a child at a more advanced reproductive age, often seemingly oblivious to the risk of infertility and the limited success rates of in vitro fertilisation above age 40 (e.g., [62]). Fertility rates past age 40 have been rising rapidly in most parts of Europe since the 1980s–90s. In the past decade, when overall fertility rates fell in most countries in Europe, women around age 40 and older were often the only group with increasing fertility; this was the case, for instance, in Sweden and Denmark [63]. The profile of late fertility has shifted, with a typical 'late mother' now having her first or second child rather than adding one last birth to a larger family, as was typical in the past.

Biological age limits to motherhood are gradually being redrawn as more women use donor eggs to get pregnant in their mid- or late 40s and a rising number of women have been freezing their eggs. Those might later be thawed and used at ages which were in the past considered to be 'post-reproductive'. Correspondingly, the number of births to women in their late 40s and even 50s has been rising fast across Europe, although from a very low initial base. Continuous childbearing postponement is also eroding the normative age deadlines to parenthood. Verweij et al. [64] show that in the Netherlands the desired age of becoming a parent has increased over time, and this increase is partly driven by many people not having children by their initially desired age and, subsequently, updating their desired age for parenthood upwards.

Women with a degree lead the trend toward late reproduction. They take longer to establish themselves in the labour market and find a partner and they have most to lose in terms of their career, wages and employment if they start a family earlier in life [65,66]. Selected data on education-specific patterns in late reproduction in Europe, which we presented in this chapter, indeed show that highly educated women are more likely to plan having their first or second child at around age 40 and to actually realise these plans when compared with their lower-educated counterparts. By contrast, women with a lower education attainment more often follow the 'traditional' pathway of late reproduction, having their third or later child at ages 40 and older. More of them have a larger family, but they also experience more frequent partnership dissolution and complex partnership trajectories, with some having another child with a new partner at late reproductive age [15].

There is considerable diversity in this broadbrush picture across Europe, with Southern European countries displaying the most pronounced pattern of delayed reproduction and countries in Central and Eastern Europe generally showing fewer women having children past age 40. Nonetheless, the basic contours of the trends in late reproduction sketched out here hold across different parts of Europe. The shifts we have discussed are set to continue, or even accelerate in the future. Late reproduction may become one of the defining social trends in the highly developed countries. In most countries, the Millennials born in the 1980s–early 1990s had fewer children in their 20s and 30s than any of the previous generations. All the social and cultural forces that have driven the shift to delayed parenthood – from the massive spread of university education and the 'gender revolution' in women's roles through the rise of employment uncertainty and the shortage of affordable housing up to the changes in partnerships and more ambiguous attitudes towards parenthood – continue affecting the lives of Millennials and also of the younger members of Generation Z born past 1995. The COVID-19 pandemic and its repercussions, including limits to social contacts, family stress and the looming economic and labour market costs, is likely to further speed up the trend to delayed reproduction. The clash between the social and cultural 'motivation' to postpone reproduction to ever later ages and the biological rationale for having children earlier in life [67] will further intensify.

What are the likely long-term consequences of the future rise in late reproduction? We can foresee significant individual costs and repercussions, especially in the form of more pregnancy complications, miscarriages and higher psychological and monetary costs of infertility treatments in later reproductive ages. Fertility plans of many women and couples will not be realised, and more of them will remain involuntary childless. In addition, postponement of parenthood to late reproductive ages narrows the space couples have to flexibly respond to changing life events and circumstances: they may not have extra time left for additional postponement of childbearing if they encounter health problems, partnership breakup or if they lose their job. In contrast, some positive consequences include lower income loss, higher family stability and more engaged and mature parenting practices [2]. At a societal level, late reproduction will be responsible for a higher share of total fertility, likely to increase from the current range of 2–7% to well above 10% during the next two decades. Medically assisted reproduction will take an ever more important role in helping women and couples to achieve their fertility plans later in life and will also increasingly contribute to future fertility trends. Egg freezing technology may take off on a grander scale, but this might also create new inequalities between women who can afford it and the others, who will be left out.

Societal costs of late reproduction will include smaller families due to later start of parenthood and rising infertility due to unfulfilled fertility plans among the 'intended' late parents. The societal-level fertility postponement is likely to become an important factor depressing fertility rates in Europe and other highly developed regions as more of the postponed births will turn into births foregone. The confluence of societal conditions favouring late reproduction and individual obstacles to realising these fertility plans may become a powerful drag on future fertility rates especially among highly educated women and in less family-friendly societies.

Acknowledgements

Eva Beaujouan's contribution was funded by the Austrian Science Fund (FWF), project 'Later Fertility in Europe' (Grant agreement no. P31171-G29); The Office for National Statistics provided access to the British General Household Survey series (originally constructed by the ESRC Centre for Population Change).

Appendix A

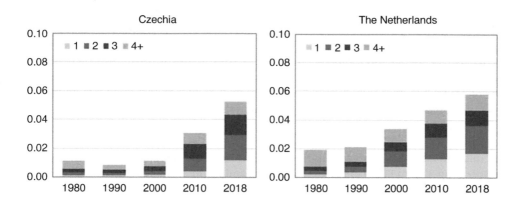

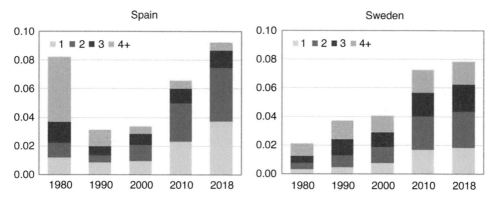

Figure A1.1 Cumulative fertility rates at ages 40+ by birth order, selected European countries, 1980–2018.
Source: Computations based on Human Fertility Database [42]: data on period and cohort fertility rates by age and birth order, period fertility tables by age and parity.

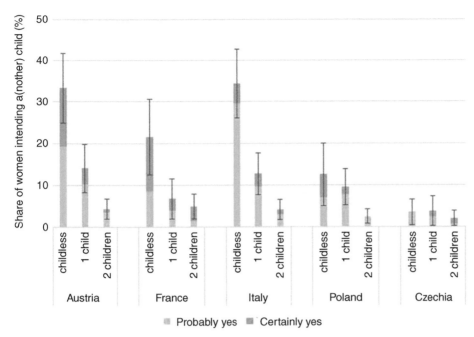

Figure A1.2 Share of women aged 40–44 who intend to have a child, by year and parity, selected European countries, 2005–11.
Source: Generations and Gender Surveys [58], first wave collected between 2005 and 2011 depending on the country.
Note: Figure displays 95% confidence intervals, results are weighted with survey weights.

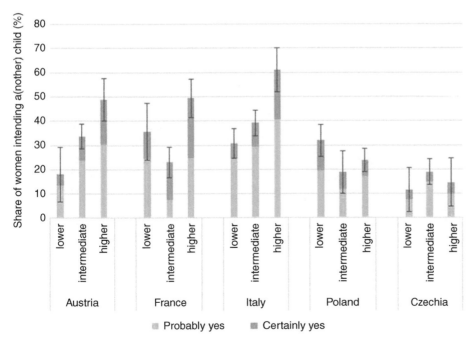

Figure A1.3 Share of women aged 35–44 with no or one child who intend to have a child, by level of education; selected countries in Europe.
Source and notes: see Figure A1.2. Low education corresponds to ISCED 0–2, medium education to ISCED 3–4, and high education to ISCED 5–6 in the International Standard Classification of Education 1997.

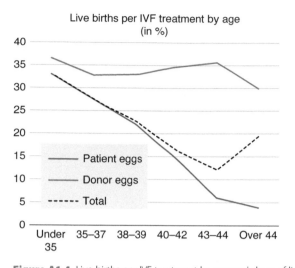
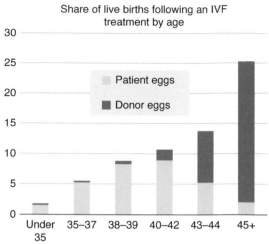

Figure A1.4 Live births per IVF treatment by age and share of live births following in vitro fertilisation by age, United Kingdom, 2018.
Source: Computations based on IVF data published by HFEA [68] and data on live births by age in the Human Fertility database (2021).

References

1. Kohler H-P, Billari FC, Ortega JA. The emergence of lowest-low fertility in Europe during the 1990s. Popul Dev Rev 2002;**28**(4):641–80. DOI http://dx.doi.org/10.1111/j.1728-4457.2002.00641.x

2. Sobotka T, Beaujouan É. Late motherhood in low-fertility countries: reproductive intentions, trends and consequences. In: Stoop D, ed., *Preventing age related fertility loss* (Switzerland: Springer International Publishing, 2018) pp. 11–29.

3. Beaujouan É. Latest-late fertility? Decline and resurgence of late parenthood across the low-fertility countries. Popul Dev Rev 2020;**46**(2):219–47. DOI https://onlinelibrary.wiley.com/doi/10.1111/padr.12334

4. Mills MC, Rindfuss RR, Mcdonald P, Velde ET, Force ERST. Why do people postpone parenthood? Reasons and social policy incentives. Hum Reprod Update 2011;**17**(6):848–60.

5. Sobotka T, Beaujouan É. Two is best? The persistence of a two-child family ideal in Europe. Popul Dev Rev 2014;**40**(3):391–419. DOI http://onlinelibrary.wiley.com/doi/10.1111/j.1728-4457.2014.00691.x/abstract

6. Frejka T. Parity distribution and completed family size in Europe: Incipient decline of the two-child family model? Demogr Res (Special Collect 7) 2008;**19**(4):47–72.

7. Habbema JDF, Eijkemans MJC, Leridon H, te Velde ER. Realizing a desired family size: When

should couples start? Hum Reprod 2015;**30**(9):2215–21. DOI http://doi.org/10.1093/humrep/dev148

8. Beaujouan É, Toulemon L. European countries with delayed childbearing are not those with lower fertility. Genus 2021;**77**(2).

9. Menken JA, Trussell J, Larsen U. Age and infertility. Science 1986;**233**(4771):1389–93.

10. Schmidt L, Sobotka T, Bentzen JG, Nyboe Andersen A-M. Demographic and medical consequences of the postponement of parenthood. Hum Reprod Update 2012;**18**(1):29–43. DOI http://doi.org/10.1093/humupd/dmr040

11. Ní Bhrolcháin M, Beaujouan É. Fertility postponement is largely due to rising educational enrolment. Popul Stud (NY) 2012;**66**(3):311–27. DOI http://dx.doi.org/10.1080/00324728.2012.697569

12. Nicoletti C, Tanturri ML. Differences in delaying motherhood across European countries: Empirical evidence from the ECHP. Eur J Popul / Rev Eur Démographie 2008;**24**(2):157–83.

13. Beaujouan É, Brzozowska Z, Zeman K. The limited effect of increasing educational attainment on childlessness trends in twentieth-century Europe, women born 1916–65. Popul Stud (NY) 2016;**70**(3):275–91. DOI https://www.tandfonline.com/doi/full/10.1080/00324728.2016.1206210

14. Jalovaara M, Neyer G, Andersson G, Dahlberg J, Dommermuth L, Fallesen P, et al. Education, gender, and cohort fertility in the Nordic countries. Eur J Popul 2019;**35**:563–86. DOI https://doi.org/10.1007/s10680-018-9492-2

15. Jalovaara M, Andersson L, Miettinen A. Parity disparity: Educational differences in Nordic fertility across parities and number of reproductive partners. Popul Stud (Camb) 2021; DOI http://doi.org/10.1080/00324728.2021.1887506

16. Prioux F. Late fertility in Europe: some comparative and historical data. Rev Epidemiol Sante Publique 2005;53 **Spec No 2**:3–12.

17. Billari FC, Kohler H-P, Andersson G, Lundström H. Approaching the limit: Long-term trends in late and very late fertility. Popul Dev Rev 2007;33(1):149–70.

18. Sobotka T. Postponement of childbearing and low fertility in Europe. PhD thesis, University of Groningen. (Amsterdam: Dutch University Press, 2004).

19. Goldin C. The quiet revolution that transformed women's employment, education, and family. Am Econ Rev 2006;96(2):1–21.

20. Guzzo KB, Hayford SR. Pathways to parenthood in social and family contexts: decade in review, 2020. J Marriage Fam 2020;82(1):117–44.

21. Neels K, Murphy M, Ní Bhrolcháin M, Beaujouan É. Rising educational participation and the trend to later childbearing. Popul Dev Rev 2017;43(4):667–93. DOI http://doi.wiley.com/10.1111/padr.12112

22. Blossfeld H, Huinink J. Human capital investments or norms of role transition? How women's schooling and career affect the process of family formation. Am J Sociol 1991;97 (1):143–68.

23. Organisation for Economic Co-operation and Development (OECD). Education at a glance 2020. 2020; DOI https://doi.org/10.1787/69096873-en

24. Adserà A. Education and fertility in the context of rising inequality. Vienna Yearb Popul Res 2017;15:63–92.

25. Rahman F, Tomlinson D. (2018). Cross countries: international comparisons of intergenerational trends. Resolution Foundation. www.resolutionfoundation.org/publications/cross-countries-international-comparisons-of-intergenerational-trends/

26. Clark WAV. Do women delay family formation in expensive housing markets? Demogr Res 2012;27 (1):1–24.

27. Eurostat. (2020). Statistics on young people neither in employment nor in education or training. Eurostat. https://ec.europa.eu/eurostat/statistics-explained/index.php/Statistics_on_young_people_neither_in_employment_nor_in_education_or_training

28. Lesthaeghe RJ. The unfolding story of the second demographic transition. Popul Dev Rev 2010;36 (2):211–51.

29. Mikolai J. Partnership histories and the transition to motherhood in later reproductive ages in Europe. Population 2017;72(1):123–54.

30. Wagner M, Huinink J, Liefbroer AC. Running out of time? Understanding the consequences of the biological clock for the dynamics of fertility intentions and union formation. Demogr Res 2019;40:1–26. DOI 10.4054/DemRes.2019.40.1

31. Raymo JM, Park H, Xie Y, Yeung WJ. Marriage and family in East Asia: continuity and change. Annu Rev Sociol 2015;41:471–92. DOI http://doi.org/10.1146/annurev-soc-073014-112428

32. Cheng YA. Ultra-low fertility in East Asia : Confucianism and its discontents. Vienna Yearb Popul Res 2020;18: 83–120. DOI http://doi.org/10.1553/populationyearbook2020.rev01

33. Rotkirch A. The wish for a child. Vienna Yearb Popul Res 2020;18:49–61. DOI http://doi.org/10.1553/populationyearbook2020.deb05

34. Buber-Ennser I, Fliegenschnee K. Being ready for a child: a mixed-methods investigation of fertility intentions. Fam Sci 2013;4(1):139–47. DOI www.tandfonline.com/doi/abs/10.1080/19424620.2013.871739

35. Liefbroer AC, Billari FC. Bringing norms back in: a theoretical and empirical discussion of their importance for understanding demographic behaviour. Popul Sp Place 2010;16(4):287–305.

36. Mynarska M. Deadline for Parenthood: Fertility Postponement and Age Norms in Poland. Eur J Popul / Rev Eur Démographie 2009;26(3):351–73. DOI http://doi.org/10.1007/s10680-009-9194-x

37. Thévenon O, Gauthier AH. Family policies in developed countries: A "fertility-booster" with side-effects. Community Work Fam 2011;14 (2):197–216.

38. OECD. Doing better for families. OECD Publishing; 2011. ISBN No: 978-92-64-09872-5.

39. Präg P, Mills MC. Cultural determinants influence assisted reproduction usage in Europe more than economic and demographic factors. Hum Reprod 2017;32(11):2305–14.

40. Eurostat. (2021). Eurostat online database. Eurostat. http://ec.europa.eu/eurostat/data/database

41. Rendall MS, Aracil E, Bagavos C, Couet C, De Rose A, Di Giulio P, et al. Increasingly heterogeneous ages at first birth by education in Southern European and Anglo-American family-policy regimes: a seven-country comparison by birth cohort. Popul Stud (NY) 2010;64(3):209–27. DOI http://doi.org/10.1080/00324728.2010.512392

42. Max Planck Institute for Demographic Research (Germany) and Vienna Institute of Demography

(Austria). (2021) Human Fertility Database; www .humanfertility.org

43. Beaujouan É, Ní Bhrolcháin M, Berrington A, Falkingham J. (2015). Centre for Population Change General Household Survey Database, 1979–2009: Special Licence Access. UK Data Service. http://discover.ukdataservice.ac.uk/ catalogue?sn=7666

44. Beaujouan É, Brown JJ, Ní Bhrolcháin M. Reweighting the General Household Survey 1979–2007. Popul Trends 2011;**145**:115–41. http://doi .org/DOI 10.1057/pt.2011.21

45. Frejka T, Sardon J-P. First birth trends in developed countries: persistent parenthood postponement. Demogr Res 2006;**15**:147–80.

46. INSEE. (2011) Survey on family and housing. INSEE. www.insee.fr/en/metadonnees/source/serie/s1233

47. Gnoth C, Maxrath B, Skonieczny T, Friol K, Godehardt E, Tigges J. Final ART success rates: a 10 years survey. Hum Reprod 2011;**26**(8):2239–46.

48. Luke B, Brown MB, Wantman E, Lederman A, Gibbons W, Schattman GL, et al. Cumulative birth rates with linked assisted reproductive technology cycles. N Engl J Med 2012;**366**:2483–91.

49. Becker G. The elusive embryo: how women and men approach new reproductive technologies. (Berkeley: University of California Press; 2000).

50. Friese C, Becker G, Nachtigall RD. Rethinking the biological clock: eleventh-hour moms, miracle moms and meanings of age-related infertility. Soc Sci Med 2006;**63**(6):1550–60.

51. Präg P, Mills MC, Tanturri ML, Monden C, Pison G. The demographic consequences of assisted reproductive technologies. SocArXiv 2017; DOI http://doi.org/10.31235/osf.io/su49v

52. Wyns C, Bergh C, Calhaz-Jorge C, De Geyter C, Kupka MS, Motrenko T, et al. ART in Europe, 2016: results generated from European registries by ESHRE. *Hum Reprod Open* 2021;**3**:hoab026. DOI http://doi.org/10 .1093/hropen/hoab026

53. Beaujouan É, Sobotka T. Late childbearing continues to increase in developed countries. Popul Soc 2019;**562**(1):1–4.

54. Beaujouan É, Reimondos A, Gray E, Evans A, Sobotka T. Declining realisation of reproductive intentions with age. Hum Reprod 2019;**34**(10):1906–14. https://doi.org/10.1093/humrep/dez150/5575324

55. Leridon H. Can assisted reproduction technology compensate for the natural decline in fertility with age? A model assessment. Hum Reprod 2004;**19** (7):1548–53. DOI http://doi.org/10.1093/humrep/ deh304.

56. Frank O, Bianchi PG, Campana A. The end of fertility – age, fecundity and fecundability in women. J Biosoc Sci 1994;**26**(3):349–68.

57. Towner MC, Nenko I, Walton SE. Why do women stop reproducing before menopause? A life-history approach to age at last birth. Philos Trans R Soc B Biol Sci 2016;**371**(1692):20150147.

58. Settersten RA, Hägestag GO. What's the latest? Cultural age deadlines for family transitions. Gerontologist 1996;**36**(2):178–88.

59. GGP. (2021) Generations & Gender Programme. GGP. https://www.ggp-i.org/

60. Beaujouan É. Late fertility intentions and fertility in Austria. *Vienna Institute of Demography Working Papers, No. 06/2018* (Vienna: Austrian Academy of Sciences (ÖAW), Vienna Institute of Demography (VID), 2018). http://dx.doi.org/ 10.1553/0x003ccd3c

61. Billari FC, Goisis A, Liefbroer AC, Settersten RA, Aassve A, Hagestad GO, et al. Social age deadlines for the childbearing of women and men. Hum Reprod 2011;**26**(3):616–22. DOI http://doi.org/10 .1093/humrep/deq360.

62. Wyndham N, Marin Figueira PG, Patrizio P. A persistent misperception: assisted reproductive technology can reverse the "aged biological clock. Fertil Steril 2012;**97**(5):1044–7. DOI http://dx .doi.org/10.1016/j.fertnstert.2012.02.015

63. Hellstrand J, Nisén J, Miranda V, Fallesen P, Dommermuth L, Myrskylä M. Not just later, but fewer: novel trends in cohort fertility in the Nordic countries. *MPIDR Working Paper* 2020;WP 2020–007. https://doi.org/10.4054/MPIDR-WP-2020-007

64. Verweij R, Mills M, Snieder H, Stulp G. Three facets of planning and postponement of parenthood in the Netherlands. Demogr Res 2020;**43**(September):659–72.

65. Miller AR. The effects of motherhood timing on career path. J Popul Econ 2011;**24**(3):1071–100.

66. Bratti M, Cavalli L. Delayed first birth and new mothers' labor market outcomes: evidence from biological fertility shocks. Eur J Popul 2014;**30** (1):35–63.

67. Sobotka T. Shifting parenthood to advanced reproductive ages: trends, causes and consequences. In: A young generation under pressure? (Springer Berlin / Heidelberg; 2010) pp. 129–54.

68. HFEA. (2020) Information on Fertility treatments 2018: trends and figures. Human Fertilisation and Embryology Authority. www .hfea.gov.uk/about-us/publications/research-and-data/fertility-treatment-2018-trends-and-figures/

2

Biological Basis of Female Reproductive Aging: What Happens to the Ovaries and Uterus as They Age?

Jacquelyn Shaw, Jennifer K. Blakemore, and David L. Keefe

Introduction

The impact of age on female fecundability is well known [1,2]. As the number of women in the workforce continues to grow, the number delaying childbearing is climbing simultaneously [3]. Thus, more women than ever experience the difficulties of reproductive aging and age-related fertility decline. Aging has extensive effects on reproduction in women. Perhaps its most recognized effect is loss of oocytes via atresia, resulting in diminishing ovarian reserve over the course of a woman's lifetime [4,5]. However, the process of reproductive aging supersedes just declining number of oocytes. Oocyte developmental competence declines with age, reflected in decreased implantation rates, increased miscarriage rates, and marked genomic instability [6], as depicted in Figure 2.1. Age-related decreases in fecundity traditionally were attributed to aneuploidy, but oocyte aging is accompanied by a host of other cellular effects, including mitochondrial DNA mutations, cellular fragmentation, and cell cycle arrest in embryos. The molecular and cellular basis of these remain poorly understood [7]. Fertility decreases throughout the life of the woman, even while the ovary contains primordial follicles. Indeed, the average age of last child occurs roughly 10 years prior to menopause [8].

Age-related subfertility is a major contributor to reproductive success in couples trying to conceive, but may show subtle if any signs or symptoms [8]. The lack of overt symptomology and the lack of patient appreciation of reproductive aging [9] contributes to a high rate of unintended childlessness, even with the assistance of fertility treatment and assisted reproductive technology (ART).

Aging affects all tissues, including reproductive tissues, but the ovary is especially susceptible to its effects. The ovary is a complex organ comprising follicles, stroma, blood vessels, and nerves. Each follicle contains a single oocyte. The oocyte must be the locus of reproductive aging because donation of oocytes from younger women abrogates the effects of reproductive aging on recipients. The oocyte is a single, long-lived cell, uniquely susceptible to aging, so studies of its biology should bring insights into the fundamental mechanisms of aging.

Reciprocal nuclear transfer between oocytes from older and younger females enabled further localization of the aging effect into the nucleus [10], consistent with extensive data supporting a central role for aneuploidy in reproductive aging. Elucidation of the mechanisms underlying aneuploidy is an urgent priority. The follicular microenvironment [11], cumulus-oophorus complex, granulosa cells, gap junctions, and gonadotropin receptors are all required for developmental competence. Presumably, each of these could unravel with age. Moreover, once a healthy blastocyst forms, the uterine environment must additionally be suitable for implantation. Several studies have highlighted that implantation rates improve when a donor oocyte is utilized, circumventing the age effect on the egg [12]. However, increased risks and poor obstetrical outcomes are still seen in pregnancies of women with advanced maternal age [13] – suggesting that the uterus and/or the endometrium may also contribute to reproductive aging.

In this chapter we review the major theories of female reproductive aging. First, we will examine the principal mechanisms underlying oocyte aging, which include chiasmata formation, cohesin defects, telomere attrition, reactive oxygen species and mitochondria, alterations in blood flow, and the production line. We also will evaluate promising new theories for oocyte and/or ovarian aging including amyloid-like substance infiltration, sirtuins, and possible protection by resveratrol. The second section of the chapter

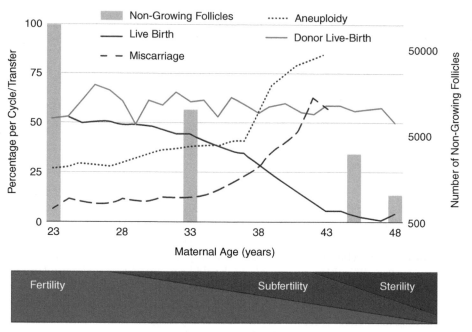

Figure 2.1 Characteristics of age-related fertility decline in patients of fertility centers in the United States. With advanced maternal age, the number of follicles available for recruitment declines. In addition, the quality of oocytes is reduced, as demonstrated by exponentially decreased ongoing pregnancy rates and increased risk of aneuploid embryos and miscarriage. Modified from CDC, SART 2012–13. Figure reprinted from original article [8] with permission.

will highlight some of the important signs of uterine aging seen in animal models as well as the adverse obstetric outcomes seen in women of advanced maternal age despite use of a "young oocyte." We conclude by summarizing the evidence for the aging female reproductive tract and the importance of continuing research to further our understanding of the impacts of age on reproduction.

Theories of Ovarian Aging

Maternal age is the best predictor of oocyte and embryo developmental capacity. Mammalian oocytes halt oogenesis before the birth of the girl, at about 20 weeks' gestation. Primordial follicles contain oocytes arrested at the diplotene stage of the first meiotic division, and remain in a state of partial metabolic quiescence throughout the reproductive lifespan – upward to 50 years [14,15]. The known sharp decline in fertility with age takes place while primordial follicles remain in the ovary, and manifests as decreasing oocyte developmental competence [16].

Maternal age predisposes to meiotic nondisjunction and embryonic aneuploidy [17]. How does the predilection for aneuploidy increase with age?

Chiasmata Formation

Within the oocyte, the nucleus is more sensitive to aging than the cytoplasm or mitochondria [10]. Nuclear factors must be examined individually, including meiotic spindles and chromosomes. It is estimated that 80% of meiotic aneuploidies are of maternal origin, with 30–80% of oocytes from women of all ages containing a detectable genetic abnormality, compared with less than 10% of mature sperm [15]. The majority of maternal nondisjunction arises during meiosis I [15]. Older oocytes more commonly have meiotic spindle abnormalities with defects in chromosome alignment, as well as spindle structure and architecture [18]. Spindles from oocytes of older women lose symmetry and microtubule density. Chiasmata are the physical sites of chromosome recombination during meiosis and they play essential roles in chromosome segregations. They ensure proper chromosome segregation by countering the spindle pulling forces [19,20]. The number and location of chiasmata along the chromosome play an essential role in preventing nondisjunction; too many or few cause errors in chromosomal number [15,21], as is seen in upwards of 80% of oocytes from women over 40 years old [8].

Cohesin Defects

Cohesins hold sister chromatids together during meiosis and mitosis, facilitating segregation of homologous chromosome pairs during meiosis I in reproduction. Disruptions of meiotic cohesins increase with age [22,23]. The consequences of cohesin defects are high rates of premature sister chromatid separation, seen with oocytes from older females [24]. Oocytes from an aging mouse model show reduction in cohesins with age [25]. Experimental depletion of cohesin subunit Smc1beta in a mouse model progressively disrupts chromosomal integrity during prophase [26]. Mice deficient in REC8 cohesin are sterile, lacking oocytes at birth [27], further highlighting the essential role of functioning cohesins in reproduction.

Telomere Attrition

Telomeres, repetitive DNA sequences, work in conjunction with protein complexes called shelterin, to protect the ends of chromosomes and maintain structural and genetic stability [28]. Extensive evidence supports a role for telomere attrition in reproductive aging. Mice have very long telomeres and very little oocyte aneuploidy. Genetic or biochemical shortening of telomeres reduces synapsis and chiasmata, increases the proportion of fragmented and arrested embryos apoptosis and spindle dysmorphologies [29–32]. Telomeres are maintained primarily by the enzyme telomerase, but this enzyme is inactive in most adult cells, including the adult female germline [33]. Support for the telomere theory of reproductive aging was generated originally in mouse models, but growing evidence from human studies confirms a central role for telomeres in reproductive aging in women. Women with dyskeratosis congenital, a canonical human telomeropathy, develop precocious follicular depletion, short oocyte telomeres, and arrested and aneuploidy embryos [34]. Oocytes have among the shortest telomeres in the body. Professor Robert Edwards previously demonstrated that oocytes ovulating late in the life of the female were the last to exit germ line proliferation during fetal life, a process he termed "the production line." These late exiting oocytes have undergone more telomere attrition as oocyte precursors traverse more mitotic cell cycles

before entering meiosis than oocytes ovulated from younger females. Furthermore, older oocytes accumulate additional exposure to reactive oxygen species from prolonged arrest in the adult ovary [7,35].

Mitochondria DNA and Reactive Oxygen Species

Mutations in mitochondrial DNA (mtDNA) have been implicated in oocyte aging. mtDNA is especially susceptible to damage from exposure to reactive oxygen species. It lacks protective histones and has limited capacity for DNA damage repair. However, oocytes contain a very high copy number of mtDNA, and the possible proportion of those with mutations remains low, even in aged oocytes [36]. Women with decreased ovarian reserve may have lower mtDNA copy number [37], but oocytes with poor development potential have been found to have both low and high quantities of mtDNA [38], weakening the argument of mtDNA as a strong contributor to aging. This argument is further conflicted by studies modeling mitochondrial dysfunction and showing increased oocyte and embryo death [39], while others show negligible effect from mitochondria disruption [40]. A mouse model of reproductive aging with senescence-accelerated mice (SAM) supports that reproductive aging segregates with the nucleus, rather than the mitochondria or cytoplasm [10]. Finally, mitochondria within oocytes are remarkably quiescent. Oocytes consume very little oxygen and oxidative phosphorylation increases only at the morula and blastocyst stages. These physiological facts likely explain why women with high enough levels of mitochondrial mutations to transmit mitochondrial disease to offspring do not typically experience infertility.

The Production Line

Professor Robert Edwards demonstrated in a mouse model that oocytes ovulated late in life traversed more cell cycles during fetal oogenesis [41], a process he called "the production line." According to the production line hypothesis, germ cells in female mammals become committed to meiosis and enter prophase sequentially in fetal life – and then are released as mature oocytes in the same sequence postpuberty [42]. This theory suggests that a portion of maternal age-dependent errors at the first meiotic division might be seeded prenatally. Shorter telomeres, from additional cycles of replication during fetal life, would be exacerbated by environmental conditions in the postnatal ovary.

Altered Blood Flow

Blood flow is crucial to the health of the ovary, and alterations in basal ovarian stromal blood flow provide a marker for low ovarian reserve. Multiple studies have evaluated intraovarian vasculature at different points within natural and ART stimulation cycles, with conflicting results [43–45]. Undetectable ovarian stromal blood flow at cycle baseline has predicted poor ovarian reserve markers, lower response to controlled ovarian stimulation – and decreased pregnancy rates [46]. The mechanism of basal ovarian stromal blood flow is not fully understood; is the size of follicular pool a driver of blood flow, or is the limited hematologic infrastructure prohibiting the existing follicular pool from being stimulated?

Amyloid-like Substance Infiltration

Amyloid plaques provide the basis of aging of most long-lived tissues, including the brain, and are considered to have toxic and degenerative roles. The ovary is no exception. In buddying yeast, amyloids are involved in oocyte maturation and cell division [47]. Amyloid-like substances are present in mammalian oocytes and embryos at varying levels according to stage of development, with a speculated role in oocyte maturation [48]. Early studies also show a correlation between levels of amyloid-like substances and good prognoses clinical characteristics in patients undergoing assisted reproductive technology [48–50], suggesting these could play a role as a marker for embryo development.

Sirtuins

In practically every species examined to date, caloric restriction prolongs lifespan and healthy lifespan. Caloric restriction in mice also prolongs reproductive lifespan. Sirtuins (silent information regulator 2 (Sir2) proteins) have emerged as potential mediators of the beneficial effect of caloric restriction on aging [51,52]. Early evidence suggests that sirtuins play a primary role for the oocyte, rather than fertilization events, in the adaptive response to oxidative stress [53]. Sirtuins also may protect the oocyte against loss of developmental competence with reproductive and postovulatory aging [54]. These findings suggest that direct or indirect modulation of sirtuin activity by nutritional interventions may have beneficial effects on ovarian physiology [55,56].

Resveratrol

The accumulation of free radicals over time is toxic to cells, leading to DNA mutations, protein damage, telomere shortening, apoptosis, and accelerated ovarian aging. Antioxidants reduce damage induced by reactive oxygen species, including in oocytes and follicles. Antioxidants have been demonstrated to prevent maternal aging-associated oocyte aneuploidy and meiotic spindle defects in mice [57]. Resveratrol is a polyphenolic compound found in the skin of red grapes, red wine, and other botanical extracts and has gained popularity for its biological activities, including activation of sirtuins, putative mediation of the caloric restriction effect, anticarcinogenic, anti-inflammatory, and telomerase-enhancing activities, and inhibition of cell senescence. In mice, long-term administration of oral resveratrol and the antioxidant cysteine protected against the reduction of fertility with reproductive aging, as demonstrated by increased litter size, follicle number, telomere length and telomerase activity, and oocyte quantity and quality [58]. While hopeful, the data obtained by mouse models does not extrapolate directly to human reproduction and further studies are required.

The Aging Uterus

The depth and breadth of investigation into the understanding of ovarian aging, as seen in the previous section, is staggering. In contrast, much less is known about aging and its effect on the uterus. It can be debated how much uterine aging matters, if at all, as evidenced by the high pregnancy rates in women of advanced maternal age who utilize donor oocytes [12]. However, the uterus is one of the most dynamic organs in the body. A comparison of menopausal with premenopausal endometria, both with morphology and with steroid receptor concentration and cell proliferation indices, shows that while the endometrium itself involutes with age, the steroid and cellular indices intimate continued activity [59], suggesting that perhaps the uterus becomes quiescent due to age but not necessarily atrophic. So, does the uterus age differently or separately from the ovary? Or is it less susceptible?

While the impact of uterine aging remains controversial, it does impact obstetric outcomes [13]. Given the trend to delay childbearing, aged uteri will likely continue to be utilized. Therefore, this section will discuss the evidence of uterine aging from animal models, the effect on clinical outcomes seen in ART as well as on obstetric outcomes, and, lastly, some exciting discoveries related to uterine biomarkers.

Animal models show that the uterus does display signs of biological aging [60]. Indeed, in rodents the uterus ages before the ovary. In the rat, density of endometrial stromal cells changes [61], concentration of estrogen receptors decreases [62], and uterine collagen content increases with age [63]. Mouse studies show that endometrial mitotic activity decreases [64], and stromal mitotic activity increases with age [65]. Uterine epithelial microvilli in response to estrogen [65] also decrease with age. Pigs develop intimal thickening of the endometrial arteries and glandular cyst formation within the endometrium [66] with aging. The presence of such age-related uterine changes in women has not been well studied.

Signs of uterine aging are also seen in the infertility clinic and in ART outcomes. The armamentarium of treatment and protocols used in ART is vast. However, good evidence suggests that certain endometrial preparation protocols are more successful for hormone replacement for embryo transfer in women of advanced age [67]. Women at the extremes of age have difficulty with endometrial development [68]. Beyond endometrial preparation, there is literature to support a higher incidence of luteal phase deficiency in women of older age, especially in the extremes of age [69]. While the diagnoses and incidence of luteal phase deficiency is often debated, further research has shown that older women need higher doses of progesterone for ART success [70]. Moreover, older women undergoing donor oocyte therapy seem to require higher doses of progesterone [70], consistent with a role for the "aging luteal phase." Clearly, the uterus is capable of performing its reproductive age functions later in life but studies provide strong evidence of a clinical impact of uterine aging.

Pregnancy outcomes also show effects of uterine aging. Thin endometrium has been associated with poor obstetric outcomes [71]. A meta-analysis of women pregnant at advanced age showed increased risk of stillbirth, even after controlling for maternal comorbidities [72]. Further, pregnancies in women over 40 are at higher risk for many poor obstetric outcomes including preterm birth, pre-eclampsia or hypertensive disorders of pregnancy, gestational diabetes, and cesarean delivery [13]. Perhaps the most convincing evidence of uterine aging is that the highest obstetric risks are seen in women of the most advanced age, over 45 years old [73]. Pregnant women in this extreme age category also are at higher risk of postpartum hemorrhage, thrombosis, and hysterectomy [73]. While many older women have uncomplicated pregnancies, the effects of age on obstetrical outcome must inform the counseling of older women contemplating infertility treatment.

Several biomarkers may help measure uterine aging and its potential effects on implantation. The endometrium has remarkable ability to regenerate with each ovarian cycle. Adult progenitor cells within the endometrium express telomerase. Telomerase active has dynamic activity within the uterus across the menstrual cycle and is necessary for endometrial regeneration [74]. Endometrial telomerase has also been implicated in several endometrial conditions [74]. Another biomarker that may help characterize uterine age is endometrial stem cells. Older women have higher rates of miscarriage, which coincide with the age-related loss of endometrial stem cells. Stem cells are located in the basal layer of the endometrium and assist with the cyclic regeneration of the endometrium [75]. The loss of these cells over time may be implicated in recurrent pregnancy loss, miscarriage [75], and Asherman's syndrome.

Abundant evidence shows that the oocyte is the primary driver of age-related decline in fertility yet the uterus clearly does age and likely contributes to reproductive aging. Further investigation of uterine aging will be necessary as social trends show women continue to build their families later in life, with older reproductive systems.

Summary

The loss of oocytes and reduced oocyte quality contribute to age-associated ovarian decline and decreased fertility, which is at odds with the social trend toward delayed family-building. Females are born with a finite cohort of germ cells, arrested from midgestation, and they progressively lose them throughout their reproductive lifespan, reaching a state of near depletion at menopause. Declining oocyte number, however, is not the sole culprit for age-related infertility. Oocyte competence, the ability to fertilize, develop, implant, and produce a live offspring, deteriorates more or less in concert with declining ovarian reserve. The uterus likely also plays a role, further hindering reproduction later in life, although additional studies are needed.

References

1. Schwartz D, Mayaux MJ. Female fecundity as a function of age: results of artificial insemination in 2193 nulliparous women with azoospermic husbands. Federation CECOS. N Engl J Med. 1982;306(7):404–6.

2. Gosden RG. Maternal age: a major factor affecting the prospects and outcome of pregnancy. Ann N Y Acad Sci. 1985;442:45–57.

3. Matthews TJ, Hamilton BE. Delayed childbearing: more women are having their first child later in life. NCHS Data Brief. 2009(21):1–8.

4. Hurwitz A, Adashi EY. Ovarian follicular atresia as an apoptotic process: a paradigm for programmed cell death in endocrine tissues. Mol Cell Endocrinol. 1992;84(1–2):C19–23.

5. Marcozzi S, Rossi V, Salustri A, De Felici M, Klinger FG. Programmed cell death in the human ovary. Minerva Ginecol. 2018;70(5):549–60.

6. Keefe DL. Telomeres, reproductive aging, and genomic instability during early development. Reprod Sci. 2016;23(12):1612–5.

7. Keefe DL, Liu L. Telomeres and reproductive aging. Reprod Fertil Dev. 2009;21(1):10–4.

8. Kalmbach KH, Antunes DM, Kohlrausch F, Keefe DL. Telomeres and female reproductive aging. Semin Reprod Med. 2015;33(6):389–95.

9. Lemoine ME, Ravitsky V. Sleepwalking into infertility: the need for a public health approach toward advanced maternal age. Am J Bioeth. 2015;15(11):37–48.

10. Liu L, Keefe DL. Nuclear origin of aging-associated meiotic defects in senescence-accelerated mice. Biol Reprod. 2004;71(5):1724–9.

11. Tatone C, Amicarelli F. The aging ovary–the poor granulosa cells. Fertil Steril. 2013;99(1):12–7.

12. Forman EJ, Treff NR, Scott RT, Jr. Fertility after age 45: From natural conception to assisted reproductive technology and beyond. Maturitas. 2011;70(3):216–21.

13. Bouzaglou A, Aubenas I, Abbou H, Rouanet S, Carbonnel M, Pirtea P, et al. Pregnancy at 40 years old and above: obstetrical, fetal, and neonatal outcomes. Is age an independent risk factor for those complications? Front Med (Lausanne). 2020;7:208.

14. Adhikari D, Zheng W, Shen Y, Gorre N, Hamalainen T, Cooney AJ, et al. Tsc/mTORC1 signaling in oocytes governs the quiescence and activation of primordial follicles. Hum Mol Genet. 2010;19(3):397–410.

15. Nagaoka SI, Hassold TJ, Hunt PA. Human aneuploidy: mechanisms and new insights into an age-old problem. Nat Rev Genet. 2012;13(7):493–504.

16. Broekmans FJ, Kwee J, Hendriks DJ, Mol BW, Lambalk CB. A systematic review of tests predicting ovarian reserve and IVF outcome. Hum Reprod Update. 2006;12(6):685–718.

17. Munné S, Cohen J. Advanced maternal age patients benefit from preimplantation genetic diagnosis of aneuploidy. Fertil Steril. 2017;107(5):1145–6.

18. Battaglia DE, Goodwin P, Klein NA, Soules MR. Fertilization and early embryology: Influence of maternal age on meiotic spindle assembly oocytes from naturally cycling women. Hum Reprod. 1996;11(10):2217–22.

19. Cromie GA, Smith GR. Branching out: meiotic recombination and its regulation. Trends Cell Biol. 2007;17(9):448–55.

20. Maguire MP. Is the synaptonemal complex a disjunction machine? J Hered. 1995;86(5):330–40.

21. Hassold T, Hunt P. To err (meiotically) is human: the genesis of human aneuploidy. Nat Rev Genet. 2001;2(4):280–91.

22. Jessberger R. Deterioration without replenishment–the misery of oocyte cohesin. Genes Dev. 2010;24(23):2587–91.

23. Liu L, Keefe DL. Defective cohesin is associated with age-dependent misaligned chromosomes in oocytes. Reprod Biomed Online. 2008;16(1):103–12.

24. Handyside AH, Montag M, Magli MC, Repping S, Harper J, Schmutzler A, et al. Multiple meiotic errors caused by predivision of chromatids in women of advanced maternal age undergoing in vitro fertilisation. Eur J Hum Genet. 2012;20(7):742–7.

25. Liu L. Ageing-associated aberration in meiosis of oocytes from senescence-accelerated mice. Hum Reprod. 2002;17(10):2678–85.

26. Hodges CA, Revenkova E, Jessberger R, Hassold TJ, Hunt PA. SMC1β-deficient female

mice provide evidence that cohesins are a missing link in age-related nondisjunction. Nat Genet. 2005;37(12):1351–5.

27. Xu H, Beasley MD, Warren WD, Van Der Horst GTJ, McKay MJ. Absence of mouse REC8 cohesin promotes synapsis of sister chromatids in meiosis. Dev Cell. 2005;8(6):949–61.

28. De Lange T. Shelterin: the protein complex that shapes and safeguards human telomeres. Genes Dev. 2005;19(18):2100–10.

29. Kalmbach KH, Fontes Antunes DM, Dracxler RC, Knier TW, Seth-Smith ML, Wang F, et al. Telomeres and human reproduction. Fertil Steril. 2013;99(1):23–9.

30. Keefe DL, Franco S, Liu L, Trimarchi J, Cao B, Weitzen S, et al. Telomere length predicts embryo fragmentation after in vitro fertilization in women—toward a telomere theory of reproductive aging in women. Am J Obstet Gynecol. 2005;192(4):1256–60.

31. Keefe DL, Liu L, Marquard K. Telomeres and meiosis in health and disease. Cell Mol Life Sci. 2007;64(2):139–43.

32. Keefe DL. Telomeres and genomic instability during early development. Eur J Med Genet. 2020;63(2):103638.

33. Wright DL, Jones EL, Mayer JF, Oehninger S, Gibbons WE, Lanzendorf SE. Characterization of telomerase activity in the human oocyte and preimplantation embryo. Mol Hum Reprod. 2001;7(10):947–55.

34. Robinson LG, Jr., Pimentel R, Wang F, Kramer YG, Gonullu DC, Agarwal S, et al. Impaired reproductive function and fertility preservation in a woman with a dyskeratosis congenita. J Assist Reprod Genet. 2020;37(5):1221–5.

35. Keefe DL, Marquard K, Liu L. The telomere theory of reproductive senescence in women. Curr Opin Obstet Gynecol. 2006;18(3):280–5.

36. Keefe DL, Niven-Fairchild T, Powell S, Buradagunta S. Mitochondrial deoxyribonucleic acid deletions in oocytes and reproductive aging in women. Fertil Steril. 1995;64(3):577–83.

37. Reynier P, May-Panloup P, Chretien MF, Morgan CJ, Jean M, Savagner F, et al. Mitochondrial DNA content affects the fertilizability of human oocytes. Mol Hum Reprod. 2001;7(5):425–9.

38. May-Panloup P, Chrétien MF, Jacques C, Vasseur C, Malthièry Y, Reynier P. Low oocyte mitochondrial DNA content in ovarian insufficiency. Hum Reprod. 2005;20(3):593–7.

39. Navarro PAAS, Liu L, Keefe DL. In vivo effects of arsenite on meiosis, preimplantation

development, and apoptosis in the mouse. Biol Reprod. 2004;70(4):980–5.

40. Bentov Y, Yavorska T, Esfandiari N, Jurisicova A, Casper RF. The contribution of mitochondrial function to reproductive aging. J Assist Reprod Genet. 2011;28(9):773–83.

41. Henderson SA, Edwards RG. Chiasma frequency and maternal age in mammals. Nature. 1968;218(5136):22–8.

42. Polani P, Crolla J. A test of the production line hypothesis of mammalian oogenesis. Hum Genet. 1991;88(1):64–70.

43. Engmann L, Sladkevicius P, Agrawal R, Bekir J, Campbell S, Tan S. Value of ovarian stromal blood flow velocity measurement after pituitary suppression in the prediction of ovarian responsiveness and outcome of in vitro fertilization treatment. Fertil Steril. 1999;71(1):22–9.

44. Ng EHY, Tang OS, Chan CCW, Ho PC. Ovarian stromal blood flow in the prediction of ovarian response during in vitro fertilization treatment. Hum Reprod. 2005;20(11):3147–51.

45. Lunenfeld E, Schwartz I, Meizner I, Potashnik G, Glezerman M. Ovary and ovulation: intraovarian blood flow during spontaneous and stimulated cycles. 1996;11(11):2481–3.

46. Younis JS, Haddad S, Matilsky M, Radin O, Ben-Ami M. Undetectable basal ovarian stromal blood flow in infertile women is related to low ovarian reserve. Gynecol Endocrinol. 2007;23(5):284–9.

47. Berchowitz LE, Kabachinski G, Walker MR, Carlile TM, Gilbert WV, Schwartz TU, et al. Regulated formation of an amyloid-like translational repressor governs gametogenesis. Cell. 2015;163(2):406–18.

48. Pimentel RN, Navarro PA, Wang F, Robinson LG, Jr., Cammer M, Liang F, et al. Amyloid-like substance in mice and human oocytes and embryos. J Assisted Reprod Genet. 2019;36(9):1877–90.

49. Duan F-H, Chen S-L, Chen X, Niu J, Li P, Liu Y-D, et al. Follicular fluid Aβ40 concentrations may be associated with ongoing pregnancy following in vitro fertilization. J Assisted Reprod Genet. 2014;31(12):1611–20.

50. Urieli-Shoval S, Finci-Yeheskel Z, Eldar I, Linke RP, Levin M, Prus D, et al. Serum amyloid A: expression throughout human ovarian folliculogenesis and levels in follicular fluid of women undergoing controlled ovarian stimulation. J Clin Endocrinol Metab. 2013;98(12):4970–8.

51. Michan S, Sinclair D. Sirtuins in mammals: insights into their biological function. Biochem J. 2007;404(1):1–13.

25

52. Morris BJ. Seven sirtuins for seven deadly diseases of aging. Free Radic Biol Med. 2013;**56**:133–71.

53. Di Emidio G, Falone S, Vitti M, D'Alessandro AM, Vento M, Di Pietro C, et al. SIRT1 signalling protects mouse oocytes against oxidative stress and is deregulated during aging. Hum Reprod. 2014;**29**(9):2006–17.

54. Manosalva I, González A. Aging changes the chromatin configuration and histone methylation of mouse oocytes at germinal vesicle stage. Theriogenology. 2010;**74**(9):1539–47.

55. Tatone C, Di Emidio G, Vitti M, Di Carlo M, Santini S, D'Alessandro AM, et al. Sirtuin functions in female fertility: possible role in oxidative stress and aging. Oxid Med Cell Longev. 2015;**2015**:659687.

56. Tatone C, Di Emidio G, Barbonetti A, Carta G, Luciano AM, Falone S, et al. Sirtuins in gamete biology and reproductive physiology: emerging roles and therapeutic potential in female and male infertility. Hum Reprod Update. 2018;**24**(3):267–89.

57. Selesniemi K, Lee HJ, Muhlhauser A, Tilly JL. Prevention of maternal aging-associated oocyte aneuploidy and meiotic spindle defects in mice by dietary and genetic strategies. Proc Natl Acad Sci U S A. 2011;**108**(30):12319–24.

58. Liu M, Yin Y, Ye X, Zeng M, Zhao Q, Keefe DL, et al. Resveratrol protects against age-associated infertility in mice. Hum Reprod. 2013;**28**(3):707–17.

59. Noci I, Borri P, Scarselli G, Chieffi O, Bucciantini S, Biagiotti R, et al. Morphological and functional aspects of the endometrium of asymptomatic post-menopausal women: does the endometrium really age? Hum Reprod. 1996;**11**(10):2246–50.

60. Klein J, Sauer MV. Assessing fertility in women of advanced reproductive age. Am J Obstet Gynecol. 2001;**185**(3):758–70.

61. Craig SS, Jollie WP. Age changes in density of endometrial stromal cells of the rat. Exp Gerontol. 1985;**20**(2):93–7.

62. Hsueh AJ, Erickson GF, Lu KH. Changes in uterine estrogen receptor and morphology in aging female rats. Biol Reprod. 1979;**21**(4):793–800.

63. Burack E, Wolfe JM, Lansing W, Wright AW. The effect of age upon the connective tissue of the uterus, cervix, and vagina of the rat. Cancer Res. 1941;**1**(3):227–35.

64. Finn CA, Martin L. The cellular response of the uterus of the aged mouse to oestrogen and progesterone. J Reprod Fertil. 1969;**20**(3):545–7.

65. Smith AF. Ultrastructure of the uterine luminal epithelium at the time of implantation in ageing mice. J Reprod Fertil. 1975;**42**(1):183–5.

66. Bal HS, Getty R. Changes in the histomorphology of the uterus of the domestic pig (Sus scrofa domesticus) with advancing age. J Gerontol. 1973;**28**(2):160–72.

67. Adams SM, Terry V, Hosie MJ, Gayer N, Murphy CR. Endometrial response to IVF hormonal manipulation: comparative analysis of menopausal, down regulated and natural cycles. Reprod Biol Endocrinol. 2004;**2**:21.

68. Amir W, Micha B, Ariel H, Liat LG, Jehoshua D, Adrian S. Predicting factors for endometrial thickness during treatment with assisted reproductive technology. Fertil Steril. 2007;**87**(4):799–804.

69. Lenton EA, Landgren BM, Sexton L. Normal variation in the length of the luteal phase of the menstrual cycle: identification of the short luteal phase. Br J Obstet Gynaecol. 1984;**91**(7):685–9.

70. Meldrum DR. Female reproductive aging–ovarian and uterine factors. Fertil Steril. 1993;**59**(1):1–5.

71. Oron G, Hiersch L, Rona S, Prag-Rosenberg R, Sapir O, Tuttnauer-Hamburger M, et al. Endometrial thickness of less than 7.5 mm is associated with obstetric complications in fresh IVF cycles: a retrospective cohort study. Reprod Biomed Online. 2018;**37**(3):341–8.

72. Lean SC, Derricott H, Jones RL, Heazell AEP. Advanced maternal age and adverse pregnancy outcomes: A systematic review and meta-analysis. PLoS One. 2017;**12**(10):e0186287.

73. Sheen JJ, Wright JD, Goffman D, Kern-Goldberger AR, Booker W, Siddiq Z, et al. Maternal age and risk for adverse outcomes. Am J Obstet Gynecol. 2018;**219**(4):390.e1-.e15.

74. Hapangama DK, Kamal A, Saretzki G. Implications of telomeres and telomerase in endometrial pathology. Hum Reprod Update. 2017;**23**(2):166–87.

75. Cho A, Park SR, Kim SR, Nam S, Lim S, Park CH, et al. An endogenous anti-aging factor, sonic hedgehog, suppresses endometrial stem cell aging through SERPINB2. Mol Ther. 2019;**27**(7):1286–98.

What Lifestyle Adjustments Can Maximize the Chance of a Natural Conception and Healthy Pregnancy in Women over 40?

Alexandra Kermack

Introduction

In 2017, one in 23 babies was born to a woman over the age of 40 in the UK; this is approximately 29,000 births, and a significant proportion of these are as a result of assisted reproductive treatments. It is well documented that the chance of natural conception decreases dramatically as a woman approaches her 40s; from a cumulative chance per annum of up to 80% and 90% in her 20s to less than 50% over 35. With the increasing movement in social, educational and economic expectations, women continue to delay having a family. Some women may have limited knowledge of the effect of age or their pre-conception health on their fecundity. A large observational study demonstrated that couples who had more than four negative lifestyle variables (such as raised body mass index (BMI), increased alcohol intake and smoking) took seven times longer to conceive than those who had a healthier lifestyle [1]. Reproductive life plan counselling may encourage women to reflect on their reproduction and negative behaviours that may disrupt their fertility; increasing their knowledge about the effect of age and lifestyle factors on fecundity [2]. Furthermore, pre-conception lifestyle counselling has been shown to decrease the prevalence of harmful activities and improve couples' diets and physical activity levels in the short term [3]. This counselling may be particularly important in women whose reproductive window is short and in whom modification of lifestyle factors may be a relatively quick, easy and cost-effective method of increasing their chances of conception and improving pregnancy outcomes.

There is a paucity of data examining lifestyle factors that can be modified to increase the chance of conceiving naturally for women with an increased maternal age. In fact, many of the studies exclude women above the age of 40 as the lower chance of conceiving means that research requires larger numbers of participants and is more time consuming and expensive than if it is carried out in younger women; advice can, however, be extrapolated.

Body Mass Index

There is a linear decline in fertility with increasing BMI (greater than 29 kg/m^2); with each unit increase, women have a 4% lower conception rate. This is observed even in those with no ovulatory disorders [4]. Women with a raised BMI are also more likely to suffer with anovulatory infertility. This is thought to be mainly attributed to endocrine mechanisms which interfere with ovarian function [5]. In addition, in a small study examining fertility, age, BMI and ovarian volume, ovarian volume has been shown to decrease in fertile, older women with increasing BMI [6]. In women over 40, who already have a decreased chance of conception compared with their younger counterparts, this finding is especially important. Studies from America demonstrate that risk of obesity increases with age, between the ages of 20 and 60 [7]. Therefore, women who are overweight and trying to conceive after the age of 40 need adequate counselling and help to reduce their weight.

Women who become pregnant with a raised BMI have an increased risk of miscarriage, gestational diabetes [8], hypertensive disorders of pregnancy [9], and thrombotic disease [10]. Fetal complications such as intrauterine death and consequences arising from macrosomia [11] are also more common as well as an increase in difficulties diagnosing growth restriction and congenital anomalies, as body habitus impedes the ultrasound process.

There is a lack of well-designed and high-quality studies examining methods of targeting and recruiting these women to weight loss programmes and the impact of interventions. Women should be educated on the detrimental effects of obesity and the benefits of weight reduction, including improvement in pregnancy rates. According to a meta-analysis, a reduction in calories by decreasing both fat and refined carbohydrate intake and increasing aerobic exercise should form the basis of weight loss programmes, but this must be tailored to the individual [12].

Obesity is not the only way that BMI can affect a woman's fertility; those with a very low BMI (less than 18.5 kg/m^2) can also suffer from ovulatory dysfunction with one study demonstrating a relative risk of infertility of 1.6 compared with women with a normal BMI [13]. Furthermore, in a US study, 20% of women seeking intrauterine insemination met the criteria to be diagnosed with an eating disorder [14]. Unfortunately, eating disorders are on the rise in women between the ages of 40 and 50, with 1 in every 28 women in this age group suffering from anorexia or bulimia [15]. Women with very low BMI should be encouraged to optimize this prior to embarking on fertility treatment. This may involve a multidisciplinary approach with involvement from a psychiatrist, dietitian and counsellor [16]. Eating disorders are only screened for in a third of fertility consultations and nearly all clinicians feel they would benefit from more training in this area [17]. Given the growing prevalence in this age group, accurate and swift diagnosis and treatment is particularly important to increase the woman's chance of conceiving in the future and going on to have a healthy, term pregnancy.

Healthy interventions to optimize BMI often take many weeks or months and this must be balanced against the declining fertility of this age group. However, the benefits to obstetric, maternal and neonatal outcomes should not be underestimated and therefore weight loss or gain should be continued, irrespective of the result of the fertility treatment. As lack of compliance is a key barrier to BMI optimization, coached sessions may be offered to improve understanding and motivation [12].

Diet

There is evidence to suggest that women planning a pregnancy or those who are pregnant are not given adequate, high-quality nutritional advice from reputable sources to enable healthy food choices. When nutritional information is given, it is often provided too late at the 12 week appointment and not pre-conceptionally. More research is needed in how to educate women on the importance of diet, the effectiveness of public health campaigns and how to impart information to sub-sectors of society such as migrants who may have cultural and language barriers [18].

Currently, women trying to conceive are encouraged to increase their consumption of whole grains, omega-3 fatty acids, fish and soy and reduce their consumption of *trans* fats and red meat [19]. A more Mediterranean diet (comprising high fruit and vegetable intake, fish and poultry and olive oil) has also been shown to be associated with increased fecundity in women who have previously had difficulty conceiving [20]. A higher vegetable intake is observed in older women who are better educated and with a higher income [21]; however, reiterating the importance of a healthy diet when women attend for pre-conception counselling and lifestyle advice is still imperative to optimize their health.

There is currently no evidence regarding testing a woman's nutritional profile either via blood or hair prior to embarking on fertility treatment; however, if there is a particular nutritional deficiency, for example vitamin D, that the woman may be at risk of, then testing and repletion may be of benefit. Further research is needed to ascertain whether nutritional assessment and advice for certain sub-groups of women undergoing fertility treatments, such as those over the age of 40, would improve outcomes.

Vitamin Supplementation

Women who are aged over 40 are at increased risk of having a baby with a neural tube defect [22], therefore the importance of taking folic acid supplements should be reiterated to anyone seeking pre-conceptional advice [23]. Furthermore, folic acid supplementation has consistently been shown to increase the chances of conceiving as it is considered important for oocyte quality and maturation and implantation as well as the normal continuation of a pregnancy [24]. As oocyte quality is a cause of age-related decline in fertility [25], folic acid supplementation may be of increased benefit to women of advanced maternal age.

There is a growing body of evidence pointing to the importance of vitamin D in female fertility. Vitamin D insufficiency (levels of between 50 and 75 nmol/L) and deficiency (<50 nmol/L) are highly prevalent (86.9%) in healthy, pre-menopausal women aged between 40 and 52 [26]. Deficiency in vitamin D has been associated with a decreased probability of live birth following fertility treatments [27]. Vitamin D has multiple roles within the ovary including stimulating steroidogenesis. It is suggested that vitamin D and its receptors in the granulosa cells regulate the expression and activity of key enzymes [28]. There is emerging evidence that vitamin D deficiency may impact on endometrial receptivity. In a study of outcomes after oocyte donation treatment, pregnancy rates in vitamin D-depleted oocyte donor recipients, assessed by measuring serum levels using radioimmunoassay, were significantly decreased (37%) when compared with vitamin D-repleted recipients (78%) [29]. Further prospective studies are required to prove benefit. However, in women who have a deficiency, the data seem to indicate improved outcomes with supplementation. Vitamin D has also been shown to be important to the wellbeing of the offspring. Maternal vitamin D insufficiency during pregnancy is associated with reduced bone-mineral accrual of the offspring during childhood and supplementation of the mothers may have long lasting benefits in reducing osteoporotic fractures in their adult children [30].

As a woman becomes older, her oocyte quality deteriorates and this may, in part, be secondary to oxidative stress. Oxidative stress causes damage to the cellular components including mitochondria and DNA, leading to increased apoptosis. Direct evidence on the protective mechanism of antioxidants, such as vitamin E and C against the effects of oxidative stress on the ageing process of human oocytes is still required [31]. One study has previously demonstrated that in women over the age of 35, vitamin E supplementation decreases the time to conceive [32]. The study did not look specifically at the mechanisms of action but hypothesized that as an antioxidant, vitamin E may prevent damage to the ovarian surface epithelium and protect the ageing ovary during luteolysis. However, other research has shown that despite a decrease in oxidative stress levels following supplementation with vitamin C and E, no improvement in fertility was seen in women suffering with endometriosis [33]. The 2017 Cochrane review concluded that there is low-quality evidence to show that taking an antioxidant may provide benefit for sub-fertile women [34].

In addition to adverse changes in the oocyte as a woman ages, cumulus granulosa cells also demonstrate adverse alterations linked to a reduction in mitochondrial activity and decreased expression of enzymes that produce coenzyme Q10. Supplementation with coenzyme Q10 has been shown to improve mitochondrial function in cumulus cells; stimulating glucose uptake and increasing progesterone production [35]. This counteraction of mitochondrial ovarian ageing may be the mechanism by which supplementation with coenzyme Q10 protects ovarian reserve [36]. Further research is required to elucidate whether the benefits result in an increase in fecundity and live birth rates in women over 40, but to date no adverse effects have been noted and therefore further research in this area is needed.

There is growing interest in the supplementation of omega-3, and although women in this age group are not particularly at risk of insufficiency compared with the general population, the intake is low in women of childbearing age [37]. Studies in mice have demonstrated prolonged reproductive function and improved oocyte quality with omega-3 supplementation in those with advancing maternal age [38]. Omega-3 fatty acids (FA) supplementation (4 g EPA and DHA daily for one month) has also been shown to reduce serum FSH levels in women with a normal BMI, but not in obese women [39]. These findings could potentially imply that omega-3 FA supplementation may extend a woman's reproductive lifespan; however, further research is needed to examine the effect on older women with a poor ovarian reserve. In addition, cohort studies have suggested that increased dietary intake of DHA and EPA is associated with improved embryo morphology [3]. A prospective, randomized controlled trial examining the effect of omega-3 supplementation in couples undergoing IVF showed improved morphokinetic markers of embryo quality. Whether this translates to improved live birth rates still needs to be investigated [40].

29

In addition to the above vitamins, zinc and selenium are thought to be important for female fertility and are amongst the most prevalent micronutrient deficiencies [41]. Women with lower selenium levels are at greater risk (RR 1.46) of sub-fertility and those with lower levels of zinc and selenium experienced longer times to pregnancy [42]. It is believed that selenium is involved in the growth and maturation of oocytes; however, the mechanism of action is not yet fully understood [43]. Likewise, the mechanism by which zinc affects female fertility is unknown; however, it may be part of a protein that plays a role in mRNA turnover in early embryonic development [44].

Another supplement that some research has shown as a potential treatment for women with poor ovarian reserve, or older women, is dehydroepiandrosterone acetate (DHEA). Further research is needed to draw definite conclusions on the benefits, but early meta-analyses show some evidence of improved pregnancy rates (OR=1.47, 95% CI: 1.09–1.99) [45] and endometrial thickness and live birth [46]. Furthermore, DHEA has been shown to upregulate the HOXA-10 mRNA expression, which is believed to have a positive effect on endometrial receptivity [47]. Further randomized controlled clinical trials are currently ongoing to ascertain if there is a benefit, and if so who benefits and to what extent.

Women trying to conceive should ensure that they are taking 400 µg of folic acid daily, ideally for at least three months prior to conception. They should also ensure they are vitamin D-replete and, if not, take appropriate supplements and measures. Other supplements are more controversial but ensuring a healthy balanced diet and considering a multivitamin or supplement if the diet is deplete in certain vitamins may increase the chance of conception and improve maternal and fetal health during pregnancy and for the offspring.

Smoking, Alcohol and Caffeine

It is well recognized that smoking has an effect on fertility. The American Society for Reproductive Medicine has published a committee opinion assessing the effect of smoking on fecundity; within that article they cite several, large-scale studies demonstrating the negative impact on fertility, independent of other factors [48]. Studies have demonstrated that smoking accelerates ovarian follicular depletion and women who smoke, on average, go through menopause one to four years earlier than non-smokers. All women undergoing fertility treatment need to be non-smokers for at least six months prior to fertility treatment; however, women aged over 40 should be urged to stop smoking as soon as possible, in order to not delay their treatment further or suffer further follicle depletion. In addition, smoking has been shown to alter oocyte morphology and increasing maternal age is associated with poorer oocyte quality. This further emphasizes the importance of smoking cessation support in these women [49].

The studies examining alcohol use and fertility are more inconsistent [50]. The Danish cohort study concluded that low to moderate alcohol use during fertility treatment did not adversely affect the outcome [51]. Furthermore, a study examining the effect of binge drinking on ovarian reserve demonstrated a 26% lower anti-mullerian hormone level in women who binged alcohol twice per week compared with those who had moderate alcohol intake but did not binge drink [52]. This will resonate with those women over 40, who are likely to already have low ovarian reserve. Conversely, a prospective cohort study demonstrated a dose–response inverse relationship between alcohol intake and fecundability. They suggested that even moderate alcohol intake had a significant effect on fertility [53]. Women embarking on fertility treatment should be given up to date information on alcohol intake, in order to make informed decisions about their consumption.

The role of caffeine in fertility and early pregnancy has also been examined; however, for every study demonstrating a deleterious effect, there is another claiming no correlation [54]. A recent murine study demonstrated that caffeine increased pronucleus formation of aged oocytes and decreased fragmentation after fertilization [55]. Further work is needed to ascertain the safety and efficacy of caffeine in women over the age of 40 undergoing fertility treatments.

Physical Activity

The Active Lives Survey published by Sport England demonstrated that 66% of people between the ages of 35 and 44 were classed as physically active – that is, they did 150 minutes or more of moderate intensity physical activity per week. This was compared with 76% of those between the ages 16 and 24 years, demonstrating a trend of decreasing physical activity with age.

In young women with a normal BMI, high physical activity levels have been shown to decrease the risk of infertility, suggesting that improving physical activity levels could be an affordable strategy to reduce fertility problems in women trying to conceive [56]. Conversely, vigorous exercise (either daily or to exhaustion) has been associated with higher rates of sub-fertility [57] and a 50% reduction in live births compared with women who reported no exercise following in vitro fertilization (IVF) [58].

Physical activity not only affects fertility but also pregnancy outcome; women who participated minimally in exercise had an increased risk of preterm birth, hypertensive disorders of pregnancy and gestational diabetes compared with those who reported higher levels. Interestingly, if the woman increased her physical activity levels early in pregnancy then her risk of gestational diabetes was similar to those who reported high levels throughout, indicating that modifying behaviour in the early stages can improve pregnancy outcome [59]. The upper safe limit of exercise in pregnancy is not known and in fact, most women decrease their physical activity during pregnancy due to nausea, tiredness and changing body shape. It is advised, however, that the benefits of moderate exercise during pregnancy far outweigh any risks, provided the woman is adequately hydrated, remains cool and limits contact or high-risk sports [60].

Current guidelines should be followed by women trying to conceive and who are pregnant. The American College of Obstetricians and Gynaecologists advises 20 to 30 minutes of moderate exercise on most or all days of the week (in the absence of contraindications).

Sleep

As female age increases women are more likely to complain of poor sleep [61] but the reported prevalence varies greatly, with one study reporting 17% of women aged 35 to 47 complaining of poor sleep [62] and another reporting that 40% of those aged between 40 and 44 suffer from poor sleep [61]. An inverse correlation has been observed between a short sleep duration (of less than eight hours) and fecundity [63]. Furthermore, women

with sleep disorders (not including sleep apnoea) are three times more likely to experience infertility compared with their counterparts who do not have difficulty sleeping [64]. Despite this, there is limited research examining the relationship between sleep and fertility. The majority of research that has been performed has examined the diminished reproductive capacity of shift workers. Shift workers have increased rates of menstrual dysfunction (16.05% compared with non-shift workers 13.05%) and infertility (11.3% compared with 9.9%) [65]. Mechanisms by which sleep affects fertility are likely to be multifactorial and complex and a number of hypotheses have been proposed:

1. Activation of the hypothalamic-pituitary-adrenal axis altering hormone secretion including luteinizing hormone (LH), follicle stimulating hormone (FSH) and progesterone, leading to changes in follicle stimulation and menstruation.

2. The LH surge is controlled by circadian rhythm to ensure that ovulation can occur at a time when mating can also occur. Furthermore, the rhythmic oscillations of clock genes in the ovaries cause variation in ovarian sensitivity to gonadotrophins. Clock gene expression is also found in the uterus and is thought to affect embryo implantation [66].

3. Compromised immunity. An increased inflammatory response including tumour necrosis factor (TNF) [67], interleukin-6 (IL6) [68] and C-reactive protein (CRP) [69] has been demonstrated in people with sleep loss. A plausible causative effect has therefore been posited as infertile women have a greater production of intracellular TNF-α [70] and higher IL-6 levels [71] compared with a fertile group.

It has also been postulated that the relationship between sleep and fecundity may be a reciprocal one, with women who are struggling to conceive, including those over the age of 40, suffering from sleep disturbances and disruptions in their circadian rhythm due to this [72]. This causality dilemma is further established by the fact that 34% of women suffering from sub-fertility report difficulty sleeping. Women with diminished ovarian reserve are significantly more likely to manifest disturbed sleep than those with infertility but normal ovarian reserve [73].

For women with polycystic ovarian syndrome (PCOS), sleep may play a more important role; a recent Australian cohort study demonstrated that women with PCOS reported similar sleep duration but were more likely to experience difficulty sleeping and restless sleep. This had previously been thought to be due to the effects on sleep of obesity and depression (associated with PCOS). However, an independent relationship was found when adjusting for BMI and depression, raising the hypothesis that PCOS is involved in disrupting sleep [74].

Sleep quality and duration is important for female reproduction. Women trying to conceive should be advised to aim for eight hours of good-quality sleep per night. They should avoid screen-light (particularly short wave light emitted by computers, tablets and mobile phones) prior to bed as these have been shown to disrupt sleep continuity and quality [75]. Although there is no evidence that treating sleep disorders will increase a woman's chance of conceiving, healthy sleep habits and/or treatment may help and are unlikely to cause any harm. Further research is required to examine this relationship in more detail, its temporality and the potential mechanistic pathways [76].

Stress Reduction

Infertile women are three times more likely to suffer with anxiety and nine times more likely to suffer with depression than fertile women [77]. Anecdotally, these findings may become more pronounced as a woman nears the end of her reproductive window. It is well recognized that sub-fertility can cause depression and stress. What remains debated is the effect of these conditions on a woman's fertility [78]. Higher levels of stress in the pre-conception period, measured by salivary alpha-amylase, have been associated with a longer time to conceive and an increased risk of sub-fertility [79]. It is plausible that the negative impact of stress on fertility is caused by a number of different mechanisms including an increased risk of anovulation, hyperprolactinaemia, low progesterone levels, tubal spasm and abnormal gamete transport [80]. Reducing stress and anxiety using psychological interventions may therefore be beneficial and has been associated with less psychological distress, higher pregnancy rates and improved marital satisfaction

[81]. Many of the trials examining stress reduction methods and fertility have investigated these with regards to improving artificial reproductive treatment outcomes. Despite the lack of data in women trying to conceive naturally, these interventions are extremely unlikely to cause harm and may have some benefit.

In addition to the possible difficulties in conceiving caused by stress, there is some evidence that stress may have a negative impact on pregnancy outcomes; increasing hypertensive disorders of pregnancy including pre-eclampsia and pre-term birth [82]. Other research has shown associations between acute and chronic stress and low birth weight. One study demonstrated an odds ratio of 4.70 (95% CI: 1.53–13.38) for low birth weight in expectant mothers who reported household strain at 20 weeks' gestation [83]. There may be confounding factors, such as lower nutritional intake in women who are experiencing stress and anxiety, that explain these findings. However, reducing the stress experienced by a mother-to-be and improving her social support will be advantageous and possibly improve pregnancy outcomes.

Stress-related illness and anxiety is increasing across Europe, with one third of women (36%) reporting high levels of stress in 2015, increased from 17% in 2004 [84]. We are also becoming more aware of methods to reduce stress and improve our wellbeing such as mindfulness. Mindfulness is the psychological process of purposely bringing one's attention to experiences occurring at the present time and acknowledging feelings. Mindfulness-based stress reduction programmes are now widely available and participants have reported that they provide both relief from and more acceptance of their anxiety, leading them to feel more at ease [85]. In addition to improvement in their mental health symptoms, couples who have practiced mindfulness during treatment for sub-fertility have shown higher pregnancy rates [86]. Mindfulness during pregnancy has also been shown to reduce anxiety and depression during the perinatal period [87], reduce the risk of postnatal depression [88] and, in one study, modulate the parasympathetic and sympathetic nervous systems thereby reducing blood pressure response in stressful situations [89]. Further research is needed to ascertain any potential benefit on fetal growth, hypertensive disorders of pregnancy and preterm birth.

Other alternative therapies thought to reduce stress include acupuncture and meditation. Research has demonstrated that these are used by over a third of patients in both the UK and USA [90]. The evidence in this area is limited. However, out of 44 studies examining the effect of acupuncture on fertility, two showed an improvement on female fertility, two showed an improvement on male fertility and there was an improvement in mental health [91].

Conclusion

Key Points

- Women over 40 who are hoping to conceive should optimize their lifestyle as quickly as possible in order to improve their fecundity and chance of having a healthy baby.
- There is a paucity of data regarding lifestyle factors and fertility and pregnancy.
- Women should be informed of the areas in which there is extensive evidence, such as the need for pre-conception folic acid and optimizing BMI, and be counselled on the matters that are less clear cut, for instance physical activity.
- Raised BMI has a negative impact on fertility and pregnancy outcomes. Women should be given help and support to ensure their BMI is within the healthy range prior to trying to conceive or to limit weight gain if they become pregnant with a raised BMI.
- A Mediterranean diet has been shown to improve fecundity in women who had previously had difficulty conceiving.
- Women should be counselled on taking folic acid whilst trying to conceive, and vitamin D if they are found to be deplete.
- All women undergoing fertility treatment should not smoke and should be educated about possible risks of alcohol and caffeine consumption.
- The importance of sleep and stress reduction should be recognized and women over 40 planning to undergo fertility treatments should manage these as best as possible.

References

1. Hassan MAM, Killick SR. Negative lifestyle is associated with a significant reduction in fecundity. Fertil Steril. 2004;81(2):384–92.

2. Skogsdal Y, Fadl H, Cao Y, Karlsson J, Tydén T. An intervention in contraceptive counseling increased the knowledge about fertility and awareness of preconception health-a randomized controlled trial. Ups J Med Sci. 2019;124(3):203–12.

3. Hammiche F, Laven JSE, van Mil N, de Cock M, de Vries JH, Lindemans J, et al. Tailored preconceptional dietary and lifestyle counselling in a tertiary outpatient clinic in the Netherlands. Hum Reprod. 2011;26(9):2432–41.

4. van der Steeg JW, Steures P, Eijkemans MJ, Habbema JD, Hompes PG, Burggraaff JM, et al. Obesity affects spontaneous pregnancy chances in subfertile, ovulatory women. Hum Reprod. 2008;23(2):324–8.

5. Giviziez CR, Sanchez EGM, Approbato MS, Maia MCS, Fleury EAB, Sasaki RSA. Obesity and anovulatory infertility: a review. JBRA Assist Reprod. 2016;20(4):240–5.

6. Zaidi S, Usmani A, Shokh IS, Alam SE. Ovarian reserve and BMI between fertile and subfertile women. J Coll Physicians Surg Pak. 2009;19(1):21–4.

7. Villareal DT, Apovian CM, Kushner RF, Klein S. Obesity in older adults: technical review and position statement of the American Society for Nutrition and NAASO, The Obesity Society. Am J Clin Nutr. 2005;82(5):923–34.

8. Poblete JA, Olmos P. Obesity and gestational diabetes in pregnant care and clinical practice. Curr Vasc Pharmacol. 2021;19(2):154–64.

9. Lopez-Jaramillo P, Barajas J, Rueda-Quijano SM, Lopez-Lopez C, Felix C. Obesity and preeclampsia: common pathophysiological mechanisms. Front Physiol. 2018;9:1838.

10. Sirimi N, Goulis DG. Obesity in pregnancy. Hormones. 2010;9(4):299–306.

11. Yogev Y, Catalano PM. Pregnancy and obesity. Obstet Gynecol Clin North Am. 2009;36(2):285–300.

12. Best D, Avenell A, Bhattacharya S. How effective are weight-loss interventions for improving fertility in women and men who are overweight or obese? A systematic review and meta-analysis of the evidence. Hum Reprod Update. 2017;23(6):681–705.

13. Grodstein F, Goldman MB, Cramer DW. Body mass index and ovulatory infertility. Epidemiology. 1994;5(2):247–50.

14. Freizinger M, Franko DL, Dacey M, Okun B, Domar AD. The prevalence of eating disorders in infertile women. Fertil Steril. 2010;93(1):72–8.

15. Micali N, Martini MG, Thomas JJ, Eddy KT, Kothari R, Russell E, et al. Lifetime and 12-month

prevalence of eating disorders amongst women in mid-life: a population-based study of diagnoses and risk factors. BMC Med. 2017;**15**(1):12.

16. Boutari C, Pappas PD, Mintziori G, Nigdelis MP, Athanasiadis L, Goulis DG, et al. The effect of underweight on female and male reproduction. Metabolism. 2020;**107**:154229.

17. Rodino IS, Byrne SM, Sanders KA. Eating disorders in the context of preconception care: fertility specialists' knowledge, attitudes, and clinical practices. Fertil Steril. 2017;**107**(2):494–501.

18. Lucas C, Charlton KE, Yeatman H. Nutrition advice during pregnancy: do women receive it and can health professionals provide it? Matern Child Health J. 2014;**18**(10):2465–78.

19. Chiu Y-H, Chavarro JE, Souter I. Diet and female fertility: doctor, what should I eat? Fertil Steril. 2018;**110**(4):560–9.

20. Toledo E, Lopez-del Burgo C, Ruiz-Zambrana A, Donazar M, Navarro-Blasco Í, Martínez-González MA, et al. Dietary patterns and difficulty conceiving: a nested case–control study. Fertil Steril. 2011;**96**(5):1149–53.

21. Bodnar LM, Siega-Riz AM. A Diet Quality Index for Pregnancy detects variation in diet and differences by sociodemographic factors. Public Health Nutr. 2002;**5**(6):801–9.

22. Vieira A, Taucher S. Maternal age and neural tube defects: evidence for a greater effect in spina bifida than in anencephaly. Revista médica de Chile. 2005;**133**:62–70.

23. Tamura T, Picciano MF. Folate and human reproduction. Am J Clin Nutr. 2006;**83**(5):993–1016.

24. Ebisch I, Thomas C, Peters W, Braat D, Steegers-Theunissen R. The importance of folate, zinc and antioxidants in the pathogenesis and prevention of subfertility. Hum Reprod Update. 2007;**13**(2):163–74.

25. Navot D, Bergh RA, Williams MA, Garrisi GJ, Guzman I, Sandler B, et al. Poor oocyte quality rather than implantation failure as a cause of age-related decline in female fertility. Lancet. 1991;**337**(8754):1375–7.

26. Grineva EN, Karonova T, Micheeva E, Belyaeva O, Nikitina IL. Vitamin D deficiency is a risk factor for obesity and diabetes type 2 in women at late reproductive age. Aging (Albany NY). 2013;**5**(7):575–81.

27. Zhao J, Huang X, Xu B, Yan Y, Zhang Q, Li Y. Whether vitamin D was associated with clinical outcome after IVF/ICSI: a systematic review and meta-analysis. Reprod Biol Endocrinol. 2018;**16**(1):13.

28. Parikh G, Varadinova M, Suwandhi P, Araki T, Rosenwaks Z, Poretsky L, et al. Vitamin D regulates steroidogenesis and insulin-like growth factor binding protein-1 (IGFBP-1) production in human ovarian cells. Horm Metab Res. 2010;**42**(10):754–7.

29. Rudick BJ, Ingles SA, Chung K, Stanczyk FZ, Paulson RJ, Bendikson KA. Influence of vitamin D levels on in vitro fertilization outcomes in donor-recipient cycles. Fertil Steril. 2014;**101**(2):447–52.

30. Javaid MK, Crozier SR, Harvey NC, Gale CR, Dennison EM, Boucher BJ, et al. Maternal vitamin D status during pregnancy and childhood bone mass at age 9 years: a longitudinal study. Lancet. 2006;**367**(9504):36–43.

31. Sasaki H, Hamatani T, Kamijo S, Iwai M, Kobanawa M, Ogawa S, et al. Impact of oxidative stress on age-associated decline in oocyte developmental competence. Front Endocrinol (Lausanne). 2019;**10**(811).

32. Ruder EH, Hartman TJ, Reindollar RH, Goldman MB. Female dietary antioxidant intake and time to pregnancy among couples treated for unexplained infertility. Fertil Steril. 2014;**101**(3):759–66.

33. Mier-Cabrera J, Genera-García M, De la Jara-Díaz J, Perichart-Perera O, Vadillo-Ortega F, Hernández-Guerrero C. Effect of vitamins C and E supplementation on peripheral oxidative stress markers and pregnancy rate in women with endometriosis. Int J Gynecol Obstet. 2008;**100**(3):252–6.

34. Showell MG, Mackenzie-Proctor R, Jordan V, Hart RJ. Antioxidants for female subfertility. Cochrane Database Syst Rev. 2017;7(7):Cd007807.

35. Ben-Meir A, Kim K, McQuaid R, Esfandiari N, Bentov Y, Casper RF, et al. Co-enzyme Q10 supplementation rescues cumulus cells dysfunction in a maternal aging model. Antioxidants (Basel). 2019;**8**(3).

36. Özcan P, Fıçıcıoğlu C, Kizilkale O, Yesiladali M, Tok OE, Ozkan F, et al. Can coenzyme Q10 supplementation protect the ovarian reserve against oxidative damage? J Assist Reprod Genet. 2016;**33**(9):1223–30.

37. Miles EA, Noakes PS, Kremmyda LS, Vlachava M, Diaper ND, Rosenlund G, et al. The Salmon in Pregnancy Study: study design, subject characteristics, maternal fish and marine n-3 fatty acid intake, and marine n-3 fatty acid status in maternal and umbilical cord blood. Am J Clin Nutr. 2011;**94**(6 Suppl):1986s-92s.

38. Nehra D, Le HD, Fallon EM, Carlson SJ, Woods D, White YA, et al. Prolonging the female

reproductive lifespan and improving egg quality with dietary omega-3 fatty acids. Aging Cell. 2012;11(6):1046–54.

39. Al-Safi ZA, Liu H, Carlson NE, Chosich J, Harris M, Bradford AP, et al. Omega-3 fatty acid supplementation lowers serum FSH in normal weight but not obese women. J Clin Endocrinol Metab. 2016;101(1):324–33.

40. Kermack AJ, Lowen P, Wellstead SJ, Fisk HL, Montag M, Cheong Y, et al. Effect of a 6-week "Mediterranean" dietary intervention on in vitro human embryo development: the Preconception Dietary Supplements in Assisted Reproduction double-blinded randomized controlled trial. Fertil Steril. 2020;113(2):260–9.

41. Dizdar OS, Baspınar O, Kocer D, Dursun ZB, Avcı D, Karakükcü C, et al. Nutritional risk, micronutrient status and clinical outcomes: a prospective observational study in an infectious disease clinic. Nutrients. 2016;8(3):124.

42. Grieger JA, Grzeskowiak LE, Wilson RL, Bianco-Miotto T, Leemaqz SY, Jankovic-Karasoulos T, et al. Maternal selenium, copper and zinc concentrations in early pregnancy, and the association with fertility. Nutrients. 2019;11(7):1609.

43. Mintziori G, Mousiolis A, Duntas LH, Goulis DG. Evidence for a manifold role of selenium in infertility. Hormones (Athens). 2020;19(1):55–9.

44. Ramos SB, Stumpo DJ, Kennington EA, Phillips RS, Bock CB, Ribeiro-Neto F, et al. The CCCH tandem zinc-finger protein Zfp36l2 is crucial for female fertility and early embryonic development. Development. 2004;131(19):4883–93.

45. Qin JC, Fan L, Qin AP. The effect of dehydroepiandrosterone (DHEA) supplementation on women with diminished ovarian reserve (DOR) in IVF cycle: Evidence from a meta-analysis. J Gynecol Obstet Hum Reprod. 2017;46(1):1–7.

46. Liu Y, Hu L, Fan L, Wang F. Efficacy of dehydroepiandrosterone (DHEA) supplementation for in vitro fertilization and embryo transfer cycles: a systematic review and meta-analysis. Gynecol Endocrinol. 2018;34(3):178–83.

47. Çelik Ö, Acet M, İmren A, Çelik N, Erşahin A, Aktun LH, et al. DHEA supplementation improves endometrial HOXA-10 mRNA expression in poor responders. J Turk Ger Gynecol Assoc. 2017;18(4):160–6.

48. Practice Committee of the American Society for Reproductive Medicine. Smoking and infertility: a committee opinion. Fertil Steril. 2018;110(4):611–8.

49. Ozbakir B, Tulay P. Does cigarette smoking really have a clinical effect on folliculogenesis and oocyte maturation? Zygote. 2020;28(4):318–21.

50. de Angelis C, Nardone A, Garifalos F, Pivonello C, Sansone A, Conforti A, et al. Smoke, alcohol and drug addiction and female fertility. Reprod Biol Endocrinol. 2020;18(1):21.

51. Lyngsø J, Ramlau-Hansen CH, Bay B, Ingerslev HJ, Strandberg-Larsen K, Kesmodel US. Low-to-moderate alcohol consumption and success in fertility treatment: a Danish cohort study. Hum Reprod. 2019;34(7):1334–44.

52. Hawkins Bressler L, Bernardi LA, De Chavez PJ, Baird DD, Carnethon MR, Marsh EE. Alcohol, cigarette smoking, and ovarian reserve in reproductive-age African-American women. Am J Obstet Gynecol. 2016;215(6):758.e1-.e9.

53. Jensen TK, Hjollund NH, Henriksen TB, Scheike T, Kolstad H, Giwercman A, et al. Does moderate alcohol consumption affect fertility? Follow up study among couples planning first pregnancy. BMJ. 1998;317(7157):505–10.

54. Gaskins AJ, Chavarro JE. Diet and fertility: a review. Am J Obstet Gynecol. 2018;218(4):379–89.

55. Zhang X, Liu X, Chen L, Wu DY, Nie ZW, Gao YY, et al. Caffeine delays oocyte aging and maintains the quality of aged oocytes safely in mouse. Oncotarget. 2017;8(13):20602–11.

56. Mena GP, Mielke GI, Brown WJ. Do physical activity, sitting time and body mass index affect fertility over a 15-year period in women? Data from a large population-based cohort study. Hum Reprod. 2020;35(3):676–83.

57. Gudmundsdottir SL, Flanders WD, Augestad LB. Physical activity and fertility in women: the North-Trøndelag Health Study. Hum Reprod. 2009;24(12):3196–204.

58. Morris SN, Missmer SA, Cramer DW, Powers RD, McShane PM, Hornstein MD. Effects of lifetime exercise on the outcome of in vitro fertilization. Obstet Gynecol. 2006;108(4):938–45.

59. Catov JM, Parker CB, Gibbs BB, Bann CM, Carper B, Silver RM, et al. Patterns of leisure-time physical activity across pregnancy and adverse pregnancy outcomes. Int J Behav Nutr Phys Act. 2018;15(1):68.

60. Pivarnik JM, Chambliss HO, Clapp JF, Dugan SA, Hatch MC, Lovelady CA, et al. Impact of physical activity during pregnancy and postpartum on chronic disease risk. Med Sci Sports Exerc. 2006;38(5):989–1006.

61. Blümel JE, Cano A, Mezones-Holguín E, Barón G, Bencosme A, Benítez Z, et al. A multinational

35

study of sleep disorders during female mid-life. Maturitas. 2012;**72**(4):359–66.

62. Hollander LE, Freeman EW, Sammel MD, Berlin JA, Grisso JA, Battistini M. Sleep quality, estradiol levels, and behavioral factors in late reproductive age women. Obstet Gynecol. 2001;**98**(3):391–7.

63. Willis SK, Hatch EE, Wesselink AK, Rothman KJ, Mikkelsen EM, Wise LA. Female sleep patterns, shift work, and fecundability in a North American preconception cohort study. Fertil Steril. 2019;**111**(6):1201–10.e1.

64. Wang I-D, Liu Y-L, Peng C-K, Chung C-H, Chang S-Y, Tsao C-H, et al. Non-apnea sleep disorder increases the risk of subsequent female infertility—a nationwide population-based cohort study. Sleep. 2017;**41**(1).

65. Stocker LJ, Macklon NS, Cheong YC, Bewley SJ. Influence of shift work on early reproductive outcomes: a systematic review and meta-analysis. Obstet Gynecol. 2014;**124**(1):99–110.

66. Goldstein CA, Smith YR. Sleep, circadian rhythms, and fertility. Curr Sleep Med Rep. 2016;**2**(4):206–17.

67. Vgontzas AN, Zoumakis E, Bixler EO, Lin H-M, Follett H, Kales A, et al. Adverse effects of modest sleep restriction on sleepiness, performance, and inflammatory cytokines. J Clin Endocrinol Metab. 2004;**89**(5):2119–26.

68. von Känel R, Dimsdale JE, Ancoli-Israel S, Mills PJ, Patterson TL, McKibbin CL, et al. Poor sleep is associated with higher plasma proinflammatory cytokine interleukin-6 and procoagulant marker fibrin D-dimer in older caregivers of people with Alzheimer's disease. J Am Geriatr Soc. 2006;**54**(3):431–7.

69. Okun ML, Coussons-Read M, Hall M. Disturbed sleep is associated with increased C-reactive protein in young women. Brain Behav Immun. 2009;**23**(3):351–4.

70. Alijotas-Reig J, Esteve-Valverde E, Ferrer-Oliveras R, Llurba E, Gris JM. Tumor necrosis factor-alpha and pregnancy: focus on biologics. An updated and comprehensive review. Clin Rev Allergy Immunol. 2017;**53**(1):40–53.

71. Gica N, Panaitescu AM, Iancu G, Botezatu R, Peltecu G, Gica C. The role of biological markers in predicting infertility associated with non-obstructive endometriosis. Ginekol Pol. 2020;**91**(4):189–92.

72. Kloss JD, Perlis ML, Zamzow JA, Culnan EJ, Gracia CR. Sleep, sleep disturbance, and fertility in women. Sleep Med Rev. 2015;**22**:78–87.

73. Pal L, Bevilacqua K, Zeitlian G, Shu J, Santoro N. Implications of diminished ovarian reserve (DOR) extend well beyond reproductive concerns. Menopause. 2008;**15**(6).

74. Mo L, Mansfield DR, Joham A, Cain SW, Bennett C, Blumfield M, et al. Sleep disturbances in women with and without polycystic ovary syndrome in an Australian National Cohort. Clin Endocrinol. 2019;**90**(4):570–8.

75. Green A, Cohen-Zion M, Haim A, Dagan Y. Evening light exposure to computer screens disrupts human sleep, biological rhythms, and attention abilities. Chronobiol Int. 2017;**34**(7):855–65.

76. Willis SK, Hatch EE, Wise LA. Sleep and female reproduction. Curr Opin Obstet Gynecol. 2019;**31**(4):222–7.

77. Fallahzadeh H, Zareei Mahmood Abadi H, Momayyezi M, Malaki Moghadam H, Keyghobadi N. The comparison of depression and anxiety between fertile and infertile couples: a meta-analysis study. Int J Reprod Biomed (Yazd). 2019;**17**(3):153–62.

78. Szkodziak F, Krzyżanowski J, Szkodziak P. Psychological aspects of infertility. A systematic review. J Int Med Res. 2020;**48**(6):0300060520932403.

79. Lynch CD, Sundaram R, Maisog JM, Sweeney AM, Buck Louis GM. Preconception stress increases the risk of infertility: results from a couple-based prospective cohort study—the LIFE study. Hum Reprod. 2014;**29**(5):1067–75.

80. Patel A, Sharma PSVN, Kumar P. Application of mindfulness-based psychological interventions in infertility. J Hum Reprod Sci. 2020;**13**(1):3–21.

81. Chow KM, Cheung MC, Cheung IK. Psychosocial interventions for infertile couples: a critical review. J Clin Nurs. 2016;**25**(15–16):2101–13.

82. Morgan N, Christensen K, Skedros G, Kim S, Schliep K. Life stressors, hypertensive disorders of pregnancy, and preterm birth. J Psychosom Obstet Gynaecol. 2020:1–9.

83. Hobel CJ, Goldstein AMY, Barrett ES. Psychosocial stress and pregnancy outcome. Clin Obstet Gynecol. 2008;**51**(2).

84. Wiegner L, Hange D, Björkelund C, Ahlborg G. Prevalence of perceived stress and associations to symptoms of exhaustion, depression and anxiety in a working age population seeking primary care – an observational study. BMC Fam Pract. 2015;**16**(1):38.

85. Schanche E, Vøllestad J, Binder P-E, Hjeltnes A, Dundas I, Nielsen GH. Participant experiences of change in mindfulness-based stress reduction for

anxiety disorders. Int J Qual Stud Health Well-being. 2020;**15**(1):1776094.

86. Li J, Long L, Liu Y, He W, Li M. Effects of a mindfulness-based intervention on fertility quality of life and pregnancy rates among women subjected to first in vitro fertilization treatment. Behav Res Ther. 2016;**77**:96–104.

87. Dhillon A, Sparkes E, Duarte RV. Mindfulness-based interventions during pregnancy: a systematic review and meta-analysis. Mindfulness (N Y). 2017;**8**(6):1421–37.

88. Duncan LG, Cohn MA, Chao MT, Cook JG, Riccobono J, Bardacke N. Benefits of preparing for childbirth with mindfulness training: a randomized controlled trial with active comparison. BMC Pregnancy Childbirth. 2017;**17**(1):140.

89. Muthukrishnan S, Jain R, Kohli S, Batra S. Effect of mindfulness meditation on perceived stress scores and autonomic function tests of pregnant Indian women. J Clin Diagn Res. 2016;**10**(4):CC05–8.

90. Smith JF, Eisenberg ML, Millstein SG, Nachtigall RD, Shindel AW, Wing H, et al. The use of complementary and alternative fertility treatment in couples seeking fertility care: data from a prospective cohort in the United States. Fertil Steril. 2010;**93**(7):2169–74.

91. Miner SA, Robins S, Zhu YJ, Keeren K, Gu V, Read SC, et al. Evidence for the use of complementary and alternative medicines during fertility treatment: a scoping review. BMC Complement Altern Med. 2018;**18**(1):158.

Diagnostic Testing of Reproductive Aging

Tanya L. Glenn and David B. Seifer

Introduction: Why Do We Care?

Although the term "reproductive aging" may not be a widely understood concept within the general population, it is a common reality that many women are facing today. Throughout the last several decades women have been delaying childbearing; in fact, these changes have been fairly recent with each advancing generation. One study quoted the average age of first birth in 1980 as 22.7, which rose to 28.2 in 2013, while another reported that one in five women in the western hemisphere have not attempted to have a child by age 35 [1,2]. A Canadian study reported similar results, in that 4% of women having their first child in 1987 were over 35 years of age, with this percentage almost tripling in 2013 [3]. This drastic demographic change in childbearing age has led to new challenges associated with fertility, such as compromised ovarian reserve, that were not seen in previous generations.

This delay in childbearing has coincided with an increased frequency of age-related infertility and has led to the expanding area of research known as "reproductive aging." Unlike their male counterparts, women are biologically unable to replace oocytes. The maximum number of oocytes a woman has is as a fetus at 20 weeks of gestation with 6–7 million oocytes, declining to 2 million at birth, 400,000 at puberty, 25,000 at age 37, and 1,000 at the average age of menopause (51 years) [3,4]. Although the number of oocytes remaining appears impressively large, it is important to remember that approximately 99% of primordial follicles will become irreversibly atretic, regardless of the age at which a woman may try to conceive [4].

Similar to egg quantity, quality may also decrease over time. Although there is a lack of consensus to truly define egg quality, one way to determine this is through monthly fecundity or the ability to conceive per menstrual cycle [5].

Monthly fecundity declines after the age of 35; however, small decreases occur much earlier than this. There is a 6% decrease in monthly fecundity in women age 25–29, when compared with those aged 20–24 [6]. This declines by 14% in women age 30–34 and by 31% in individuals over 35 [6]. The monthly fecundability in the 10 years prior to menopause (approximately age 41) is significantly decreased. Importantly, these changes are also seen in artificial reproduction [3,6].

Another way to assess egg quality is through aneuploidy rate, which also naturally increases with age. Women under the age of 35 have an aneuploidy rate of approximately 10%, which rises to over 50% at age 40, and reaches nearly 99% by age 45 [3]. This increased aneuploidy rate increases the miscarriage rate, as well as reducing the chances of achieving a live birth.

What Is Ovarian Reserve?

Knowing that natural fertility and successful outcomes of assisted reproductive technologies (ART) decrease earlier than often realized emphasizes the importance of identifying individuals with reduced fecundability, regardless of age. This can be accomplished through ovarian reserve testing, to assess the approximate number of remaining oocytes. By obtaining this information, a physician is better able to counsel a woman about her chances of conceiving with the assistance of various therapies such as timed intrauterine insemination, ovulation induction, or in vitro fertilization (IVF). The ultimate goal with ovarian reserve testing is to create more personalized medicine by tailoring fertility treatment to each individual, while lowering the risk of ovarian hyperstimulation syndrome (OHSS), a potentially life-threatening condition, and providing better expectation for the onset of menopause [4]. However, ovarian reserve assesses *ovarian quantity*, but not necessarily *ovarian quality*. Thus, therein lies the opportunity, and the challenge, of identifying how many oocytes remain in the ovaries, with limited information on whether these oocytes will create an embryo and can achieve a live birth.

Ovarian reserve is also a way to identify individuals with diminished ovarian reserve (DOR). Although there is no universal definition for DOR, it can be thought of as a woman who has a lower number of oocytes than would be expected from other women of similar age. In order to attempt to categorize this, the Bologna criteria were created, in which two of the three following criteria are met for an individual to have DOR: age ≥40, low antral follicle count (AFC) with <5–7 follicles or anti-Mullerian hormone (AMH) of <0.5–1.1 ng/ml, or a poor ovarian response (POR) categorized by either a cancelled cycle or less than four oocytes retrieved. Some studies have characterized DOR by a follicle stimulating hormone (FSH) level >12 mIU/ml; however, no standard has been universally accepted. Women with DOR have a much lower fertility rate, with one study reporting a 6.7% live birth rate (LBR) in women who were older than 40 with an FSH >12 mIU/ml [7]. Recently, a 37% increase in DOR cases was noted from 2004 to 2011, even though minimal change was seen in the age of women attempting to conceive between these time periods [7]. These observations highlight that chronological age is only one factor when assessing ovarian reserve.

Historical and Limited Value Tests

Prior to reviewing our current tests, it is prudent to determine both historical and limited value tests. One of the traditional stimulation tests is the clomiphene citrate challenge test (CCCT), in which a patient takes a 100 mg dose of clomiphene on cycle day 5–9, and an FSH level is drawn on days 3 and 10. If an appropriate response is generated through the hypothalamic pituitary ovarian (HPO) axis, this results in suppression of FSH between days 3 and 10 [3]. An increased rate of detection of DOR with an abnormal CCCT has been noted in certain studies, but not all. However, even a limited increase in rate of detection was accomplished at greater expense, patient risk, clinical effort, and time. Additionally, a basal FSH or antral follicle count (AFC) is of equivalent clinical value [3].

Inhibin B was also studied as a potential marker of ovarian reserve. Inhibin B acts upon the negative feedback system of the HPO axis, thus preventing FSH levels from becoming elevated throughout the early part of the follicular cycle. However, Inhibin B is produced by antral follicles, and thus is gonadotrophin dependent, responding to FSH levels, unlike primordial follicles which are gonadotrophin independent [8]. Furthermore, previous assays showed a high amount of variance between laboratories, making interpretation challenging [8]. Estradiol was postulated as an indicator of ovarian reserve, yet studies displayed mixed results when investigating the relationship between estradiol levels and age, and therefore this is of limited benefit [9]. Today estradiol is mainly used to place the findings of FSH in clinical context.

Other tests that have been studied but are limited and not very informative in clinical practice include the gonadotropin (GnRH) stimulation and exogenous FSH ovarian reserve test. The GnRH stimulation test requires individuals to activate the HPO axis with leuprolide acetate, then estradiol levels are checked on days 2, 3, and 4. Researchers calculated the change in estrogen from day 2–3 and day 3–4. In their results, they saw multiple patterns of estrogen rise, but the most prudent results were in individuals who did not have a doubling of estrogen on day 3 and then limited rise on day 4. Individuals with these characteristics had the lowest number of mature follicles and the lowest pregnancy rate [10]. The exogenous FSH ovarian reserve test requires estradiol and FSH levels to be drawn at baseline, then FSH hormones to be administered, and estradiol levels drawn 24 hours later. The combination of the change in estradiol from baseline with a basal FSH level was seen to be predictive of who would have an appropriate response to IVF stimulation [11]. Although these stimulation tests appear to be of benefit, just like the CCCT, they require additional time, cost, are staff intensive, and provide little information about what patients truly are looking for in an ovarian reserve test – their chances of a live birth.

Ideal Test

The above-mentioned tests have been shown to be of limited value, are expensive, time consuming, and lack the ability to identify an individual's reproductive potential. This begs the question of what makes up an ideal ovarian reserve test? What can be highlighted as most important is the ability to identify not only quantity but also the quality of a woman's remaining eggs. We now have a better understanding of fertility decline and egg reserve, yet this does not necessarily mean that the remaining eggs have low quality. Additionally, tests should be reproducible, independent of the menstrual cycle, noninvasive, rapid, and highly specific. What would be most ideal is a test that would enable physicians to counsel women as they age about their chances for pregnancy/live birth, and to utilize these tests and/or algorithms to provide direct care for the timing and type of stimulation protocol, with decreased risk of complications such as OHSS. Results should also have age-specific values for improved counseling of women to enable realistic reproductive expectations for family planning.

Where Are We Now?

Age

There are several tests that physicians utilize currently to help women through their reproductive journey, the first being not a test but a simple fact: chronologic age. Age is one of the best predictors for reproductive outcomes, not only to counsel about expectations of ovarian reserve but also aneuploidy, birth complications, and outcomes. It is also considered the most important predictor of IVF success [3].

The relationship of time to conception when compared with age has also been noted to increase with age. One study examined nearly 3,500 natural cycles from over 900 women and noted that in the cohort of individuals who became pregnant, the time to conception was much longer in women over 40. On average, it took 8 months to become pregnant in individuals age >40 and 12 months for those age >42, compared with only 4 months in women who were 38–39 years old [2]. When utilizing this information to compare monthly fecundability versus women aged 30–31, the average reduction of fecundability was 53% in women age 40–41 and 59% in women aged 42–44. Of note, only 5% of the population in this study was aged >40 [2]. Uniquely, these findings did not change with body mass index (BMI). The other important part of this

study was the relationship between nulliparity and age. Nulliparous women had a higher risk for infertility compared with their multiparous counterparts, regardless of age. Nulliparous women over 40 had a 50% reduction in fertility compared with other women over 40 who had previously had a live birth [2].

Although the statistics seem to be challenging for older women who are attempting to conceive, there are several important counseling matters to consider and to place in perspective. One is that results suggest it takes longer to conceive, not that older women were incapable of conceiving. Additionally, age has no impact on endometrial receptivity, therefore the use of donor eggs remains a viable and commonly available but more costly option [3].

Follicle Stimulating Hormone

Analysis of follicle stimulating hormone was the first test used to determine ovarian reserve in the late 1980s. This test requires an intact HPO axis to have a meaningful value, as it responds to the secretion of hormones by ovarian follicles, estradiol, and inhibin b, which are being recruited during follicular development. Follicle stimulating hormone is only clinically significant if collected during the early portion of the follicular phase, days 2–5 of the menstrual cycle, at which time hormones created from growing follicles normally suppress pituitary secretion of FSH. Therefore, the test is only reflective of the current stimulated follicles, not the preantral follicles. Values of FSH are often coupled with estradiol levels to determine validity, as an elevated estradiol (>80 pg/ml) in the setting of a normal FSH indicates early recruitment of follicles, likely through a reduction in the ovarian pool and consistent with DOR [1]. McTavish et al., through their work with transgenic FSH mice, postulated that it may be the elevation of FSH itself that causes detrimental effects on the ovary and uterus, even when the female has oocytes remaining and regular ovulatory pattern [12].

Advantages of determining FSH include ease of use, standardization across labs, and, because of use since the late 1980s, a considerable amount of relevant research. In addition, markedly elevated FSH levels can be helpful to determine the onset of menopausal status after it has occurred and DOR [1,3]. Yet there are numerous limitations to use of

FSH levels as an ovarian reserve test. These include high intracycle and intercycle variability, dependence on intact HPO axis, inaccuracy in those taking oral contraceptives, high false positive rates in younger patient populations, and inability to use results to determine IVF protocols, to predict OHSS, or to predict a normal ovarian response to gonadotropins. There is also variation in the medical literature in terms of a cut-off value for an abnormal test, which can be anywhere between 10 and 20 IU/l. Therefore, the sensitivity to rule out DOR varies anywhere between 11% and 86% when the cut-off value changes [1].

Antral Follicle Count

Antral follicle count uses an ultrasound to calculate the number of follicles measuring between 2 and 10 mm (antral follicles) as a reflection of the ovarian pool on days 2–5 of the menstrual cycle [1,3]. Its use as a predictor for IVF outcomes was not established until the late 1990s, even though correlation between ovarian volume and menopausal status was investigated almost a decade before [13,14]. Although ultrasound limitation prevents identification of preantral follicles, the theory is that the current small antral follicle count is a reflection of the remaining ovarian follicular primordial pool. Yet, it is not possible to use AFC to assign a numerical value to determine the actual remaining ovarian pool. It is also limited because it is vulnerable to subjective bias and depends upon the ultrasonographer's technique, sensitivity of the machine and body habitus of the patient. Studies have shown that AFC may be helpful in determining ovarian response to ART or menopausal transition but its applicability is limited in quantifying ovarian quality or LBR [3,4].

Numerous studies have been conducted analyzing the associations between AFC and clinical pregnancy rate (CPR), ovarian response in IVF cycles, embryo quality, LBR, and miscarriage rate. One study that analyzed pregnancy and miscarriage rates in unstimulated cycles with male factor infertility found that AFC did not correlate with CPR or miscarriage rates, when comparing individuals with low (0–12), medium (13–23), or high (>24) AFC. They also investigated a subset of individuals with AFC <6 and results did not change. Importantly, AFC and miscarriage or CPR *did not alter with age*. This led the authors

to suggest that lower cost options for fertility treatments should not be withheld because of a low AFC in women of advanced reproductive age [5]. However, their cut-off values for low (0–12) or very low (<6) AFC, were much higher than current criteria for DOR, in which patients have <3–4 follicles [1].

Importantly, research has shown a correlation between AFC and ovarian response in stimulated cycles. A linear response has been noted between the AFC and how the ovaries respond to exogenous gonadotropins, and the number of eggs at time of retrieval, identifying those at higher risk of cycle cancellation because of DOR. One study reported a specificity of 73–97% of <3–4 eggs at retrieval when the AFC was 3–4 at the baseline [1,4]. Notably, response to a cycle is not equivalent to pregnancy rates, therefore AFC may be beneficial for advising older patients with lower AFC concerning risk of cycle cancellation, yet has limited value in determining LBR [1,5].

There are numerous advantages to use of AFC for ovarian reserve testing and education of patients: the test is easy to perform, provides immediate results, and is overall noninvasive. It also may be helpful when choosing stimulation protocols, particularly in individuals who are at high risk for OHSS [1,5]. Although some interobserver variability has been noted, this was not statistically significant in one study that compared ultrasounds from six different reproductive endocrinology physicians [15]. Furthermore, the highest variability was noted in individuals who had an elevated AFC, not individuals at risk for DOR. That same report also analyzed cycle variability in individuals from different cycles of the same year. Similar to interobserver variability, intercycle variability was only significant when the AFC was >15 and was not dependent on age [15].

Several disadvantages have already been mentioned concerning AFC, specifically its lack of predictive value of CPR/LBR and egg quality, all factors listed in consideration of an ideal test of ovarian reserve. Moreover, AFC is limited to a specific time in the menstrual cycle, it is affected by exogenous hormones (such as oral contraceptive pills), and is limited by the quality of the ultrasound machine and body habitus (i.e., obesity). As the current US patient population has a 66% overweight or obesity rate, this is detrimental to the predictive value of AFC. Although previous studies have not shown large interobserver variability, reliability of tests is also dependent on the sonographer's training and how many different sonographers are doing the assessment of AFC at an institution. Essentially, the greater the number of sonographers that perform AFC, the greater the variability and the greater the coefficient of variation, therefore reducing precision, accuracy and predictive value of the test. Overall, AFC tends to be overestimated, often because of an inability to differentiate between atretic follicles from the previous cycle and new follicles being recruited. Additionally, the use of hormonal contraceptives (combined oral, progesterone only oral, and progesterone-based intrauterine devices) likely temporarily reduces AFC [16]. Last, although relatively noninvasive in the sexually active population, it is inappropriate to conduct in the pediatric/adolescent population [4].

Most notably, when considering AFC in women of advanced reproductive age, a low AFC is reflective of low ovarian response to medication but not of low quality of oocytes or embryos. Additionally, although a decline in AFC is predictive of menopausal status, no cut-off value has been determined. Thus, AFC should be taken under advisement, and should not be used as an indicator to prevent the pursuit of fertility treatment [3].

Anti-Mullerian Hormone

Anti-Mullerian hormone is the most recently developed ovarian reserve test, discovered as clinically relevant in 2002 [17] and soon after developed as a marker for ovarian reserve. Unlike its predecessors, it is reflective of the small and large preantral follicle count found in the gonadotropin independent portion of early folliculogenesis, and small antral follicles of the gonadotropin dependent portion of late folliculogenesis. Anti-Mullerian hormone is a glycoprotein produced by the granulosa cells of early follicles (small and large preantral and small antral) that prevents the over-recruitment of primordial follicles [17]. Therefore, unlike FSH, estradiol, and inhibin B, it reflects the ovarian pool that is independent of gonadotropin influence and is relatively stable across and between menstrual cycles [1]. Anti-Mullerian hormone does decrease during a stimulated cycle; however, the rate of decline does not correlate with LBR and has not been found to be particularly

useful to assess and/or follow during a stimulated cycle [18]. Additionally, because it is not dependent on an intact HPO axis, AMH has clinical use across a variety of ages and reproductive pathologies such as polycystic ovary syndrome (PCOS) [17].

Caution is required when determining cut-off values for low, normal, and high AMH levels, as, similar to FSH, there may be a wide range of "normal" that changes the sensitivity and specificity of the test. Moreover, over the years, the type of assay has changed from manual to automated and automated values were noted to be lower and more specific than those that were manually determined. Therefore, previous research values must be taken under some consideration [19]. Additionally, some fluctuations can be noted in calibration from a single lab, let alone the variations and standards between labs. Thus, it is crucial that physicians understand which assay they are using to allow comparison of values [20]. In older assays, the median AMH value in one study of >1,000 healthy women with male factor infertility was 1.27 ng/ml by the age of 40, whereas another study of >17,000 women who presented for a variety of fertility problems was 0.7 ng/ml [21]. In a review by Tal and Seifer cut-off values for DOR for gonadotropins were defined between 0.1 and 1.66 ng/ml, which corresponds to sensitivity of 44–97% [1]. In similar fashion, this review delved into the concept that conservative age-related normal values of an individual at 40 would be 1.0 ng/ml, whereas a value of 0.5 ng/ml at the age of 45 would be anticipated. Yet even though these values would be considered "normal," they still reflect a declining ovarian pool and thus a reduction in ovarian response in stimulated cycles [1]. Importantly, it is difficult to obtain true baseline AMH values in a healthy patient population, as the majority of the women who undergo AMH testing do so as a result of a history of infertility. However, numerous independent studies globally have clearly shown that AMH values decline over time, even during peak reproductive years, with one study reporting the decline at a rate of 0.2 ng/ml per year until the age of 35 and continuing at 0.1 ng/ml per year thereafter [9,21]. It has been highlighted several times that AMH testing is most applicable to the infertility population for counseling purposes, therefore a low AMH in a noninfertile population of women presently has limited clinical value [1].

Anti-Mullerian hormone is traditionally measured in nanograms per milliliter and current assays often have a lower detection limit of around 0.08 ng/ml [22]. Therefore, women of advanced reproductive age or those with DOR may receive a generic <0.08 ng/ml result rather than an actual value for AMH. A small study evaluated 48 women with DOR who were undergoing IVF and calculated their AMH values in picograms/ml (pg/ml). They found that women with an AMH of >500 pg/ml had an 83% sensitivity of obtaining at least three oocytes at the time of retrieval, whereas no oocytes were retrieved from any woman with an AMH <100 pg/ml [22]. Only 21 of these women had embryo transfers, of whom four had clinical pregnancies and two delivered. However, one of the clinical pregnancies had an AMH of 142 pg/ml, further supporting the notion that our current tests must be used to counsel patients and not as an indication to refuse care [22]. Another study of ultralow AMH levels, defined as ≤ 0.16 ng/ml (the lowest level of detection with the most highly used AMH kit of the time, Beckman-Coulter), reviewed over 5,000 fresh and 243 frozen cycles taken from the Society for Assisted Reproductive Technology Clinic Outcome Reporting System (SART CORS) between 2012 and 2013 [23]. When comparing women of the same age with ultralow AMH to normal AMH (defined as 1.0–1.2 ng/ml), women with ultralow AMH had a lower LBR per fresh cycle (9.5% versus 28.7%), increased risk of cycle cancellation after start (38.6% versus 7.5%), and were less likely to have extra embryos for cryopreservation (5.7% versus 26.8%). Thus, women with ultralow AMH need to be counseled about a higher possibility of cycle cancellation, less oocytes retrieved, less embryos cryopreserved, and a lower LBR. Yet, if an individual is successful in making it to embryo transfer, results indicate a LBR of over 20% [23].

Unlike other ovarian reserve labs, AMH can be drawn at any time of the cycle, as it is relatively stable throughout the cycle because of its indirect reflection of the primordial pool and not follicles that are currently under the influence of gonadotropins. However, it is influenced by other factors that should be taken into consideration. Use of hormones (≥3 months), such as oral contraceptives, should be discontinued for at least 2 months so as not to falsely lower AMH values [16]. A recent retrospective Danish study showed that not only could AMH be affected by current use of combined oral contraceptives (31.1% reduction in AMH) but also by use of progesterone only oral contraceptives (35.6% reduction), and progesterone intrauterine devices (17.1% reduction). However, such a decrease was not seen with the contraceptive vaginal ring. As a result of these findings, caution is proposed when testing ovarian reserve in any individual who has taken hormonally based contraceptives for >3 months. Other factors that can affect AMH levels include tobacco use, obesity, anovulation/PCOS, low vitamin D levels, and race/ethnicity [1]. One study examining AMH and race/ethnicity showed that compared with white women, black and Hispanic women had AMH levels that were 25% lower, despite controlling for differences in age, BMI, HIV status, and tobacco use [24].

The predictive nature of AMH in determining ovarian reserve has been noted as particularly robust. Some of the earliest research on AMH identified the ability to better predict an adequate response to ovarian stimulation compared with early follicular FSH. This initial study in 2002, which established a relationship between AMH and egg yield in ovulation induction, analyzed AMH levels from frozen day 3 serum samples and levels were compared in women with <6 versus >11 oocytes retrieved. Anti-Mullerian hormone values of those with >11 oocytes averaged 2.5 ± 0.3 ng/ml versus 1.0 ± 0.4 ng/ml in individuals with <6 oocytes, even though FSH in all of these women was <10 IU/l. Additionally, higher AMH was associated with more mature oocytes [17].

Similar to its predecessors, AMH has not been proven to have a powerful predictive value for pregnancy, LBR in a single specific IVF cycle, or quality of remaining oocyte pool [1,3]. The specificity of nonpregnancy rates changes with various AMH cut-off values, with ranges anywhere between 55% and 89%, with a sensitivity of 19–66% [1]. However, one study did report that extremely abnormal levels correlated with a pregnancy rate of <5%, yet these values occurred in only 3% of their patient population [3]. One large review of data from the SART CORS database showed that AMH was a very weak predictor of LBR after ART, both for fresh and frozen embryo transfers [25]. In this review, over 50,000 fresh and 15,000 frozen cycles were analyzed, taking into consideration confounders such as age, BMI, race, day of transfer, and FSH. When using a multiple logistic regression model, the area under the curve (AUC) for fresh transfer was only 0.63 and for frozen transfer was 0.54. The investigators stressed in their conclusion that although there may be a weak association, AMH alone should not be used to prevent individuals undergoing ART [25]. Smaller reviews also showed similar results, with a meta-analysis of AMH levels and CPR with an AUC for CPR of only 0.63 for all women and 0.70 in individuals with DOR [26]. However, recent analysis of the SART CORS database from 2014 to 2016 of women with DOR, defined as AMH <1.0 ng/ml, showed that AMH is prognostic of cumulative LBR independent of age [27]. Cumulative live birth rate is the most clinically relevant measure of success of an IVF cycle because it accounts for the rate of live birth resulting from a single individual egg retrieval whether or not the transfer is from a fresh or a frozen cycle. This most recent information suggests that AMH is of greatest clinical value when setting realistic patient expectations in counseling within the context of DOR (Table 4.1).

One potential way to analyze the quality of oocytes is by studying miscarriage rates. A few studies have noted a link between miscarriage rates and AMH values, and this observation could be particularly useful when counseling women of advanced reproductive age. In one study by Lyttle Schumacher et al., of over 500

naturally conceived pregnancies, individuals with recurrent pregnancy loss or whose current pregnancies ended in miscarriage were noted to have lower AMH values, with similar results seen in McCormack's study that specifically analyzed 182 women with recurrent pregnancy loss [28,29]. Additionally, Lyttle Schumacher et al.'s study determined that the relative risk for miscarriage decreased with each unit increase in AMH, even after adjusting for numerous confounders such as age, race, and BMI was 0.83 (95% CI 0.73; 0.94) [28]. Importantly, those with a modest decrease in AMH, 0.40–1.0 ng/ml, did not have an elevated risk of miscarriage compared with individuals with AMH >1.0 ng/ml. However, a 50% miscarriage rate was noted in those with AMH <0.40 ng/ml [28]. Yet, in McCormack's study, miscarriage rate was fairly consistent across low, normal, and high values of AMH values, although the authors did note a significantly decreased AMH value in those with recurrent pregnancy loss compared with controls and a wide variance of normal values [29,30]. A recent study by Tarasconi et al. examined women undergoing IVF and ongoing pregnancy rates (>12 weeks) were compared with AMH values (low 0.08–1.60; medium 1.61–5.59; high 5.6–35.0 ng/ml) [31]. The authors performed a regression analysis to remove confounding factors, such as response to medication and age. It was determined that in women age 33 and over, a lower AMH incurred a higher chance of miscarriage than did medium or high AMH values.

Table 4.1 Cumulative live birth rate (CLBR) (%) in women with diminished ovarian reserve stratified by anti-Mullerian hormone (AMH) and age

AMH (ng/ml)	Age (years)				
	<35	35–37	38–40	41–42	43+
0.00–0.10	22.1	18.7	9.2	6.1	1.2
0.11–0.20	29.1	19.8	12.5	6.4	1.7
0.21–0.30	30.3	26.1	16.3	7.9	1.9
0.31–0.40	32.0	26.1	17.8	7.4	2.4
0.41–0.50	35.9	27.6	17.7	7.3	3.2
0.51–0.60	34.0	26.7	19.1	9.2	3.9
0.61–0.70	36.7	30.8	18.9	10.1	2.6
0.71–0.80	38.2	31.2	21.8	11.1	3.2
0.81–0.90	42.7	30.2	19.0	10.7	4.1
0.91–<1.00	41.2	34.0	20.6	9.5	4.1

From: Tal R, Seifer DB, Tal R, Granger E, Wantman E, Tal O. AMH highly correlates with cumulative live birth rate in women with diminished ovarian reserve independent of age. *J Clin Endocrinol Metab* 2021;106(9):2754–66.

Thus, it was postulated that AMH production is lower in the follicles containing inadequate oocytes, leading to a higher rate of miscarriage. Notably, all of these studies were completed in women undergoing IVF cycles and may not be reflective of natural conception cycles [28,29,31]. In contrast, Zarek et al. found no correlation between AMH values and miscarriage rate. They looked at 1,202 women with a history of one to two losses and found that the miscarriage rates in unassisted pregnancies were not statistically different in those with AMH <1.0, 1.0–3.5, or >3.5 (15.3%, 10.3%, 10.4%, respectively), although the majority of women who achieved CPR had normal (48.9%) or high (40.8%) AMH versus low AMH (10.3%). Additionally, there were no differences in aneuploidy rate with the various AMH levels [32]. More research is needed to determine the relationship between miscarriage rate and AMH, and whether it is pertinent to women naturally conceiving, as well as conceiving through ART with extremely abnormal values.

Previously, it has not been possible to estimate menopausal transition by any laboratory test. However, Freeman et al. reported that AMH values can be helpful to determine an approximate time to menopause, which alters with an individual's age [33]. An AMH value of <0.20 ng/ml in those who are 35–39 years old could estimate 10 years to menopause, while the same value in those who are 40–44 years old would predict menopause in under 8 years [33]. In the review article by Leader et al., they pointed out that research has shown some statistical significance between AMH value and the timing of menopause; however, this is also impacted by race and BMI, and the confidence intervals vary widely [20]. Thus, AMH may be better used to predict a later onset of menopause or an earlier onset in individuals whose AMH values are at the extremes, either high or low, respectively, compared with age-related normal ranges [20]. At this time, more information is required to assist with the creation of algorithms or established values for age and time to menopause.

The use of AMH as a predictor for ovulatory reserve has been widespread and impactful in the field of infertility. It has improved the ability of physicians to choose the timing of appropriate stimulation protocols and medications, as well as reduce the risk of OHSS. There is limited variability throughout the cycle, AMH does not require an intact HPO axis, testing is relatively noninvasive, and the test itself has an outstanding turnaround time if using an automated assay (i.e., 20 minutes). Although strict cut-off values are difficult to ascertain, age-specific normal ranges are available and AMH is sensitive to change (decrease) over time with age. Additionally, testing for AMH has utility outside of infertility, such as suggesting a timeframe for the menopausal transition and assisting in diagnosis of PCOS.

For all of its advantages, there should be consideration of multiple observations with regard to AMH. Although AMH can be taken at any time of the menstrual cycle, slight fluctuations may be noted, the values can be altered by external exposures and no generalized cut-offs have been identified as recommendations that fertility treatment cannot be pursued. Additionally, like any laboratory test, this test requires sample handling, appropriate laboratory technique, and there are variations between lab standards/values. Last, and most importantly, low AMH does not mean low egg quality or that a live birth cannot occur, and thus low AMH should not be used as an indication of sterility [1,4,20,22].

Decisions, Decisions

After reviewing the numerous ways to estimate ovarian reserve – whether through hormone levels, age, or ultrasound – which is the most informative? In part the choice of test is dependent on the body habitus of the patient and resources available to the clinician, for example trained sonographers and available laboratories; however, the majority of fertility centers have these tools at their fingertips (Table 4.2).

When comparing AMH with AFC, both have the advantage of being predictors of a poor response or an over-response (OHSS) to gonadotropins. Additionally, both show a decline with age; as AMH is predicted to decrease by 6% each year and AFC by 4.5% each year, regardless of whether an individual is fertile or infertile [34]. Although high AFC can be suspicious for an exaggerated response, especially in PCOS individuals, AMH is better able to predict a high response. Measurement of AMH can also be used to estimate ovarian reserve more accurately, as it indirectly measures the primordial follicular pool via preantral and early small antral follicles,

Table 4.2 Comparison of ovarian reserve markers: follicle stimulating hormone, antral follicular count, and anti-Mullerian hormone

Test	Basal FSH	AFC	AMH
Year described	1988	1997	2002
Timing	Day 2–5 of menstrual cycle	Day 2–5 of menstrual cycle	Any day
Temporal change indicating ovarian aging	Latest	Early	Earliest
Intracycle variability	Clinically significant	Clinically significant	Minimal
Intracycle variability	Clinically significant	Minimal	Minimal
Methodology	Automated	Ultrasound	ELISA/automated
Cost. $	95–125	300–500	76–95
Advantages	Widespread use	Immediate results; good predictive value for stimulation ovarian response, including predicting OHSS	Reliable; high sensitivity; good predictive value for stimulation ovarian response, including predicting OHSS
Limitations	Reliability; low sensitivity; dependent on functional HPO axis; less precision because of intercycle and intracycle variability; does not predict OHSS	Interobserver variability (sonographer dependent); requires cost of ultrasound technician and availability of ultrasound machine; significant intercycle variation in overweight and obese	Lack of international standardized assay; requires careful sample preparation and storage
Cut-offs used for determining sensitivities and specificities	10–20 IU/l	<3–4 follicles (total)	0.1–1.66[a] ng/ml or <0.1–<0.3[b] ng/ml
Sensitivity for poor response, %	11–86 [14]	9–73 [14]	44–97 [4]
Specificity for poor response, %	45–100 [14]	73–97 [14]	41–100 [4]
AUC for poor response	0.68 (95% CI 0.61–0.71) [42]	0.76 (95% CI 0.70–0.82) [42]	0.78 (95% CI 0.72–0.84) [42]
Sensitivity for nonpregnancy, %	3–65 [14]	7–34 [14]	19–66 [32]
Specificity for nonpregnancy, %	50–100 [14]	64–98 [14]	55–89 [32]

AFC, antral follicular count; AMH, anti-Mullerian hormone; AUC, area under the curve; CI, confidence interval; ELISA, enzyme-linked immunosorbent assay; FSH, follicle stimulating hormone; HPO, hypothalamus-pituitary-ovarian; OHSS, ovarian hyperstimulation syndrome.

[a] Cut-offs used for calculating sensitivities and specificities for prediction of poor ovarian response;

[b] Cut-offs used for calculating sensitivities and specificities for prediction of nonpregnancy.

From "Ovarian reserve testing: a user's guide," by R. Tal and D.B. Seifer, 2017, *American Journal of Obstetrics & Gynecology*, pp. 129–140. Copyright 2017 by Elsevier Inc. Reprinted with permission.

rather than only late antral follicles as is the case when measuring AFC [4,9].

When comparing AMH with FSH, researchers noted that protocols driven by AMH values had higher embryo transfers, CPR, LBR, and cumulative live birth rates when compared with those that used FSH [4]. Similar to when comparing AMH to AFC, AMH predicts high response better than AFC, while predicting lower response with improved accuracy.

Discordant Tests

Although a direct comparison of ovarian reserve tests often shows that AMH may be slightly more predictive and helpful for protocol choice, it is rare for a physician to obtain just one of these tests. Often, when counseling a patient and deciding on timing and type of treatment course, all three may be performed and age is taken into consideration. Therefore, it can be a common dilemma to have discordant tests, where one test

Table 4.3 AMH and FSH discrepancies

Frequency of discordance between FSH and AMH >40 years old	LBR with AMH normal (≥0.8 ng/ml) FSH abnormal (>10 mIU/ml)	LBR with AMH abnormal (<0.8 ng/ml) FSH normal (≤10 mIU/ml)
33.3% [35] **20% for women >38 years old** **9.1% for women <35 years old**	22.8–39% [34,37]	15.6–26% [34,37]

AMH, anti-Mullerian hormone; FSH, follicle stimulating hormone, LBR, live birth rate.

states ovarian reserve is compromised and another shows an age-appropriate value.

Only a few studies have specifically compared outcomes when AMH and AFC are discordant, and these found that the results are often between what would be expected when both are age-appropriate or both are low. Thus, patients may be counseled that they can anticipate oocyte numbers to be less than normal, but not necessarily an inadequate response.

A significant amount of research has gone into investigating outcomes when AMH and FSH are discordant. When looking at oocyte yield, the majority of studies have shown that AMH is more predictive of an appropriate or inadequate outcome than FSH. This is especially true as a women ages, as noted in Leader et al.'s study in 2012 of over 5,000 women specifically looking at outcomes in concordant and discordant values [35,36]. In women <35 years old, 1/11 had discordant values (AMH <0.8 ng/ml and FSH >10 mIU/ml); however, this changed to 1/5 in women older than 38 and 1/3 in those aged >40 [36]. In Wang's study of nearly 14,000 cycles, they found that a reassuring AMH (>1.0 ng/ml) was more predictive than a reassuring FSH (≤10 mIU/ml), in all age groups [35]. Additionally, when lab values were discordant, those with a reassuring AMH and nonreassuring FSH had higher LBR (22.8%) versus those with only a reassuring FSH (15.6%, p<0.005). Moreover, the average ages of those who had concordant nonreassuring values and individuals with only a reassuring FSH were older than those with both normal or with only a reassuring AMH (38.0, 37.3 versus 34.1, 35.6, respectively; p<0.001) [35]. In a larger, retrospective study of over 44,000 women, 25% had discordant AMH and FSH, in which LBR was lower for women with a normal FSH (<10 mIU/ml) and low AMH (<1.0 ng/dl), when compared with those with a normal AMH and high FSH (26% versus

39%, respectively) [37]. A recent editorial nicely summarized many of the above findings, highlighting the conundrum physicians often face, as discordant AMH/FSH values confuse matters for nearly one in five women seen for fertility issues [38]. Again, they feature that LBR is much higher in women with normal AMH and abnormal FSH than the opposite (39% versus 26%). However, limitations of each of these studies were reviewed, such as the exclusion of freeze all studies and lack of knowledge of confounding factors (prior pregnancies, losses, embryos frozen). In all, this reflection focused on how ovarian reserve testing can assist with patient care; however, the patient's prior history and other laboratory values are crucial when counseling on reproductive issues (Table 4.3) [38].

New Kids On the Block: Algorithms

It is apparent that we are far from having a test that is able to reach all of the established goals previously discussed. Thus, providers often use multiple tests, as previously mentioned, to counsel patients on their reproductive capacity and drive decisions surrounding treatment type and medication choices. But this can be especially challenging when current tests may not have well-defined cut-off values, vary between labs, and results from different tests have conflicting conclusions. This is why multiple commercial diagnostic companies have created algorithms that examine several values at once and use these values to help with education and decision purposes. Additionally, there are online calculators that patients or providers may use to help predict success (Table 4.4).

There are currently at least three online calculators available to the public. One of these is on the Center for Disease Control's (CDC) website. This IVF success estimator allows patients/providers to

Table 4.4 Ovarian reserve algorithms

Lab test	Purpose	Factors assessed	Cons	Uses
SART Patient Predictor [43]	Estimate LBR after one, two, or three ART cycles Estimates LBR and risks of multiples with two embryos after one cycle	Age AMH BMI Prior full-term pregnancies Some diagnostic information concerning infertility	Limited information on infertility diagnosis Prior ART cycles not assessed	Counseling
CDC IVF Success Outcome [39]	Estimate LBR after one, two, or three ART cycles Estimates LBR and risks of multiples with two embryos after one cycle	Age BMI Fertility history including prior ART Autologous or donor eggs	Hormone levels not assessed Ovarian reserve not assessed	Counseling
Med Calc Egg Freezing Tool [42]	Estimate LBR pending age and number frozen oocytes	Age Oocytes cryopreserved	Limited information for patients who have not undergone ART	Counseling
Ovarian Age Algorithm (OvAge) [44]	Linear model to assess ovarian age	Hormone levels Age Ovarian volume Vascular flow index	Not prospectively tested	Counseling
ReproSource: Ovarian assessment report (OAR) [45]	Algorithm to estimate number of oocytes at retrieval	Hormone levels Age	Does not consider previous ART cycles, BMI, fertility history	Reduces number of independent variables while counseling
Unify [46]	Algorithm to estimate various IVF outcomes (LBR)	Multi-factorial (10–20 variables) pending center-specific data	Requires site enrollment into program	Site-specific counseling

AMH, anti-Mullerian hormone; ART, assisted reproductive technologies; BMI, body mass index; FSH, follicle stimulating hormone; IVF, in vitro fertilization; LBR, live birth rate.

calculate their predicted LBR after one, two, or three ART cycles. This is based on history and anthropomorphic data, such as age, BMI, and fertility/infertility history [39]. A paper published in 2017 critiqued the database the CDC uses to report ART outcomes as their LBR does not consider embryo or oocyte banking. This inflates the LBR for practices that predominantly oocyte/embryo bank because of the lower denominator [40]. From the most recent database in 2017, it is reported that success rates (i.e., LBR) are now considered for the 12 months surrounding the retrieval and not just in the consecutive year. However, it is not specified whether the LBR includes banking cycles or not [41]. This has the potential to falsely elevate the LBR in the calculator. A second online calculator is MedCalc, which has an Egg Freezing Counseling Tool, which can estimate how many live births can be expected with age and number of eggs already frozen. It is important to note, both websites do counsel against using this information as medical advice [42].

Along with these online calculators, the Society for Assisted Reproductive Technology (SART) has used over 10 years of data and 500,000 cycles to put together an algorithm on its website to help estimate LBR after one, two, or three ART cycles based on age, BMI, infertility diagnosis, and prior live births. Unlike the other two sites, this algorithm can also estimate the LBR with the risk of multiples after a single two embryo transfer [43] (Table 4.3). All of these calculators assist with counseling, yet often fall short of the true ability to predict LBR to account for an individual's entire history.

A last noncommercial algorithm to consider was created by Venturella et al. who established an ovarian age algorithm (OvAge) by analyzing several variables, for example, hormone levels, age, ovarian volume, and vascular flow index, and incorporated these into a linear model to see which created a best fit. Data from over 600 women were used to create this model; however, it has yet to be prospectively tested and has limited use at this time. Additionally, it states nothing about fertility and considers only ovarian age [44].

Companies have also started to market specific algorithms to estimate various ART outcomes. One such company is ReproSource, which has established an algorithm to determine the number of oocytes anticipated at the time of retrieval, called the ovarian assessment report (OAR) [45]. This proprietary algorithm takes into consideration the patient's age and various lab values to include AMH, FSH, and inhibin B. Estradiol is used only to ensure appropriate timing of the lab values. The score provided to the clinician is a numerical value of 1–20 for number of anticipated oocytes, whereas patients get a generic response of "reduced" (1–5 oocytes), "fair" (6–10 oocytes), "good" (11–15 oocytes), and "excellent" (16–20 oocytes). To validate the algorithm, outcomes of over 250 women with more than 400 oocyte retrievals were reviewed, with mean numbers of oocytes retrieved in each of these categories (reduced, fair, good, excellent) as 5, 9, 13, and 20, respectively [45]. It was found that the OAR correlated better than any of the individual lab values for predicting the number of oocytes retrieved, although AMH was a close second (r^2 of 0.40 versus 0.36) [45]. Notably, use of this score is meant to help practitioners reduce the number of independent variables they have to consider when assessing a patient's reproductive capacity. Thus, numerous lab values are given as one score and the clinician then needs to compare this against other known variables, such as previous IVF cycles, physical exam, BMI, and reason for infertility.

Univfy is another such company that predicts IVF outcomes by creating a center-specific algorithm based on data routinely collected at the center (e.g., FSH versus AFC versus AMH, or a combination; BMI, reproductive history) (Yao M, telephone interview, December 2019). The algorithm is created from the site's electronic medical record and is based on as few as 100 cycles for a small center, or around 500 cycles for larger centers. Between 10 and 20 variables are incorporated at each site to customize the algorithm. Univfy then uses this algorithm to calculate various outcomes, such as LBR after one, two, or three cycles of ART. One of the goals of Univfy is to enable patient to take home information and data tailored to their projected outcomes after what is often an emotional and overwhelming visit (Yao M, telephone interview, December 2019). Univfy reports a greater than 95% accuracy that is standard throughout their affiliated centers, and is connected with several financial programs to assist patients with refunds when data are inaccurate [46].

As we are coming into the age of personalized medicine, several researchers have attempted to use pre-ART AMH levels to determine gonadotropin doses for IVF cycles. One randomized prospective multinational study of nearly 1,400 women showed that dosing based on pretreatment AMH levels was noninferior to conventional dosing in regards to CPR and LBR, but improved rates of "target" response (8–14 oocytes retrieved), with fewer low or high responses, and fewer cases of OHSS [47]. In contrast, a smaller study by Friis Petersen et al. reported no differences between individualized versus conventional dosing of FSH when looking at optimal oocyte number retrieved (5–14 oocytes) [48]. Additionally, those with high AMH (>24 pmol/l or 3.36 ng/ml) had an increased proportion with less than five oocytes retrieved in the individualized group (38%) over those in the standard group (6%, p = 0.029). The LBR was not different between the two groups; however, the sample sizes were powered to look specifically at oocytes retrieved [48]. Taken together, algorithms and specific lab values may help physicians take a step closer to individualized medicine to optimize dosing; however additional well-designed research is required to determine the optimal dose for each AMH range.

Patients Today

Ovarian reserve tests, algorithms, and ART prediction kits have become more prevalent in current clinical practice, especially as the population seeking fertility treatment ages. However, it is also important to take a step back and look at why people are delaying fertility, if there is any support for using ovarian reserve tests to counsel patients earlier in life, and whether it is ethical to do so. Although the reasons women delay fertility are numerous, the change in professional dynamics is likely playing a significant part. There has been a 20-fold increase in women with professional degrees in the last 20 years and women make up the majority of students pursuing masters or doctorate degrees [49].

There has been much survey-based research, mainly of women during postgraduate work, assessing knowledge of fertility, reasons for delaying fertility, and a woman's desire for information. Although such studies have attempted to answer various questions, several common themes can be elucidated. The first is that women, even highly educated women, have a limited knowledge base of how fertility declines with age. One study of medical/graduate students stated that about half knew that fertility started rapidly declining between the ages of 35 and 39, yet only 15% realized that the majority of women are infertile by the age of 45. Knowledge concerning fertility decline was more prevalent in those with a higher education, and older women tended to believe that fertility decline started later in life [49,50]. Another common theme is that the choice to delay fertility is multifactorial; women cited education, lack of a partner, career, and lack of financial security [49,51]. On the other hand, religion, ethnicity, specific type of medical field (physician or nonphysician), and having other children did not seem to impact the results [51].

The next consideration is patient awareness of ovarian reserve tests/oocyte preservation, whether they would undergo testing, and if results would cause them to change their decisions towards fertility. In the studies that analyzed patients' knowledge of ovarian reserve testing, 81.6% had knowledge of ovarian reserve and 92% understood that there were options for oocyte cryopreservation [49,51]. This varied significantly by education, and even career choice; one study analyzed obstetrics and gynecology (OBGYN) physicians versus other surgical subspecialists (OSS), and found that only 15.8% of OSS women were aware of ovarian reserve testing or fertility preservation versus 91.3% of OBGYNs [50]. Only one of the analyzed surveys specifically asked whether they would undergo ovarian reserve testing (AMH), in which nearly half (47%) of the surveyed population answered yes and believed that an appropriate age to start testing would be 35 [51]. In Hurley et al.'s study, AMH testing was offered to OBGYNs and OSS, of whom 25/42 of those surveyed accepted the opportunity [50]. When asked how knowledge of ovarian reserve would, theoretically, impact an individual's decision, responses varied widely. If faced with DOR, 21–61.3% stated that they would consider oocyte cryopreservation and 48% stated they would attempt to conceive earlier [50,51]. However, in those who actually had AMH tested, only 11.1–12.5% stated that this knowledge would change their current reproductive decisions, yet 18.8–33.3% reported interest in gaining more knowledge concerning fertility preservation [50].

The last common theme gathered from these surveys concerned the numerous barriers for oocyte cryopreservation, including financial, ethical, pain, perceived low success, and emotional; 87% of those surveyed reported at least two barriers [50,51]. Approximately 1/4 of those surveyed wanted more education on ovarian reserve, and over 1/3 wanted to discuss with their OBGYN. Additionally, 93% stated that future fertility was important to them [49].

A small study was performed in Ireland that specifically looked at the psychiatric outcomes of AMH testing by performing multiple in person interviews. Three different areas were analyzed: AMH experience/reasoning for testing, response to results, and potential lessons for health care professionals. The majority of the women (8/10) were seeking fertility treatment, and 50% were found to have DOR [52]. Those who discovered they had DOR had a very mixed response from complete dismay, to feeling "cheated" out of good years, grief, to happiness in understanding what they were going through. The impact on an individual's mental health also had a wide spectrum: some women felt a loss of their femininity, whereas others appreciated being informed and had realistic expectations. The last part of their interviews concerned lessons for health care providers. Those who had a better experience with delivery of their results reported that they were delivered in person and in words they could understand. Those who had a negative experience stated that these results were often given over the phone or at a nonoptimal time, and they were dismayed by their general practitioner's lack of knowledge concerning the test. Universal screening was also proposed to these women; the majority stated that screening should be reserved for specific people only, but some thought it could enable further education and possible adjustment of childbearing time frame, and yet some stated this causes added worry and stress [52].

Although inherent flaws are notable in survey-based studies and the majority were performed in a subset of highly educated individuals, what they highlight is extremely important. There is a variable knowledge base concerning ovarian reserve testing, oocyte cryopreservation, and patient responses to the outcomes of potential testing. Additionally, results from ovarian reserve testing can have a wide variety of psychologic and social implications for an individual, therefore advising against the idea of universal screening in women who are not pursuing fertility. A committee opinion from the American College of Obstetrics & Gynecology recently stated that AMH should be used with discretion in women with low prevalence of infertility, as in those who have never attempted to conceive or with proven, unassisted, fertility [53]. They took point in this article to review various studies that showed no difference in time to conception in women without a history of infertility who had a low versus normal AMH, which was also true in women aged 38–44 [53]. One study specifically followed 750 women, aged 30–44, without a history of infertility and collected ovarian biomarkers prior to conception (AMH, FSH, and inhibin B). They found that in women with untested fertility, these biomarkers did not show a difference to CPR at 6 or 12 cycles in women with low reserve (AMH <0.7 ng/ml and serum FSH >10 mIU/ml) versus normal (AMH >0.7 ng/ml and serum FSH <10 mIU/ml) [54]. It is the authors' opinion that women should be advised of fertility decline and the options of ovarian reserve testing and oocyte cryopreservation. However, the pursuit of testing should only be undertaken by individuals who are familiar with these tests and can properly counsel individuals on the wide variety of outcomes.

Additionally, practitioners need to change their attitudes from a contraception-based to a fertility-based thought process. Early on in a women's reproductive life, her thoughts on family planning should be identified, enabling appropriate counseling on fertility, contraception, and, if necessary, fertility preservation [55]. In this scenario, if a woman chooses not to have children, then the conversation can focus entirely on contraception, otherwise a discussion about optimal fertility, prenatal visit, and when to seek further counsel could support a well-educated patient.

Where Do We Go From Here?

As the population of fertility-seeking patients who tend to be older continues to increase, practitioners must be able to appropriately counsel patients, order and interpret ovarian reserve testing, and understand the potential ramifications of these results. It is important that these results are presented to patients as measures of ovarian reserve, thus quantity, not specifically quality, and that patients realize there has been minimal correlation between values for testing and LBR, outside of those whose values are grossly abnormal. Additionally, laboratory values should not be used to deny infertility treatment to anyone but rather to advise patients of realistic expectations and options.

As a medical community, we want to continue to determine better ways to test and counsel women of advanced reproductive age, with the mindset of analyzing both quantity and quality of oocytes to continue to increase our ability to communicate with them. Additionally, education concerning reproductive capacity and potential family planning should be raised early in a women's life as part of general obstetrics and gynecologic education, allowing each informed individual to choose her own path.

References

1. Tal R, Seifer DB. Ovarian reserve testing: a user's guide. *American Journal of Obstetrics & Gynecology*. 2017;**217**(2):129–40.

2. Steiner AZ, Jukic AM. Impact of female age and nulligravidity on fecundity in an older reproductive age cohort. *Fertility & Sterility*. 2016;**105**(6):1584–8.e1.

3. Liu KE, Case A. No. 346-Advanced reproductive age and fertility. *Journal of Obstetrics & Gynaecology Canada*. 2017;**39**(8):685–95.

4. Fleming R, Seifer DB, Frattarelli JL, Ruman J. Assessing ovarian response: antral follicle count versus anti-Mullerian hormone. *Reproductive Biomedicine Online*. 2015;**31**(4):486–96.

5. Ripley M, Lanes A, Leveille MC, Shmorgun D. Does ovarian reserve predict egg quality in unstimulated therapeutic donor insemination cycles? *Fertility & Sterility*. 2015;**103**(5):1170–5.e2.

6. Nelson SM, Telfer EE, Anderson RA. The ageing ovary and uterus: new biological insights. *Human Reproduction Update*. 2012;**19**(1):67–83.

7. Devine K, Mumford SL, Wu M, DeCherney AH, Hill MJ, Propst A. Diminished ovarian reserve in the United States assisted reproductive technology population: diagnostic trends among 181,536 cycles from the Society for Assisted Reproductive Technology Clinic Outcomes Reporting System. *Fertility & Sterility*. 2015;**104**(3):612–19.e3.

8. Toner JPS, Seifer DB Why we may abandon basal follicle-stimulating hormone testing: a sea change in determining ovarian reserve using antimullerian hormone. *Fertility & Sterility*. 2013;**99**(7):1825–30.

9. van Rooij IA, Broekmans FJ, Scheffer GJ, Looman CW, Habbema JD, de Jong FH, et al. Serum antimullerian hormone levels best reflect the reproductive decline with age in normal women with proven fertility: a longitudinal study. *Fertility & Sterility*. 2005;**83**(4):979–87.

10. Winslow KL, Toner JP, Brzyski RG, Oehninger SC, Acosta AA, Muasher SJ. The gonadotropin-releasing hormone agonist stimulation test—a sensitive predictor of performance in the flare-up in vitro fertilization cycle. *Fertility & Sterility*. 1991;**56**(4):711–7.

11. Fanchin R, de Ziegler D, Olivennes F, Taieb J, Dzik A, Frydman R. Endocrinology: Exogenous follicle stimulating hormone ovarian reserve test (EFORT): a simple and reliable screening test for detecting 'poor responders' in in-vitro fertilization. *Human Reproduction*. 1994;**9**(9):1607–11.

12. McTavish KJ, Jimenez M, Walters KA, Spaliviero J, Groome NP, Themmen AP, et al. Rising follicle-stimulating hormone levels with age accelerate female reproductive failure. *Endocrinology* 2007;**148**(9):4432–9.

13. Lass A, Skull J, McVeigh E, Margara R, Winston RM. Measurement of ovarian volume by transvaginal sonography before ovulation induction with human menopausal gonadotrophin for in-vitro fertilization can predict poor response. *Human Reproduction*. 1997;**12**(2):294–7.

14. Chang M-Y. Use of the antral follicle count to predict the outcome of assisted reproductive technologies. *Fertility & Sterility*. 1997;**69**(3):505–10.

15. Hansen KR, Morris JL, Thyer AC, Soules MR. Reproductive aging and variability in the ovarian antral follicle count: application in the clinical setting. *Fertility & Sterility*. 2003;**80**(3):577–83.

16. Landersoe SK, Birch Petersen K, Sorensen AL, Larsen EC, Martinussen T, Lunding SA, et al. Ovarian reserve markers after discontinuing long-term use of combined oral contraceptives. *Reproductive Biomedicine Online* 2020;**40**(1):176–86.

17. Seifer DB, MacLaughlin DT, Christian BP, Feng B, Shelden RM. Early follicular serum mullerian-inhibiting substance levels are associated with ovarian response during assisted reproductive technology cycles. *Fertility & Sterility*. 2002;**77**(3):468–71.

18. Styer AK, Gaskins AJ, Brady PC, Sluss PM, Chavarro JE, Hauser RB, et al. Dynamic antimullerian hormone levels during controlled ovarian hyperstimulation predict in vitro

fertilization response and pregnancy outcomes. *Fertility & Sterility*. 2015;**104**(5):1153–61.e1-7.

19. Nelson SM, Pastuszek E, Kloss G, Malinowska I, Liss J, Lukaszuk A, et al. Two new automated, compared with two enzyme-linked immunosorbent, antimüllerian hormone assays. *Fertility & Sterility*. 2015;**104**(4):1016–21.

20. Leader B, Baker VL. Maximizing the clinical utility of antimullerian hormone testing in women's health. *Current Opinion in Obstetrics & Gynecology*. 2014;**26**(4):226–36.

21. Seifer DB, Baker VL, Leader B. Age-specific serum anti-Mullerian hormone values for 17,120 women presenting to fertility centers within the United States. *Fertility & Sterility*. 2011;**95**(2):747–50.

22. Burks HR, Ross L, Opper N, Paulson E, Stanczyk FZ, Chung K. Can highly sensitive antimullerian hormone testing predict failed response to ovarian stimulation? *Fertility & Sterility*. 2015;**104**(3):643–8.

23. Seifer DB, Tal O, Wantman E, Edul P, Baker VL. Prognostic indicators of assisted reproduction technology outcomes of cycles with ultralow serum antimullerian hormone: a multivariate analysis of over 5,000 autologous cycles from the Society for Assisted Reproductive Technology Clinic Outcome Reporting System database for 2012–2013. *Fertility & Sterility*. 2016;**105**(2):385–93.e3.

24. Seifer DB, Golub ET, Lambert-Messerlian G, Benning L, Anastos K, Watts DH, et al. Variations in serum mullerian inhibiting substance between white, black, and Hispanic women. *Fertility & Sterility*. 2009;**92**(5):1674–8.

25. Tal R, Seifer DB, Wantman E, Baker V, Tal O. Antimullerian hormone as a predictor of live birth following assisted reproduction: an analysis of 85,062 fresh and thawed cycles from the Society for Assisted Reproductive Technology Clinic Outcome Reporting System database for 2012–2013. *Fertility & Sterility*. 2018;**109**(2):258–65.

26. Tal R, Tal O, Seifer BJ, Seifer DB. Antimullerian hormone as predictor of implantation and clinical pregnancy after assisted conception: a systematic review and meta-analysis. *Fertility & Sterility*. 2015;**103**(1):119–30.e3.

27. Tal R, Seifer DB, Tal R, Granger E, Wantman E, Tal O. AMH highly correlates with cumulative live birth rate in women with diminished ovarian reserve independent of age. *The Journal of Clinical Endocrinology and Metabolism*. 2021;**106**(9):2754–66.

28. Lyttle Schumacher BM, Jukic AMZ, Steiner AZ. Antimullerian hormone as a risk factor for miscarriage in naturally conceived pregnancies. *Fertility & Sterility*. 2018;**109**(6):1065–71.e1.

29. McCormack CD, Leemaqz SY, Furness DL, Dekker GA, Roberts CT. Anti-Mullerian hormone levels in recurrent embryonic miscarriage patients are frequently abnormal, and may affect pregnancy outcomes. *Journal of Obstetrics and Gynaecology*. 2019;**39**(5):623–7.

30. Shebl O, Ebner T, Sir A, Schreier-Lechner E, Mayer RB, Tews G, et al. Age-related distribution of basal serum AMH level in women of reproductive age and a presumably healthy cohort. *Fertility & Sterility*. 2011;**95**(2):832–4.

31. Tarasconi B, Tadros T, Ayoubi JM, Belloc S, de Ziegler D, Fanchin R. Serum antimullerian hormone levels are independently related to miscarriage rates after in vitro fertilization-embryo transfer. *Fertility & Sterility*. 2017;**108**(3):518–24.

32. Zarek SM, Mitchell EM, Sjaarda LA, Mumford SL, Silver RM, Stanford JB, et al. Antimüllerian hormone and pregnancy loss from the Effects of Aspirin in Gestation and Reproduction trial. *Fertility & Sterility*. 2016;**105**(4):946–52.e2.

33. Freeman EW, Sammel MD, Lin H, Gracia CR. Anti-mullerian hormone as a predictor of time to menopause in late reproductive age women. *The Journal of Clinical Endocrinology and Metabolism*. 2012;**97**(5):1673–80.

34. Khan HL, Bhatti S, Suhail S, Gul R, Awais A, Hamayun H, et al. Antral follicle count (AFC) and serum anti-Mullerian hormone (AMH) are the predictors of natural fecundability have similar trends irrespective of fertility status and menstrual characteristics among fertile and infertile women below the age of 40 years. *Reproductive Biology & Endocrinology*. 2019;**17**(1):20.

35. Wang S, Zhang Y, Mensah V, Huber WJ, 3rd, Huang YT, Alvero R. Discordant anti-mullerian hormone (AMH) and follicle stimulating hormone (FSH) among women undergoing in vitro fertilization (IVF): which one is the better predictor for live birth? *Journal of Ovarian Research*. 2018;**11**(1):60.

36. Leader B, Hegde A, Baca Q, Stone K, Lannon B, Seifer DB, et al. High frequency of discordance between antimullerian hormone and follicle-stimulating hormone levels in serum from estradiol-confirmed days 2 to 4 of the menstrual cycle from 5,354 women in U.S. fertility centers. *Fertility & Sterility*. 2012;**98**(4):1037–42.

37. Ligon S, Lustik M, Levy G, Pier B. Low antimullerian hormone (AMH) is associated with decreased live birth after in vitro fertilization when follicle-stimulating hormone and AMH are

discordant. *Fertility & Sterility*. 2019;**112**(1):73–81.
e1.

38. Hipp HS, Kawwass JF. Discordant ovarian reserve testing: what matters most? *Fertility & Sterility*. 2019;**112**(1):34.

39. Centers for Disease Control and Prevention. IVF Success Estimator. 2019. https://www.cdc.gov/art/ivf-success-estimator/index.html

40. Kushnir VA, Choi J, Darmon SK, Albertini DF, Barad DH, Gleicher N. CDC-reported assisted reproductive technology live-birth rates may mislead the public. *Reproductive Biomedicine Online*. 2017;**35**(2):161–4.

41. Centers for Disease Control and Prevention. 2017 Assisted Reproductive Technology Fertility Clinic Success Rates Report. 2018. https://www.cdc.gov/art/reports/2017/fertility-clinic.html

42. Goldman RJF. BWH Egg Freezing Counseling Tool (EFCT). MD Calc. 2019. https://www.mdcalc.com/bwh-egg-freezing-counseling-tool-efct

43. Society for Assisted Reproductive Technology. What are my chances with ART. 2020. https://www.sartcorsonline.com/Predictor/Patient

44. Venturella R, Lico D, Sarica A, Falbo MP, Gulletta E, Cannataro M, et al. A new algorithm to predict ovarian age combining clinical, biochemical and 3D-ultrasonographic parameters. *Fertility & Sterility*. 2014;**102**(3):e145.

45. ReproSource I. ReproSource Ovarian Assessment Report Clinical Data Update from Multiple US Fertility Centers. 2019.

46. Univfy Inc. Univfy PreIVF Report. 2013. https://www.univfy.com/ivf-success

47. Nyboe Andersen A, Nelson SM, Fauser BCJM, García-Velasco JA, Klein BM, Arce J-C, et al. Individualized versus conventional ovarian stimulation for in vitro fertilization: a multicenter, randomized, controlled, assessor-blinded, phase 3 noninferiority trial. *Fertility & Sterility*. 2017;**107**(2):387–96.e4.

48. Friis Petersen J, Løkkegaard E, Andersen LF, Torp K, Egeberg A, Hedegaard L, et al. A randomized controlled trial of AMH-based individualized FSH dosing in a GnRH antagonist protocol for IVF. *Human Reproduction Open*. 2019;**2019**(1):hoz003-hoz.

49. Hickman LC, Fortin C, Goodman L, Liu X, Flyckt R. Fertility and fertility preservation: knowledge, awareness and attitudes of female graduate students. *The European Journal of Contraception & Reproductive Health Care*. 2018;**23**(2):130–8.

50. Hurley EG, Ressler IB, Young S, Batcheller A, Thomas MA, DiPaola KB, et al. Postponing childbearing and fertility preservation in young professional women. *Southern Medical Journal*. 2018;**111**(4):187–91.

51. Azhar E, Seifer DB, Melzer K, Ahmed A, Weedon J, Minkoff H. Knowledge of ovarian reserve and reproductive choices. *Journal of Assisted Reproduction and Genetics*. 2015;**32**(3):409–15.

52. O'Brien Y, Kelleher C, Wingfield M. "So what happens next?" exploring the psychological and emotional impact of anti-Mullerian hormone testing. *Journal of Psychosomatic Obstetrics and Gynaecology*. 2020;**41**(1):30–7.

53. ACOG Committee. Opinion No. 773 Summary: The use of antimüllerian hormone in women not seeking fertility care. *Obstetrics and Gynecology*. 2019;**133**:e275–9.

54. Steiner AZ, Pritchard D, Stanczyk FZ, Kesner JS, Meadows JW, Herring AH, et al. Association between biomarkers of ovarian reserve and infertility among older women of reproductive age. *Journal of the American Medical Association*. 2017;**318**(14):1367–76.

55. Seifer DB, Minkoff H, Merhi Z. Putting 'family' back in family planning. *Human Reproduction*. 2015;**30**(1):16–9.

Fertility Preservation for "Social" Reasons

Timothy Bracewell-Milnes and Dimitrios S. Nikolaou

Background

Societal progression over recent decades has resulted in improved gender equality, which has led to greater educational and professional opportunities for women worldwide, particularly in western societies. This has led to a trend of women delaying having children, contributing to a rise in age of first-time motherhood worldwide. Data from the Office for National Statistics in the UK show that, since the mid-1970s, the average age of motherhood has increased from 26.4 years to 30.4 years in 2016 [1]. It is an established fact that female fertility decreases gradually but significantly after age 32, with this decline accelerating after age 35 [2]. Given this physiological decline in egg reserve with advancing maternal age, the relatively recent trend in deferring motherhood for social reasons has led to increasing rates of involuntary childlessness [3]. Leridon (2008) created a model which reported that 14% of women would be childless if they started trying to conceive at age 35 years, with this figure increasing to 34.8% if they delayed trying until age 40 [4].

Egg freezing was initially introduced as a fertility preservation measure in women without a male partner who were about to undergo gonadotoxic treatments, such as chemotherapy for cancer [5]. The use of oocyte cryopreservation for social reasons has been an increasingly popular strategy for women to preserve their fertility potential, a term most commonly referred to as 'social egg freezing' (SEF) [6]. As well as for career progression, or waiting until they are financially more secure [7], some women may be single, or may decide to egg freeze to relieve pressure on a relationship, until they decide they are ready to have children with their partner [8].

Upon introduction, success rates with SEF were low due to poor oocyte survival rates. With the advent of oocyte vitrification techniques, assisted reproductive technology (ART) procedures using

frozen oocytes have shown a similar live birth rate (LBR) to those using fresh oocytes [9]. Altruistic oocyte donation programmes, which use eggs that were collected from young women, also report high LBR using vitrified oocytes [10]. Due to this growing evidence for the efficacy of egg freezing, both the European Society for Human Reproduction and Embryology (ESHRE) and the American Society for Reproductive Medicine (ASRM) changed their stances and no longer consider oocyte freezing to be an experimental technique [11,12]. Therefore, SEF gives women the possibility of conceiving their own genetic offspring in the future. The Royal College of Obstetricians and Gynaecologists (RCOG) urge for caution and reiterate that SEF does not guarantee having a child in the future as there is the possibility of having failed future embryo transfers and exhausting the supply of stored oocytes, often at an age where ART with the patients' own eggs will not result in pregnancy [13]. In addition to this, in the UK, legislation limits cryostorage of oocytes to a maximum of 10 years, with the gametes destroyed if they are not used within this timeframe.

Optimal Age to Freeze Eggs

Perhaps unsurprisingly, studies have consistently reported that the LBR from frozen oocytes is highly dependent on the female age at which the eggs were collected [14–16]. These studies have used different models to estimate the LBR from frozen eggs. Cobo et al. (2016) reported cumulative LBR (CLBR) to be 50% in women aged ≤35 years and 22.9% in women >35 years [14]. Stratifying by the youngest and oldest age groups, the same study reported a CLBR of 100% in women aged ≤29 years and 3.7% in those aged 40–44 years [14]. Doyle et al. (2016) calculated 'oocyte efficiency' by reporting the birth rates per oocyte retrieved and reported

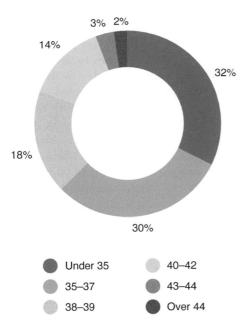

Figure 5.1 Egg freezing by age in the United Kingdom.
Source: HFEA, 2018 [17].

Legend:
- Under 35 — 32%
- 35–37 — 30%
- 38–39 — 18%
- 40–42 — 14%
- 43–44 — 3%
- Over 44 — 2%

this to be 8.7% in women aged 30–34 years, 4.5% in 38–40 years and 2.5% in women aged 41–42 years [16]. The only meta-analysis to investigate this, prior to these more recent studies, found the most significant discriminating factor for success was SEF prior to 36 years of age [15].

In the UK in 2017, 1,462 SEF cycles took place, and of these 32% were ≤35 years [17] (Figure 5.1). This is similar to studies from other western countries that have taken place, such as in Australia [18], Belgium [19], Spain [20], and the USA [21], where the average age at cryopreservation was 36.5 to 38 years.

This is supported in other studies from other western countries, showing that the average age to cryopreserve oocytes is 38 years [18,22]. This has significant consequences regarding the outcome of egg freezing treatments, and sadly it appears the majority of women are taking measures to preserve their fertility too late, as a 'last ditch' effort, instead of a planned and informed choice in their early to mid-30s [23].

Each woman considering SEF needs to have comprehensive counselling on the psychosocial and financial aspects of the procedure involved, as well as her individualised chances of having a baby through oocyte cryopreservation. This process allows her to think realistically about her chances of conceiving, therefore making an informed decision about proceeding with SEF [11].

Studies have shown that young women are not aware or concerned about the age limits of female fertility and significantly overestimate the ability of ART in helping them to conceive at an advanced age [24]. Ter Keurst et al. (2016) constructed a cross-sectional online survey surrounding the factors associated with the intentions of childless women aged 28–35 years to use fertility preservation [25]. They found that these women were overwhelmingly not considering the use of fertility preservation because they did not feel the threat of infertility [25].

Optimal Number of Eggs to Freeze

One of the most important factors regarding efficacy of egg freezing is the number of mature oocytes retrieved. Cobo et al. (2016) reported that in women under 35 years of age, CLBR was 40.8% if 8 mature oocytes were frozen, compared to 60.5% with 10 oocytes, reaching a plateau of 85.2% with 15 oocytes stored [14]. In women over 35 years using 8 or 10 eggs, a CLBR of 19.9% or 29.7% was achieved, respectively. Compared with younger women, the CLBR plateau was reached at 35.6% with 11 frozen oocytes, indicating that in this age group success is not increased with a larger frozen oocyte pool [14].

Other studies contradict these findings of a plateau in CLBR, with one reporting that women aged 35 or 38 years with 20 frozen oocytes would have a CLBR of 80% or 60%, respectively [16]. A mathematical model has been developed to predict the probability of live birth based on number of frozen oocytes, taking into account female age [26]. This model reported that women aged 34, 37 or 42 would need to freeze 10, 20 or 61 eggs, respectively, to have a 75% chance of at least one live birth [26]. This model has the potential to act as a useful counselling tool for physicians treating social egg freezers, but is limited by only including those with a normal ovarian reserve for their age. It is important to explain to women over the age of 40 that to obtain an adequate number of oocytes to realistically have any chance of having a child, multiple cycles of controlled ovarian stimulation may be required. Even at this, the chances of conceiving may be slim.

Cost-Effectiveness

Social egg freezing has the potential to reduce the costs associated with ART in the future for patients by hypothetically increasing success rates, as the gametes were frozen at an earlier reproductive age. Studies have used theoretical models to define efficacy and cost-effectiveness of SEF, simulating different scenarios regarding age when egg freezing and number of treatments.

Mesen et al. (2015) constructed a decision-tree model to determine cost-effectiveness of SEF compared with no action, when it was considered at ages 25–40 years, assuming there was an attempt for pregnancy at 3, 5 or 7 years after SEF [27]. They reported that freezing oocytes was most cost-effective at age 37 years, compared with no action [27].

van Loendersloot et al. (2011) constructed a model where women would freeze eggs at age 35 and then use them for fertility treatment age 40, compared with women trying to conceive naturally at age 40 [28]. Social egg freezing was cost-effective only if 61% of women who cryopreserved returned for IVF and paid 19,560 Euros per live birth [28].

Devine et al. (2015) reported SEF to be cost-effective if it were carried out before 38 years of age and if 49% or more of those not falling pregnant naturally returned to use their frozen oocytes [29].

Finally, Hirshfeld-Cytron et al. (2012) used a model to compare freezing oocytes at age 35 years and then using those oocytes to achieve a pregnancy when aged 40 years, and this approach was less cost-effective than a 'waiting strategy' [30].

These theoretical models have significant limitations, mainly due to the assumptions that are used to create them. Firstly, it is critical to know the realistic usage rate to allow a more accurate prediction of cost-effectiveness. Although some studies have stated the importance of usage rates in cost-effectiveness calculations, none have commented on whether the high suggested usage rates are achievable [28,29]. Secondly, the costs of fertility treatments vary significantly between different countries, so these data could not necessarily be extrapolated outside of the country in which the study was performed.

Women are advised by most specialists that the perfect time to freeze their oocytes is 30–35 years of age. Studies identified a usage rate of 49–61% required to render SEF a cost-effective procedure [28,29]. Malchau et al. (2017) attempted to discover whether these figures were achievable by analysing data from 19,884 women to assess differing utilisation rates in different female age groups [31]. In women under 35 years of age the maximum infertility rate is 15%, and 80% of these women will achieve pregnancy with fertility treatment [31]. This means in this age group the maximum 'usage rate' is only 3%. However, in women aged over 40 years, with a 60% infertility rate, the maximum usage rate would be 43.8%, which is still below a cost-effective threshold, but significantly higher than in younger women.

These data reveal a contradiction between freezing at a younger age, with good success rates but low utilisation and, and freezing at a later age, with lower potential success rates, but improved cost-effectiveness. The cost–benefit debate should consider not only the financial viewpoint but also the psychological aspects, including freedom of choice and the women's feelings of taking a pro-active role in attempting to preserve their fertility, which are impossible to assess from a monetary standpoint.

Usage of Stored Oocytes

There are sparse data available on the proportion of women who return to use their frozen eggs, which is disappointing as these data should represent a crucial part of patient counselling in women who present to fertility clinics considering SEF. Five studies have been identified that used surveys to follow up SEF patients and reported 'usage rates' for SEF patients.

Hammarberg et al. (2017) surveyed 95 SEF patients and found that 6% had returned to use their frozen oocytes [18]. They found the main reasons for not using them were (i) not wanting to be a single parent; (ii) a preference for natural conception; and (iii) reluctance to use donor sperm [18]. Of note, 34% of their SEF patients had been pregnant at least once. Of the 91% of SEF users who still had oocytes stored, 21% intended to use them, while 69% stated their personal circumstances would determine this decision. Stoop et al. (2015) conducted interviews on 86 women who had undertaken SEF one to three years prior, and found that almost all still wished to conceive a child, but only 50.8% thought they would use their eggs in the future [22]. Interestingly, this study reported that three years after oocyte cryopreservation, 29.2% of women considered using their frozen eggs less likely than when they froze them, due to an overoptimistic assessment of their fertility at an advanced maternal age [22]. Another study performed a survey of 183 women who had frozen their oocytes between 2005 and 2011 and found a usage rate of 6%, with a third stating they were 'very likely' to still use their frozen eggs [32]. Of the 23 women who had previously undergone SEF interviewed by Baldwin et al. (2015), 8.7% had used their frozen oocytes [33]. Finally, Cobo et al. (2016) performed a retrospective analysis of their SEF patients, and reported a usage rate of 9.3%, with a mean time to return of 2.1 years and a mean age of 39.2 years [14].

Gürtin et al. (2019) reported on their SEF patients who returned to use their frozen oocytes over a 10-year period [34]. Their SEF patients were all single at the time of freezing, and on average kept their eggs in storage for five years, returning to use them at an average age of 42.5 years [34]. At the time of thawing their oocytes, 43.5% were single, with 47.8% using donor sperm to fertilise their eggs [35]. However, this study did not give usage rates on their total population who had undergone SEF, focusing solely on those who returned to use their eggs.

It is important to note that the reason for the consistently reported low usage rate may well be due to data collection from a relatively recent fertility preservation programme. As the fundamental purpose of SEF is to delay motherhood, many women who stored their oocytes would still not have considered pursuing motherhood during the relatively short follow-up of these studies. This is supported by Cobo et al. (2018) who performed a large retrospective multi-centre analysis two years after their previous research, and reported a usage rate of 12.1%, compared with 9.3% from their study two years previously [14,20]. Therefore, it is very possible the usage rate will significantly increase in future; however, these data are not yet available, and merely a hypothesis. An increasing number of studies with longer follow-up are required to investigate the usage rates of SEF. This will help us understand the reproductive trajectories of SEF patients in the future and will aid in their counselling.

Motivations and Attitudes towards Social Egg Freezing

Motivations towards Social Egg Freezing

A systematic review investigating the motivations for women to freeze their eggs found that studies consistently revealed the major motivating factors as (i) not having a partner; (ii) not being ready to start a family; (iii) fear of future regret; (iv) fear of age-related fertility decline [36–38]. Neither of these last two factors were reported in surveys from the general public, perhaps indicating a lack of consideration about the consequences of delayed childbearing compared with those who use SEF.

The decline of fertility with advancing maternal age co-exists with the limited timeframe available to find a suitable partner. Studies consistently reported that women were keen to avoid committing to have a child with someone they felt might not be suitable as a life-long partner, and that SEF potentially extended their window of opportunity to find a suitable partner, easing the pressure to conceive [38,39]. It has been reported that there is an increased divorce rate in women over 35 years of age [40]. Although some women who are concerned they are running out of time to have a baby may turn to 'panic partnering' to achieve this, these findings show that an increasing proportion of women are using SEF as an alternative option, increasing their reproductive choices.

Career advancement was not found to be a direct motivating factor in studies of users of SEF [37,38,41]. This is in contrast with recent studies of the general population, with 50–63% considering SEF for 'career reasons' [19,42]. However, these studies were from women in their 20s, who represent a minority of the population of women who actually egg freeze. This implies that although women consider their career to be a possible motivating factor in the future, this does not eventually lead to them undergoing SEF.

Knowledge of Age-Related Fertility Decline and Attitudes towards Social Egg Freezing

General Public

Studies consistently revealed a lack of understanding by the general public surrounding age and reduced fertility potential, as well as overly optimistic views regarding the ability of ART to overcome their infertility [43,44]. Several studies have also reported poor awareness of the option of SEF amongst the general public [42,45,46], although other studies found that over 75% of women were aware of this option [19,47,48]. One study surveying medical students from Singapore reported that only 36.4% of participants were aware of SEF, which is lower than many studies involving the general public; this suggests a likelihood that education amongst healthcare professionals is inadequate [45]. This offers a partial explanation for why the majority of women are freezing their eggs in their late 30s, with significantly reduced success rates.

The most consistently raised concern surrounding SEF amongst the general public was the associated cost [46,49], with studies reporting that 71–73% of women would consider SEF if the cost was subsidised by their employer or the government [45,48]. The cost of freezing eggs is significant, with recurring annual storage costs, and it is therefore perhaps unsurprising that it is a deterring factor for women to go ahead with SEF. Since 2014, large companies such as Apple, Google and Facebook have offered free or heavily subsidised SEF to their female employees. Many argue that this is not altruistic but done for financial reasons, keeping their talented young female employees at work, rather than raising children, implying these companies prefer a 'productive' to a 'reproductive' workforce [50].

Data from most surveys show generally widespread support for SEF, with studies finding 58–89% of women amongst the general public in favour of SEF [46,48]. Interestingly, these studies reported that younger women were more accepting of SEF. Stoop et al. (2011) report that one in three women from Belgium would consider oocyte cryopreservation to extend their reproductive window [19].

Social Egg Freezers

Regarding actual SEF users, studies reported that those women who perceived higher levels of information and emotional support given during their treatment were less likely to regret having participated [21]. Studies of patients who undertook SEF consistently report that the vast majority did not regret this decision [38]. One of the most consistently raised arguments

against SEF is the likelihood of falling pregnant naturally in the remaining reproductive years, with the patients having therefore undergone unnecessary oocyte cryopreservation. However, studies have consistently reported that SEF patients who went on to conceive naturally did not regret their participation in the programme [38]. Unsurprisingly, one study reported that 49% of participants had mild-to-moderate regret about participating in SEF if they had a low number of oocytes stored [21]. A study examining chances of success based on age and number of oocytes stored found that only 12% of patients correctly estimated this [38]. However, in the same study only 8% overestimated and 42% underestimated their chances of success, suggesting that their pre-treatment counselling was overly cautious.

A situation unique to the UK is risk of premature disposal of frozen oocytes due to the HFEA regulations only permitting storage of frozen gametes for 10 years. A study reported that a significant minority (20%) of women were not aware of this storage limit, or that it would result in their oocytes subsequently being disposed of if they remained unused after this time period [38]. Regarding the fairness of this limit, more than 50% disagreed with it, identifying discontent within the SEF community in the UK. If this legislation remains, it will lead women to transfer their stored oocytes overseas to countries not restricted by this legislation, or to prematurely create embryos for further storage. The literature from the UK on this topic supports the momentum for the HFEA to consider its position on this legislation, which is not evidence-based, dated and not in the best interests of the women it claims to protect [51].

The Debate Surrounding SEF

Fertility preservation for social reasons is likely to remain or increase in popularity due to its inherent logic. However, opinions vary significantly about whether this option benefits women.

Those in favour have clear cut arguments that it: (i) adds to women's reproductive choices giving them the opportunity to extend their reproductive window; (ii) allows them time to find a suitable partner and avoid 'panic partnering'; (iii) allows them to pursue other life goals outside having a family, such as their education and careers;

(iv) decreases the risk of fetal aneuploidy due to advanced maternal age [52]; and finally according to some cost-effectiveness models, can reduce the cost to obtain a live birth, in women planning to delay pregnancy until 40 years [29].

Those against this practice firstly fear that SEF is encouraging women to delay their childbearing years, meaning an increasing number of women in the future could potentially have children beyond the natural reproductive lifespan, with the associated increased medical risks. Studies have found that the vast majority of women who pursue SEF are aware of the risks of pregnancy with advanced maternal age, such as pre-eclampsia, gestational diabetes mellitus and pulmonary embolism, but they are willing to accept these risks to pursue this option [38]. Reassuringly, no relevant obstetric and perinatal complications were reported in pregnancies using frozen oocytes, giving reassuring safety data for this procedure [6]. There are currently no studies reporting long-term follow-up of children born as a result of social egg freezing.

Secondly, some argue that instead of increasing women's reproductive window, SEF could lead to new pressures and ethical dilemmas, and that women are being 'misled to believe that the reproductive fountain of youth is obtainable by freezing their eggs' [53].

Thirdly, it is pointed out that SEF is at best a 'halfway house', with the oocytes in storage being of no personal value to a woman wanting pregnancy unless she chooses to reproduce using IVF. In situations where companies have paid for their employees' SEF, are they also willing to pay the costs of these fertility treatments in years to come if they are still an employee?

Fourthly, there will be a significant number of unused oocytes, due to the likelihood of natural conception in the remaining fertile years, meaning the cost and medical procedures endured would have been unnecessary. However, it should be noted that studies investigating this found that none of the women who spontaneously conceived reported regret that their oocytes were in storage. Of course, these oocytes could allow this couple the opportunity of having a second sibling, which might not have been possible without SEF.

Fifthly, SEF does nothing to correct a fundamental societal injustice experienced by professional women, who are potentially being told indirectly to choose between a career or raising a child. This is not a choice that men have to endure. Many argue it would be more helpful to implement family-friendly social policies, which support women to have children during their fertile years. This would need to include a societal change where partners share equally the responsibilities of having children, including maternity/paternity leave, and returning to work part-time.

Finally, although minimal, women should be made aware of the short-term risks associated with ovarian stimulation and trans-vaginal egg collection. These include blood loss, pelvic infection, damage to local organs and ovarian hyper-stimulation syndrome (OHSS). Approximately 1–3% of women will develop moderate or severe OHSS, and these effects are short term and can be well managed [54]. Due to ovarian stimulation protocols using an antagonist with agonist trigger injection, the risk of developing OHSS has been significantly reduced, especially in women who are egg freezing and thus not having an embryo transfer.

It is established that the majority of western countries have seen an increase in age of two to five years at first motherhood, which is now at 30 years [6]. Whilst, ideally, social and political policies should provide young families with an appropriate financial and structurally supportive package to have children, this is not currently evident in the majority of western societies. Social egg freezing could be seen as a biological fix to a sociological problem, with the debate still ongoing.

Fertility Preservation Using Donor Sperm to Cryopreserve Embryos

Women over the age of 40 who present to fertility clinics to preserve their fertility should be offered SEF, provided they are counselled about the low chance of success and the likelihood to require multiple rounds of stimulation to collect a potentially adequate number of eggs. However, they must also be informed of the option of fertilising their eggs at the time of collection with donor sperm, and then storing frozen embryos if they do not want a fresh embryo transfer at that time. The major disadvantage of this strategy is that if they were to meet a partner and want to have a genetic link of the offspring with the paternal side, it would not be possible to use these embryos. However, as

61

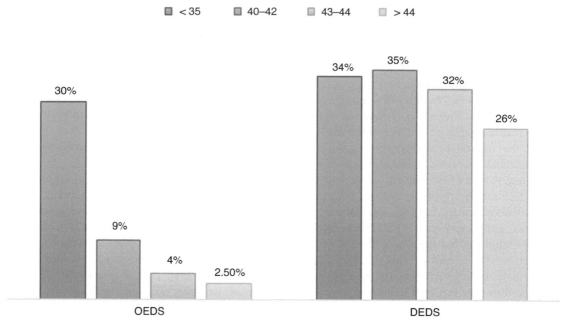

Figure 5.2 IVF birth rates per embryo transfer by age in the UK. OEDS, own egg donor sperm; DEDS, donor egg donor sperm. *Source:* HFEA, 2017 [55]

the data in Figure 5.2 show, 9% of patients will achieve a live birth in the UK using their own eggs and donor sperm (OEDS) aged 40–42. A direct comparison with frozen oocytes is difficult due to low usage rates and limited data; however, studies report that in women who freeze their eggs in this age group, LBR would be between 1% and 2.5% per frozen oocyte [16,23].

Figure 5.2 does clearly reveal, however, that in women over 40 years of age the success rates are significantly higher using a donor oocyte, with a four-fold increase in LBR in women aged 40–42 years, and a 10-fold increase in women over 44 years of age [17]. These data must be clearly communicated to women in this age group, to enable them to make an informed decision with the best available current data.

Early Ovarian Ageing

Background

The average age of menopause in western countries is 51, and the average woman would have started an accelerated decline of ovarian follicles 13 years earlier, at 38 years old [56]. Early menopause (occurring <45 years) is a common condition, affecting 10% of women. Presuming a relatively

fixed time interval between reproductive milestones, these women would have undergone accelerated decline of ovarian reserve at 32 years [56]. It has been proposed that this process should be termed 'early ovarian ageing' (EOA) [57]. In the vast majority of cases, women with EOA will be asymptomatic, until continuing follicular depletion causes the condition to deteriorate to an extent to cause infertility, irregular cycles and eventually early menopause. With a known continuing trend toward increasing maternal age at first pregnancy, the impact of EOA clinically increases, with more than 20% of patients presenting with infertility showing evidence of EOA [58].

It should be noted that EOA is not the same entity as premature ovarian insufficiency (POI), a condition at the extreme end of the ovarian ageing process, affecting 1% of the population. Patients with POI have irregular periods or secondary amenorrhoea, suffer menopausal symptoms, have very raised baseline FSH levels and are realistically not able to achieve pregnancy with their own oocytes. Based on the fact that 10% of women enter the menopause before 45 years, 10% of the population are at risk of EOA. In contrast to POI these are asymptomatic young women in the general population, rendering this a public health issue, which may be amenable to screening and prevention of involuntary childlessness through early intervention [59].

Management of Fertility in Women with Early Ovarian Ageing

If identified early, women with EOA can still have good reproductive outcomes. In women with a partner and sufficient ovarian reserve who are ready to start a family, natural conception remains an option, although early investigations and referral for fertility treatments is recommended. Nevertheless, IVF is the most commonly used fertility treatment in these cases; however, its success compared to expectant management or intrauterine insemination has not been studied.

This is especially true for younger women with EOA, as although their follicular pool may be depleted, the quality of their oocytes is usually good [57,59]. This is evidenced by the better IVF success rates in these young women with low ovarian reserve, compared with the extremely poor IVF outcome of the older women with a poor response [59]. Recent data showed that overall the LBR in women with an antral follicle count (AFC) of ≤4 was 10.7% [60]. However, when taking into account female age in those with an AFC of ≤4, the LBR was 30.0% in <35 years, 13.3% in 35–39 years, 3.9% in 40–44 years and 0% in ≥45 years [60]. The pregnancy loss also increased significantly based on AFC, with a 21.8% miscarriage rate with AFC ≥20, compared with 54.4% with an AFC ≤4, implying an increased aneuploidy rate in women with EOA. These data highlight the potential for screening, and empowering women identified with EOA to make informed choices about when to start trying to conceive or undergo SEF, before it is too late to realistically have a successful outcome.

In women undergoing IVF who already have a very low ovarian reserve, the optimal regime and pre-treatment options remain unclear. The vast majority of studies investigating poor ovarian responders are low quality with heterogeneity in their sample populations [61]. Nevertheless a recent meta-analysis investigated the effectiveness of testosterone supplementation on poor ovarian responders prior to ovarian stimulation, reporting higher LBR, total oocytes collected, total metaphase II oocytes and total embryos compared with control groups who received no supplementation [62]. Another meta-analysis investigated

the potential benefit in dehydroepiandrosterone (DHEA) with the same patient group on IVF outcome, and reported increased LBR, increased clinical pregnancy rate and lower miscarriage rate [63]. These data are encouraging and show there are treatments available that appear to optimise the follicle pool in poor responders prior to embarking on an IVF cycle. Further randomised controlled trials with more vigorous methodology and inclusion criteria are required before these treatments become more widespread.

There is currently significant debate surrounding the options of mild versus standard doses of ovarian stimulation for women with low ovarian reserve overall; however, in older women it appears increased stimulation doses are preferable [64].

Women with EOA are currently usually identified during fertility investigations and IVF treatment. After their fertility treatment, whether successful or not, these women currently have no clinical pathway regarding their reproductive health. Improving knowledge regarding this population and their risk of early menopause is imperative. These women need to be advised to seek medical advice early if they start to experience menstrual irregularity or menopausal symptoms. Ideally, women identified with EOA should be followed up in specialised clinics to help manage their future increased risks of osteoporosis and cardiovascular disease.

The key message to women with EOA is that while they are still young and asymptomatic they retain good fertility potential. However, they should be warned that this could decline at an earlier age and that they could enter the menopause earlier. Although the progression of EOA is usually slow, it is difficult to predict the rate of this decline, and women should be advised not to delay trying for a pregnancy if this is possible. Many women overestimate the effect of IVF on overcoming the effects of advanced female age and low ovarian reserve, and public health education messages should aim to address this in schools, family planning clinics and routine general practitioner consultations.

Fertility Counselling and Screening: What Do Women Want?

During the 1970s revolutionary contraceptives became available and there was widespread legalisation of terminations of pregnancy, providing monumental progress in women's ability to avoid unwanted pregnancies. Family planning clinics were set up to ease the access of women to these services. In today's society, with delayed childbearing and increasing usage of SEF, there is a need for family planning clinics to include pre-fertility initiatives.

As EOA is initially an asymptomatic condition, identifying it when the women are still young would allow the woman greater autonomy to plan having children with more available options, reduce the chances of involuntary childlessness, as well as facilitating management of the long-term health risks associated with this condition.

A survey of 663 women aged 18–44 years reported that 64.8% would be interested in having their egg reserve tested, with younger (<30 years) and single women statistically more interested [65]. Another survey of healthcare professionals reported that 86% would have treatment or take active steps to have children sooner if they were found to have poor ovarian reserve [66]. A group in Copenhagen opened such a Fertility Assessment and Counselling Clinic (FAC) in 2011, with the concept of reducing infertility and diminishing the need for subsequent fertility treatments [67]. The mean female age of the 916 women they have seen is 33.4 years, meaning the majority are attending the clinic at an appropriate age. Of the women attending, 70% attended to estimate how long they could safely postpone childbearing [67]. After consultation, 35% of women stated they would advance their decision to try to conceive, compared with 6% who said they would consider postponing [67]. It was reported that 99% of the women found the consultation useful, with two-thirds reporting improved knowledge of the impact of age of fecundity [67]. It was felt by 75% of women that the general public needed improved education about reproductive risk factors [67].

There could be different strategies for screening. One strategy would be to screen high-risk patients only, such as those with infertility, family history of POI, previous ovarian surgery or cancer treatment. A second option would be to screen the whole population at a suitable timepoint, suggested to be 25–30 years [68]. It is known that women often do not take generic advice about delaying conception beyond 30 years of age, but studies have consistently shown that by offering

personalised risk assessment tools an individual's motivation to take active steps is increased [68].

The screening test options to assess ovarian reserve include follicle stimulating hormone (FSH), AFC and anti-mullerian hormone (AMH). Large-scale population data exist for all these markers, demonstrating age-related normal values, thus making EOA screening feasible (Figure 5.3). These tests do have limitations; FSH levels have significant variability cycle to cycle, and FSH is a late marker of low ovarian reserve and has low sensitivity [69]. Antral follicle count is relatively expensive and has inter-observer variability [69]. Anti-mullerian hormone is generally considered the earliest, most reliable and cost-effective marker of ovarian reserve, but is also not without limitations. It appears not to be as stable through the menstrual cycle as first thought, especially in younger women, and is also affected by taking hormonal contraceptive pills [69]. A further hurdle is the need for international consensus to agree which cut-off values of AMH would constitute EOA per age group.

Because of the variable rate of early ovarian ageing, it is important to realise that a single assessment of ovarian reserve may be insufficient. Therefore, those identified as being at high risk of EOA should ideally be offered serial screening. Studies have suggested screening protocols, such as 'ovarian function charts', similar to the much used antenatal and paediatric growth charts. However, again the introduction of such strategies should be agreed with national and international consensus.

Those against screening of ovarian reserve firstly argue that identifying women with EOA would have a negative psychological impact and cause significant anxiety, despite not being able to definitively predict fertility potential. Secondly, women with reduced ovarian reserve may pursue treatments such as egg freezing, with the risk of this screening initiative turning clients into patients. These women may never use these eggs and could conceive naturally, meaning they have suffered a significant and unnecessary financial and psychological burden. Finally, a normal or 'high ovarian reserve' may be counterproductive, as women will be falsely reassured that they can delay having children beyond their reproductive window.

Studies surveying women have consistently shown a significant interest in screening for ovarian reserve. However, currently there are many

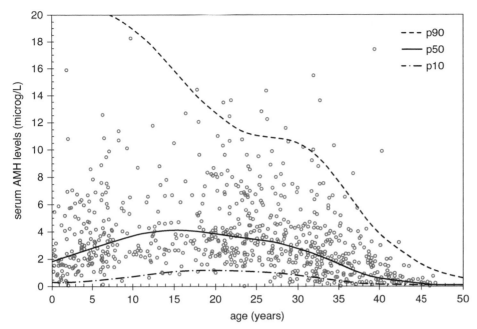

Figure 5.3 Age-related population normal values for serum anti-mullerian hormone (AMH) with reference lines for the 10th, 50th and 90th percentiles of AMH values versus age.
Source: J Clin Endocrinol Metab. 2012 Dec; 97(12): 4650–4655. Published online 2012 Sep 19. doi: 10.1210/jc.2012-1440

barriers to overcome, and studies investigating the economic costs and potential impact on public health services are required to move this programme forward.

Ovarian Cryopreservation: the Future?

An alternative to oocyte cryopreservation is ovarian cortex cryopreservation and transplantation (OCT), a procedure still considered 'experimental' by the ASRM [70]. The main body of research into this technique has centred around cancer patients prior to necessary treatment which could render women infertile. A recent large prospective study compared OCT with oocyte cryopreservation, and found a trend towards higher clinical pregnancy rates and LBR in the oocyte cryopreservation group, although this was not statistically significant [71]. Orthotopic OCT can restore ovarian function and allow natural fertility, and indeed 46.7% of pregnancies in the OCT group were conceived naturally. Another significant advantage is that if ART is required, orthotopic OCT allows multiple rounds of ovarian stimulation, as long as the graft remains active, compared with oocyte cryopreservation, where

'all of the eggs are in one basket' and the oocyte pool can be depleted.

The main indications for ovarian cortex cryopreservation are firstly in oncology patients who have very limited time to undergo ovarian stimulation prior to starting their oncology treatment; however, with random start protocols for fertility preservation this scenario would be very uncommon. Secondly, ovarian tissue cryopreservation offers a realistic, albeit invasive, option for prepubertal girls, as well as potentially restoring long-term hormonal function, improving long-term health and quality of life after cancer treatment.

Unfortunately, this new technology does not currently appear to be of benefit to older women, with Diaz-Garcia reporting no live births beyond the age of 36 years, with 6 of 16 (37.5%) patients in the egg freezing group being older than 36 years [71]. This caused this group to change their patient management algorithm, only offering oocyte tissue cryopreservation to women aged >35 years if there was proof of good ovarian reserve. This low success rate of OCT in older patients has been consistently reported by other groups [72,73].

A further significant limitation of these data is a lack of a control group in the studies. While it would be unethical to perform a randomised controlled trial on patients prior to undergoing cancer treatment, it would be of interest to investigate reproductive outcomes of fertility patients who decided not to undertake ovarian cryopreservation. It is likely that some of the pregnancies reported by Diaz-Garcia et al. (2017) may have been due to the native ovary [71].

All these published studies come from a few large fertility centres with significance experience in ovarian cryopreservation. However, the vast majority of fertility units have limited or no experience in freezing and thawing ovarian tissue, and introducing this practice would be a significant challenge for these centres. Collecting ovarian tissue requires a laparoscopy or mini-laparotomy, and although these are safe surgical procedures, they are far more invasive than trans-vaginal egg collection. Complications will still happen, particularly when procedures are performed at centres with less experience in this technique.

This technique offers an exciting alternative to egg freezing, with encouraging initial data in younger women. However, this technique has not been shown to benefit older women, and more data need to be gathered before ovarian tissue cryopreservation should be recommended in more widespread clinical practice.

Conclusion

Women worldwide are continuously improving their education, which has had a negative effect on fertility rates, raising concerns about rising involuntary childlessness and smaller families than desired due to postponement of childbearing. Women over the age of 40 who present to fertility clinics to preserve their fertility should be offered SEF, provided they are counselled about the low chance of success and the likelihood to require multiple rounds of stimulation to collect a potentially adequate number of eggs. They must also be informed of the improved success rates if they were to fertilise their eggs at the time of collection with donor sperm, and then store frozen embryos. It is known that the usage of frozen oocytes is currently low, with the majority remaining in storage unused, which means SEF is not usually a cost-effective strategy. However, the psychological impact of women taking a pro-active role to attempt to preserve their fertility cannot be assessed from a monetary standpoint.

With success rates plateauing and remaining low for women in their 40s, alternative strategies need to be developed. Family planning clinics have successfully provided advice and easy access to contraception. However, healthcare systems have a responsibility to not only advise on how to avoid unwanted pregnancy, but also to offer expert individualised advice on reproduction and when action may be required to ensure a desired family. As with all screening programmes, this would not be without risks and potential for false negative and positive findings; however, such pro-fertility initiatives currently carry far more potential to impact societal involuntary childlessness compared with technologies such as oocyte cryopreservation.

References

1. Baldwin, K., *Conceptualising women's motivations for social egg freezing and experience of reproductive delay.* Sociol Health Illn, 2018. **40**(5): p. 859–73.

2. Dunson, D.B., D.D. Baird, and B. Colombo, *Increased infertility with age in men and women.* Obstet Gynecol, 2004. **103**(1): p. 51–6.

3. Nicoletti, C. and M.L. Tanturri, *Differences in delaying motherhood across European countries: empirical evidence from the ECHP / Différences entre pays européens dans le retard à la maternité: Analyse des données de l'ECHP.* European Journal of Population / Revue Européenne de Démographie, 2008. **24**(2): p. 157–83.

4. Leridon, H., *A new estimate of permanent sterility by age: sterility defined as the inability to conceive.* Popul Stud (Camb), 2008. **62**(1): p. 15–24.

5. Goldman, K.N., *Elective oocyte cryopreservation: an ounce of prevention?* Fertil Steril, 2018. **109**(6): p. 1014–15.

6. Alteri, A., et al., *Elective egg freezing without medical indications.* Acta Obstet Gynecol Scand, 2019. **98**(5): p. 647–52.

7. Crawford, S., et al., *Cryopreserved oocyte versus fresh oocyte assisted reproductive technology cycles, United States, 2013.* Fertil Steril, 2017. **107**(1): p. 110–18.

8. Waldby, C., *'Banking time': egg freezing and the negotiation of future fertility.* Cult Health Sex, 2015. **17**(4): p. 470–82.

9. Argyle, C.E., J.C. Harper, and M.C. Davies, *Oocyte cryopreservation: where are we now?* Hum Reprod Update, 2016. **22**(4): p. 440–9.

10. Cobo, A., et al., *Six years' experience in ovum donation using vitrified oocytes: report of*

cumulative outcomes, impact of storage time, and development of a predictive model for oocyte survival rate. Fertil Steril, 2015. **104**(6): p. 1426–34. e1–8.

11. Dondorp, W., et al., *Oocyte cryopreservation for age-related fertility loss.* Hum Reprod, 2012. **27**(5): p. 1231–7.

12. *Mature oocyte cryopreservation: a guideline.* Fertil Steril, 2013. **99**(1): p. 37–43.

13. RCOG. *RCOG suggests caution over social egg freezing.* 8 August 2018; Available from: https://www.rcog.org.uk/en/news/rcog-suggests-caution-over-social-egg-freezing/.

14. Cobo, A., et al., *Oocyte vitrification as an efficient option for elective fertility preservation.* Fertil Steril, 2016. **105**(3): p. 755–764.e8.

15. Cil, A.P., H. Bang, and K. Oktay, *Age-specific probability of live birth with oocyte cryopreservation: an individual patient data meta-analysis.* Fertil Steril, 2013. **100**(2): p. 492–9.e3.

16. Doyle, J.O., et al., *Successful elective and medically indicated oocyte vitrification and warming for autologous in vitro fertilization, with predicted birth probabilities for fertility preservation according to number of cryopreserved oocytes and age at retrieval.* Fertil Steril, 2016. **105**(2): p. 459–66.e2.

17. Human Fertilisation and Embryology Authority (HFEA), *Fertility Treatment 2014-2016: trends and figures.* 2018. Available from: https://www.hfea.gov.uk/media/3188/hfea-fertility-trends-and-figures-2014-2016.pdf

18. Hammarberg, K., et al., *Reproductive experiences of women who cryopreserved oocytes for non-medical reasons.* Hum Reprod, 2017. **32**(3): p. 575–81.

19. Stoop, D., J. Nekkebroeck, and P. Devroey, *A survey on the intentions and attitudes towards oocyte cryopreservation for non-medical reasons among women of reproductive age.* Hum Reprod, 2011. **26**(3): p. 655–61.

20. Cobo, A., et al., *Elective and Onco-fertility preservation: factors related to IVF outcomes.* Hum Reprod, 2018. **33**(12): p. 2222–31.

21. Greenwood, E.A., et al., *To freeze or not to freeze: decision regret and satisfaction following elective oocyte cryopreservation.* Fertil Steril, 2018. **109**(6): p. 1097–104.e1.

22. Stoop, D., et al., *Does oocyte banking for anticipated gamete exhaustion influence future relational and reproductive choices? A follow-up of bankers and non-bankers.* Hum Reprod, 2015. **30**(2): p. 338–44.

23. Bracewell-Milnes, T., J. Norman-Taylor, and D. Nikolaou, *Social egg freezing should be offered to single women approaching their late thirties: AGAINST: Women should be freezing their eggs earlier.* BJOG, 2018. **125**(12): p. 1580.

24. Lemoine, M.E. and V. Ravitsky, *Sleepwalking into infertility: the need for a public health approach toward advanced maternal age.* Am J Bioeth, 2015. **15**(11): p. 37–48.

25. Ter Keurst, A., J. Boivin, and S. Gameiro, *Women's intentions to use fertility preservation to prevent age-related fertility decline.* Reprod Biomed Online, 2016. **32**(1): p. 121–31.

26. Goldman, R.H., et al., *Predicting the likelihood of live birth for elective oocyte cryopreservation: a counseling tool for physicians and patients.* Hum Reprod, 2017. **32**(4): p. 853–9.

27. Mesen, T.B., et al., *Optimal timing for elective egg freezing.* Fertil Steril, 2015. **103**(6): p. 1551–6.e1–4.

28. van Loendersloot, L.L., et al., *Expanding reproductive lifespan: a cost-effectiveness study on oocyte freezing.* Hum Reprod, 2011. **26**(11): p. 3054–60.

29. Devine, K., et al., *Baby budgeting: oocyte cryopreservation in women delaying reproduction can reduce cost per live birth.* Fertil Steril, 2015. **103**(6): p. 1446–53.e1–2.

30. Hirshfeld-Cytron, J., W.A. Grobman, and M.P. Milad, *Fertility preservation for social indications: a cost-based decision analysis.* Fertil Steril, 2012. **97**(3): p. 665–70.

31. Malchau, S.S., et al., *The long-term prognosis for live birth in couples initiating fertility treatments.* Hum Reprod, 2017. **32**(7): p. 1439–49.

32. Hodes-Wertz, B., et al., *What do reproductive-age women who undergo oocyte cryopreservation think about the process as a means to preserve fertility?* Fertil Steril, 2013. **100**(5): p. 1343–9.

33. Baldwin, K., et al., *Oocyte cryopreservation for social reasons: demographic profile and disposal intentions of UK users.* Reprod Biomed Online 2015. **31**(2): p. 239–45.

34. Gürtin, Z.B., et al., *For whom the egg thaws: insights from an analysis of 10 years of frozen egg thaw data from two UK clinics, 2008-2017.* J Assist Reprod Genet, 2019. **36**(6): p. 1069–80.

35. Gurtin, Z.B., K.K. Ahuja, and S. Golombok, *Emotional and relational aspects of egg-sharing: egg-share donors' and recipients' feelings about each other, each others' treatment outcome and any resulting children.* Hum Reprod, 2012. **27**(6): p. 1690–701.

36. Inhorn, M.C., et al., *Ten pathways to elective egg freezing: a binational analysis.* J Assist Reprod Genet, 2018. **35**(11): p. 2003–11.

37. Pritchard, N., et al., *Characteristics and circumstances of women in Australia who*

cryopreserved their oocytes for non-medical indications. J Reprod Infant Psychol, 2017. **35**(2): p. 108–18.

38. Jones, B.P., et al., *Perceptions, outcomes, and regret following social egg freezing in the UK; a cross-sectional survey.* Acta Obstet Gynecol Scand, 2020. **99**(3): p. 324–32.

39. Baldwin, K., et al., *Running out of time: exploring women's motivations for social egg freezing.* J Psychosom Obstet Gynaecol, 2019. **40**(2): p. 166–73.

40. Kennedy, S. and S. Ruggles, *Breaking up is hard to count: the rise of divorce in the United States, 1980-2010.* Demography, 2014. **51**(2): p. 587–98.

41. Woodtli, N., et al., *Attitude towards ovarian tissue and oocyte cryopreservation for non-medical reasons: a cross-sectional study.* Arch Gynecol Obstet, 2018. **298**(1): p. 191–8.

42. Tozzo, P., et al., *Understanding social oocyte freezing in Italy: a scoping survey on university female students' awareness and attitudes.* Life Sci Soc Policy, 2019. **15**(1): p. 3.

43. Daniluk, J.C. and E. Koert, *Fertility awareness online: the efficacy of a fertility education website in increasing knowledge and changing fertility beliefs.* Hum Reprod, 2015. **30**(2): p. 353–63.

44. Carroll, K. and C. Kroløkke, *Freezing for love: enacting 'responsible' reproductive citizenship through egg freezing.* Cult Health Sex, 2018. **20**(9): p. 992–1005.

45. Tan, S.Q., et al., *Social oocyte freezing: a survey among Singaporean female medical students.* J Obstet Gynaecol Res, 2014. **40**(5): p. 1345–52.

46. Daniluk, J.C. and E. Koert, *Childless women's beliefs and knowledge about oocyte freezing for social and medical reasons.* Hum Reprod, 2016. **31**(10): p. 2313–20.

47. Milman, L.W., et al., *Assessing reproductive choices of women and the likelihood of oocyte cryopreservation in the era of elective oocyte freezing.* Fertil Steril, 2017. **107**(5): p. 1214–22.e3.

48. Lallemant, C., et al., *Medical and social egg freezing: internet-based survey of knowledge and attitudes among women in Denmark and the UK.* Acta Obstet Gynecol Scand, 2016. **95**(12): p. 1402–10.

49. Hurley, E.G., et al., *Postponing childbearing and fertility preservation in young professional women.* South Med J, 2018. **111**(4): p. 187–91.

50. Baylis, F., *Left out in the cold: arguments against non-medical oocyte cryopreservation.* J Obstet Gynaecol Can, 2015. **37**(1): p. 64–7.

51. Bowen-Simpkins, P., J.J. Wang, and K.K. Ahuja, *The UK´s anomalous 10-year limit on oocyte storage: time to change the law.* Reprod Biomed Online, 2018. **37**(4): p. 387–9.

52. Goold, I. and J. Savulescu, *In favour of freezing eggs for non-medical reasons.* Bioethics, 2009. **23**(1): p. 47–58.

53. Schattman, G.L., *A healthy dose of reality for the egg-freezing party.* Fertil Steril, 2016. **105**(2): p. 307.

54. Gelbaya, T.A., *Short and long-term risks to women who conceive through in vitro fertilization.* Hum Fertil (Camb), 2010. **13**(1): p. 19–27.

55. Human Fertilisation and Embryology Authority (HFEA). Fertility treatment 2017: trends and figures. 2017; Available from: https://www.hfea.gov.uk/media/3189/fertility-treatment-2017-trends-and-figures.pdf

56. te Velde, E.R. and P.L. Pearson, *The variability of female reproductive ageing.* Hum Reprod Update, 2002. **8**(2): p. 141–54.

57. Nikolaou, D. and A. Templeton, *Early ovarian ageing: a hypothesis. Detection and clinical relevance.* Hum Reprod, 2003. **18**(6): p. 1137–9.

58. Nikolaou, D. and A. Templeton, *Early ovarian ageing.* Eur J Obstet Gynecol Reprod Biol, 2004. **113**(2): p. 126–33.

59. Nikolaou, D., *How old are your eggs?* Curr Opin Obstet Gynecol, 2008. **20**(6): p. 540–4.

60. Mustafa, K.B., et al., *Live birth rates are satisfactory following multiple IVF treatment cycles in poor prognosis patients.* Reprod Biol, 2017. **17**(1): p. 34–41.

61. Papathanasiou, A., et al., *Trends in 'poor responder' research: lessons learned from RCTs in assisted conception.* Hum Reprod Update, 2016. **22**(3): p. 306–19.

62. Noventa, M., et al., *Testosterone therapy for women with poor ovarian response undergoing IVF: a meta-analysis of randomized controlled trials.* J Assist Reprod Genet, 2019. **36**(4): p. 673–83.

63. Zhang, M., et al., *Dehydroepiandrosterone treatment in women with poor ovarian response undergoing IVF or ICSI: a systematic review and meta-analysis.* J Assist Reprod Genet, 2016. **33**(8): p. 981–91.

64. Haahr, T., S.C. Esteves, and P. Humaidan, *Individualized controlled ovarian stimulation in expected poor-responders: an update.* Reprod Biol Endocrinol, 2018. **16**(1): p. 20.

65. O'Brien, Y., et al., *What women want? A scoping survey on women's knowledge, attitudes and behaviours towards ovarian reserve testing and egg freezing.* Eur J Obstet Gynecol Reprod Biol, 2017. **217**: p. 71–6.

66. Azhar, E., et al., *Knowledge of ovarian reserve and reproductive choices*. J Assist Reprod Genet, 2015. **32**(3): p. 409–15.

67. Hvidman, H.W., et al., *Individual fertility assessment and pro-fertility counselling; should this be offered to women and men of reproductive age?* Hum Reprod, 2015. **30**(1): p. 9–15.

68. Tremellen, K. and J. Savulescu, *Ovarian reserve screening: a scientific and ethical analysis*. Hum Reprod, 2014. **29**(12): p. 2606–14.

69. Tal, R. and D.B. Seifer, *Ovarian reserve testing: a user's guide*. Am J Obstet Gynecol, 2017. **217**(2): p. 129–40.

70. Practice Committee of American Society for Reproductive Medicine.*Ovarian tissue cryopreservation: a committee opinion*. Fertil Steril, 2014. **101**(5): p. 1237–43.

71. Diaz-Garcia, C., et al., *Oocyte vitrification versus ovarian cortex transplantation in fertility preservation for adult women undergoing gonadotoxic treatments: a prospective cohort study*. Fertil Steril, 2018. **109**(3): p. 478–85.e2.

72. Meirow, D., et al., *Transplantations of frozen-thawed ovarian tissue demonstrate high reproductive performance and the need to revise restrictive criteria*. Fertil Steril, 2016. **106**(2): p. 467–74.

73. Donnez, J., et al., *Ovarian cortex transplantation: time to move on from experimental studies to open clinical application*. Fertil Steril, 2015. **104**(5): p. 1097–8.

When to Use ART beyond 40: How Often, How Many Attempts, When to Stop

Steven D. Spandorfer and Pietro Bortoletto

As more women delay childbearing, the proportion of women of advanced reproductive ages attempting to conceive has steadily increased [1]. The application of assisted reproductive technology (ART) in women of ages 40 and older is a fundamentally complex undertaking fraught with many challenges. Successful evaluation and management of this patient population is grounded in understanding the available peer-reviewed literature to provide an individualized plan of treatment. Initial evaluation of women over 40 who are considering the use of ART demands that two important areas are fully explored: assessment of ovarian reserve and comorbid conditions that may negatively impact a healthy gestation at advanced reproductive age.

Ovarian Reserve Assessment

Ovarian reserve is traditionally evaluated with a combination of antimullerian hormone (AMH) levels, antral follicle count (AFC), and day-3 follicle stimulating hormone (FSH) levels. The assessment of ovarian reserve with AMH is well described in the general population but can have important shortcomings in women of advanced age. Seifer and colleagues evaluated serum AMH levels in over 17,000 women in the United States [2]. They found that the median AMH level for women at 40 years of age was 0.7 ng/mL (5 pmol/L) and that the rate of decline in mean AMH values was 0.2 ng/mL/year (1.4 pmol/L) through age 40 and then diminished to 0.1 ng/mL/year thereafter (0.7 pmol/L) (Figure 6.1). With steadily decreasing AMH levels with advancing age, attempts have been made to use AMH as a prognosticator for success and to prevent women from accessing in vitro fertilization (IVF) care. Our group has previously reported on the value of AMH as a prognostic indicator of IVF outcomes and several of our

findings are pertinent to the counseling of patients choosing to attempt IVF with a poor prognosis, as so many women 40 and older are [3]. Expectation setting for these poor prognosis patients begins before the cycle start as many are likely to start more rounds of ovarian stimulation than they are complete to oocyte retrieval. We identified that women with ultra-low AMH levels (<0.17 ng/mL, 1.2 pmol/L) have a 37.3% chance of cycle cancelation, compared to women with an AMH of >1 ng/mL (7 pmol/L) who had a 5.3% chance of cycle cancelation, regardless of age group. In our study, there was a statistically significant trend toward higher pregnancy rates with increasing AMH, except for women over 40. Importantly, when analyzing a subset of women who are expected to be exceedingly poor responders, women 41–42 years old with an ultra-low AMH (<0.17 ng/mL), one in four went on to achieve a clinical pregnancy. This number fell to <4% when age was >42 years. Other groups have identified an AMH of <1.0 ng/mL in women over 40 as a threshold for prediction of poor ovarian response (with three or fewer retrieved oocytes). However, the same threshold did not predict odds of achieving a pregnancy [4]. We advise against the use of AMH as the sole criterion for withholding treatment for women with an expected poor response as the act of ovarian stimulation, and its associated response, are useful indicators of reproductive potential.

Antimullerian hormone alone does not tell the whole story of how a woman over 40 can be expected to respond to ovarian stimulation. In a classic study by Scott et al., day-3 FSH, luteinizing hormone (LH), and estradiol levels were measured in 441 patients to determine their predictive value for stimulation quality and pregnancy rates in IVF [5]. They found that women with low basal FSH levels (<15 mIU/mL) had higher pregnancy rates per attempt than those with moderate levels

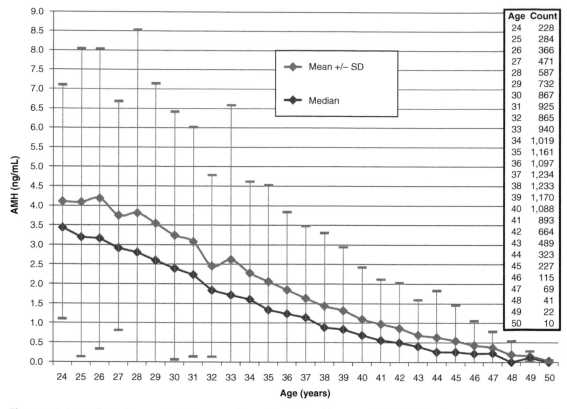

Figure 6.1 Antimullerian hormone (AMH) age-specific median values with mean ± SD AMH values for women of ages 24–50 at one year intervals.
Source: Reprinted from Seifer et al. [2], with permission from Elsevier.

(15–24.9 mIU/mL), both of which were higher than those with high FSH levels (>25 mIU/mL). In a separate study of a cohort of women 40 and older undergoing IVF, lower cycle day-3 FSH levels were associated with a higher likelihood of achieving a live birth, after adjusting for age at cycle start. Live birth rates above 5% were noted at age 40 with FSH values <12 mIU/mL. Even at FSH values of 15 mIU/mL or above, there was a 4.6% chance of pregnancy for women at 40 years of age. The highest FSH level in a woman achieving a pregnancy was 18.0 mIU/mL, at age 43 [6]. It is important that a day-3 FSH level not be considered in isolation as age is still a very important predictor of success. When comparing IVF outcomes of patients >40 years of age with FSH levels ≤15 IU/L to those <40 years of age with FSH levels ≥15 IU/L, the high FSH group had better implantation rates per embryo (34% versus 11%), higher ongoing rates per embryo transfer (ET) (40% versus 13%), and higher ongoing pregnancy rates per cycle (25% versus 10%) [7]. Lastly, our group has previously shown that ovarian response is highly

predictive of IVF outcome in women with normal and abnormal ovarian reserve, regardless of ovarian age [8]. This underscores the importance of not solely relying on age when presenting and discussing IVF outcome data.

Beyond age, incorporation of day-3 FSH and AMH levels with AFC may provide additional information to help counsel patients. In good-prognosis patients, AMH is a stronger predictor of ovarian response to gonadotropin therapy than AFC [9]. However, like AMH, AFC has been shown to decrease with age, by approximately 4.5% (95% Cl: 5–7%) per year [10]. Taken as a whole, AFC, day-3 FSH, and AMH are able to reliably differentiate among poor, normal, and high responders. A meta-analysis by Hendriks et al., identified AFC as a superior predictor of poor ovarian response when compared to day-3 FSH levels [11]. Furthermore, the number of oocytes retrieved as well as the number of embryos created have been shown to be negatively correlated with baseline FSH and positively correlated with baseline AMH and AFC, whereas AFC provides the strongest correlation [12]. While AFC retains several advantages, particularly immediacy and accessibility, international standardization of AMH assays is likely to enhance its performance in predicting poor ovarian response. Until then, AMH, holistically assessed along with other markers of ovarian reserve, such as day-3 FSH and AFC, provides a robust assessment that can be used to provide individualized counseling for this patient group.

Preconception

For any woman attempting to conceive, preconception counseling and optimization of comorbid medical conditions are vital to a healthy pregnancy. Pregnancy at advanced maternal age is not a benign undertaking, with several associated antenatal and postpartum maternal risks, including maternal death. The Center for Disease Control (CDC) estimates that approximately 65.7 out of every 100,000 live births in women 40 and older result in a maternal death. This number nearly triples to 191.6 per 100,000 for non-Hispanic Black women [13]. Among causes of pregnancy-related deaths, cardiovascular conditions (15.5%), followed by preexisting illness (14.5%), infection (12.7%), hemorrhage (11.4%), and cardiomyopathy (11.0%) were the most common. Another study using data from the CDC found that women of ages 45–54 (adjusted RR: 3.46, 95% CI: 3.15–3.80) followed by women of ages 40–44 (adjusted RR: 1.90, 95% CI: 1.84–1.97) carried the highest risk of severe maternal morbidity and pregnancy complications such as preeclampsia, postpartum hemorrhage, thrombosis, and hysterectomy [14]. It can be reasonably expected that the prevalence of comorbid conditions increases with advancing maternal age. Preconception optimization of these conditions presents an opportunity not only to counsel women regarding potential pregnancy related risks but also to risk-reduce ensuing pregnancies.

Beyond the exacerbation of existing health issues, advancing maternal age, regardless of the method of conception, is associated with a host of pregnancy-related conditions such as increased risks of hypertensive disorders of pregnancy, abnormal placentation, and low birth weight [15]. Furthermore, the use of IVF, independent of age, is also associated with an increased risk of hypertensive disorders of pregnancy, preterm

labor, and preterm delivery [16]. It is vital for women attempting to conceive at these advanced reproductive ages to understand that these risks are further heightened with increasing maternal age. At our center, women are routinely recommended to undergo preconception consultation with a maternal-fetal medicine specialist to discuss pregnancy-related risks and to address comorbid conditions prior to attempts at conception.

Lastly, a special preconception consideration for women conceiving at advanced reproductive ages is the age of the male providing sperm. Reproduction with men of advanced age has been linked to a host of childhood outcomes, particularly psychiatric disorders like autism spectrum disorders and schizophrenia but also with stillbirth and several birth defects [17]. The cause has not entirely been elucidated but it is believed to be related to the larger number of germline divisions that have occurred in older males in addition to epigenetic changes. Beyond childhood outcomes, negative effects on sperm quality and testicular function have been reported as well as reproductive and fertilization outcomes in IVF/intracytoplasmic sperm injection (ICSI) cycles [18].

How to Use ART in Women over 40

When considering the use of ART in women of ages 40 and older, an important consideration is which ART technique to utilize first. In the general infertile population, ovulation induction with oral medications such as clomiphene citrate or letrozole is used for simplicity and cost. Unfortunately, for women of advanced age, ovulation induction is associated with exceedingly low pregnancy rates, ranging from 1% to 4.3% [19]. As a result, most providers often forgo ovulation induction with oral agents and proceed with gonadotropin-stimulated cycles or IVF. In the largest reported series in women of 40 and older, ovulation induction with injectable gonadotropins and intrauterine insemination (IUI) was associated with an overall ongoing pregnancy rate of 4.5%. Pregnancy rates were highest for women age 40 (9.6%) but decreased to 5.2% and 2.4% with each advancing year. There were no pregnancies in 136 cycles in women 43 years and older [20]. Disappointingly, given the low pregnancy rates in the published studies, information on live birth rates is sorely lacking for this age group. While ovarian stimulation at this advanced age often results in monofollicular development, it has recently been shown that when more than two follicles 14 mm in size were present on the day of ovulatory trigger there is a substantially increased risk of multiple gestations without an improved chance of singleton clinical pregnancy [21]. Because of the risk of multiple gestations and low pregnancy rates with oral and injectable ovarian stimulation cycles, providers often either start with IVF or inevitably progress to it.

In vitro fertilization affords women over 40 the highest chance at achieving pregnancy. In a study of over 2,700 women 40 and older undergoing IVF with ICSI, 14.8% achieved an ultrasound-confirmed pregnancy with 9.7% going on to have a live birth per cycle start. Expectedly, the highest live birth rates were in women 40 years of age (13.9%) and decreased to 2.6% by age 44. There were no pregnancies recorded in the 17 women age 46 and older. Importantly, to achieve these pregnancy rates a mean of 3.3 embryos were transferred across all age groups with a 14.1% twin pregnancy rate for this cohort. Only 5.7% of cycles produced excess embryos for cryopreservation and future use. Our center recently published on our 20-year institutional experience caring for over 1,700 women aged 45 and older who underwent fresh autologous IVF transfer cycles [22]. In our cohort, 10% of patients never started their cycle due to elevated day-3 FSH levels above 15 mIU/mL and 28.5% of patients were canceled midcycle prior to oocyte retrieval due to poor ovarian response. Of those that did undergo oocyte retrieval and fresh embryo transfer, the overall pregnancy rate per transfer was 18.7%, of which 82.1% ended in a pregnancy loss. The overall live birth rate per transfer was 3.4%. It is important to highlight that in this cohort there were no live births recorded in any patient with four or fewer oocytes retrieved. At these advanced ages, ovarian stimulation to maximize oocyte yield is of particular importance as every additional oocyte may offer a significant reproductive advantage.

Traditionally, women with predicted poor response have been prescribed increasingly large doses of injectable gonadotropins to maximize oocyte yield. In perhaps the best designed study to evaluate whether higher FSH doses yield better cycle outcomes, van Tilborg et al., randomized 511 poor-responding women to an increased FSH dose (225 or 450 IU/day) versus a standard dose (150 IU/day). They found that despite an increase of on average one to two more oocytes with higher gonadotropins doses, there was no impact on live birth (risk difference: 0.02; 95% CI: −0.11 to 0.06) [23]. Intuitively, higher gonadotropin doses would be suspected to yield more oocytes and more pregnancies in poor responders. However, these poor-responding women, by definition, have a smaller antral follicle pool that is able to respond to FSH, regardless of the magnitude of the dose. Age, and its associated decline in quantity and quality of oocytes, continues to be the rate-limiting step in the ability of these women to achieve pregnancy.

The decision regarding which IVF stimulation protocol to use in the poor responders is subject to debate. A retrospective study of poor responders being stimulated with either a gonadotropin releasing hormone (GnRH) agonist long protocol versus a GnRH antagonist protocol found no statistical difference in clinical pregnancy rates, but the GnRH agonist long protocol had fewer cycle cancelations and higher live birth rates per retrieval when compared to the GnRH antagonist protocol [24]. When comparing the microdose GnRH agonist protocol to GnRH antagonist in poor responders, patients receiving a micro-dose GnRH agonist protocol had more mature oocyte retrieved and higher implantation rates compared to GnRH antagonist protocols [25]. The implantation and clinical pregnancy rate were not significantly different. A further variation on the theme, ultra-short GnRH agonist compared to GnRH antagonist cycles produced a higher number of oocytes retrieved and embryos transferred in patients with a history of poor ovarian response [26]. At our center, in the absence of prior ovarian stimulation cycles to review, we typically start with a GnRH antagonist protocol. In patients with a previously documented premature LH surge, commonly those with diminished ovarian reserve, we will add a GnRH antagonist twice a day [27]. Leading into the follicular phase, we also routinely utilize estradiol patching as we have previously shown that this improves ovarian stimulation and results in greater uniformity in follicular development and improved pregnancy rates [28]. For patients who have poor response to the GnRH antagonist protocol, we will often consider the addition of letrozole or clomiphene to a GnRH antagonist protocol before progressing to variations on the GnRH agonist cycle [29].

In an effort to maximize the reproductive outcomes of poor-responding women, dozens of adjunctive treatments have been proposed and studied. Perhaps the most widely used treatment has been the application of preimplantation genetic testing for aneuploidy (PGT-A). In a study by Rubio et al., 205 women aged 38–41 years were randomized to day-3 PGT-A (via comprehensive 24-chromosome screening) with blastocyst transfer versus no PGT-A. They found that women 38–41 who underwent PGT-A had lower miscarriage rates (2.7% versus 39.0%), higher live birth rates (52.9% versus 24.2%), and shorter time to pregnancy (7.7 versus 14.9 weeks) compared to women who underwent fresh transfer without PGT-A [30]. Importantly, in the PGT-A arm, one in three women did not have an embryo transfer due to failure to reach the blastocyst stage. In this poor-responding population of advanced age, a practice of uniform blastocyst stage transfer or freeze-all for PGT at the blastocyst stage does not represent the nuanced, individualized approach this challenging patient population requires. A 2020 study by Deng et al. retrospectively analyzed 353 cycles in women with poor ovarian response (four or fewer oocytes retrieved) who underwent either PGT-A or fresh/frozen transfer of day-3 or day-5 embryos [31]. They found that patients who underwent PGT-A were significantly less likely to reach embryo transfer compared with those who underwent non-PGT cycles (13.7% versus 70.6%). Furthermore, live birth rates were similar between groups (6.6% versus 5.4%) but miscarriage rate per retrieval was lower with PGT-A tested embryos (0.4% versus 3.6%). However, the number needed to treat to avoid one clinical miscarriage was 31 PGT-A cycles. It is our view that PGT-A should be selectively applied on a case-by-case basis in women of advanced age, taking into account their reproductive history, reproductive goals, and risk tolerance for miscarriage. A universal PGT-A approach for all women of advanced age undoubtedly excludes women from ever having a transfer due to poor blastocyst development or shortcomings of chromosomal assessment of embryos (i.e., damage to embryo, mosaic results, or false-positive aneuploidy).

Other adjunctive treatments aim to improve the oocyte yield and subsequent embryo quality in poor-responding women. Through its stimulation of hepatic production of insulin-like growth factor-1, growth hormone (GH) is thought to potentiate the action of FSH via folliculogenesis and granulosa cell differentiation [32]. A 2010 Cochrane Database review by Duffy et al. suggested that adjuvant use of GH in poor responders was associated with an increase in pregnancy rates and live birth and (OR: 3.28, 95% CI: 1.74–6.20; OR: 5.39, 95% CI: 1.89–15.35, respectively) [33]. The exact subgroup of poor responders who would benefit from GH augmentation is unknown as is the optimal dosing and pretreatment length of time. The findings of this Cochrane review should be taken with caution as the number of studies included were few in number, small, and with varying definitions of poor response. Furthermore, in the United States, GH is regulated by the US Food and Drug Administration and requires a provider to give justification for use; poor IVF response is not considered to be a justification for use unless an organic GH deficiency is suspected.

Dehydroepiandrosterone (DHT) and testosterone (T) have also been investigated as adjunctive treatments for poor prognosis patients undergoing IVF. Both DHT and T have been found to play an important role in maintaining adequate follicular steroidogenesis by acting as a substrate for the conversion of androgens to estrogens via aromatase. At the level of the ovary, they promote the induction and upregulation of FSH and androgen receptors in preantral and antral follicles, amplifying the effect of FSH on follicular growth during IVF [34]. A Cochrane Database review of 17 randomized controlled trials (RCTs) with mostly poor-responding women found that DHEA cotreatment was associated with higher rates of live birth or ongoing pregnancy (OR: 1.88, 95% CI: 1.30–2.71). However, when only high-quality studies with low risk of performance bias are analyzed, the statistical significance was no longer found [35]. The same pattern is seen with T cotreatment. As with many adjunctive treatments, there is a paucity of large, well-designed trials that answer these important questions for patients and clinicians alike.

Another popular adjunctive treatment for poor-responding women undergoing IVF is the antioxidant Coenzyme Q-10 (CoQ10). CoQ10 is a lipid-soluble antioxidant component of the mitochondrial respiratory chain that is thought to be involved in repairing reactive oxygen species (ROS)-induced DNA damage [36]. The resulting mitochondrial dysfunction from genomic instability of ROS-induced DNA damage has been implicated in poor oocyte quality, abnormal fertilization, and diminished ovarian reserve [37]. A recent prospective trial of 186 women with poor ovarian response randomized some to CoQ10 pretreatment for 60 days preceding IVF versus no pretreatment [38]. Women receiving CoQ10 required fewer gonadotropins, achieved higher peak estradiol levels, and had more oocytes retrieved compared to the no pretreatment group. Despite having more high-quality embryos available, there were no differences in clinical pregnancy and live birth rates per transfer, although the RCT was not powered to detect a difference in these outcomes. Importantly, this study was conducted in POSEIDON classification group 3 patients (age <35 with poor ovarian reserve parameters), not women of advanced age. The utility of CoQ10 in women of advanced age is still debated with a paucity of large, prospective randomized trials to inform decisions regarding dose, length of pretreatment, and clear clinical benefit. Our center does not routinely recommend the use of GH, DHEA, T, or CoQ10 as helpful adjuncts.

One modifiable treatment factor worthy of discussion is the timing and type of embryo transfer in a cohort of women of advanced age with predicted poor response. As previously mentioned, a practice of universal blastocyst stage cryopreservation for PGT-A is not a nuanced, individualized approach for this subgroup of patients undergoing IVF. At our center, patients of advanced age are routinely offered a fresh embryo transfer at the cleavage stage. This approach is generally employed for patients who have had poor blastocyst development in the past or with poor day-3 embryo quality during the fresh IVF cycle. Utilizing time-lapse imaging to help determine the likelihood of blastocyst development, we are able to triage patients to a fresh day-3 transfer versus prolonging culture to day-5 for transfer or cryopreservation [39]. A fresh transfer affords the patient an opportunity to achieve a pregnancy, whereas a strict blastocyst only policy often results in attrition leaving no

embryos available for transfer [40]. A recent study by Smith et al. using data from the UK's Human Fertilisation and Embryology Authority (HFEA) examined the live birth and perinatal outcomes of fresh versus freeze-all IVF cycles in over 330,000 women [41]. They concluded that a universal freeze-all approach to allow for segmentation of IVF and embryo transfer may be associated with a lower cumulative live birth rate and urged an individualized approach with a clear clinical indication for segmentation (i.e., ovarian hyperstimulation syndrome (OHSS) risk, PGT etc).

Beyond live birth rates, concerns have also been raised about the health of children born from cryopreserved embryos. Compared to fresh transfer, women who conceived following a frozen transfer were found to be at a 1.3-fold and 1.8 fold increased risk of hypertensive disorders of pregnancy and preeclampsia, respectively [42,43]. Given that maternal age over 40 in and of itself is associated with a 2.1-fold increased odds of early-onset preeclampsia (3.16-fold for women 45 and older), a fresh embryo transfer may offer additional benefits for the ensuing pregnancy [44].

Additionally, the number of embryos to transfer in women of advanced age, fresh or frozen, is debated. The American Society for Reproductive Medicine recommends that patients 41–42 years of age should plan to receive no more than four cleavage-stage embryos or three blastocysts [45]. In women ≥43 years of age, due to a paucity of evidence, they do not recommend a limit on the number of embryos to transfer. In cases where euploid embryos are available, a single-blastocyst transfer is recommended. Our center recently published our experience of 567 cycles in 464 patients aged 43–45 years to answer the question about the optimal number of cleavage-stage embryos to transfer in women ≥43 years of age [46]. In this cohort, live birth rates per transfer were 14.4%, 9.4%, and 1.3% for women aged 43, 44, and 45 years, respectively, with a twin birth rate of 16.3%, 6.7%, and 0 (of all live births) for ages 43, 44, and 45 years, respectively. We found that women aged 43 and 44 years having five or more embryos transferred experienced higher clinical pregnancy rates than those patients receiving a transfer of three or four embryos and that the cumulative pregnancy rate (CPR) for patients undergoing transfer with six or more embryos were not better than those undergoing transfer with five embryos. Regardless of age, the decision on the number of embryos transfer requires shared decision-making and careful assessment and discussion of potential maternal and neonatal risks associated with transfer of more than a single embryo at a time.

At our center, when embryos are cryopreserved at the blastocyst stage, the preference is for transfer in the natural cycle, rather than in the hormone replacement cycle, when clinically feasible. There are important distinctions between natural and programmed frozen embryo transfer (FET) cycles, namely the presence of a corpus luteum producing vasoactive substances important for early placental invasion and remodeling. Growing evidence suggests that maternal (postpartum hemorrhage, hypertensive disorders of pregnancy) and perinatal outcomes (post-term birth and macrosomia) are worse with programmed cycles [47].

How Often/How Many Attempts

As mentioned earlier in the chapter, the application of ART in women 40 and older is a fundamentally complex undertaking fraught with many challenges. While every effort is made to achieve a live birth, knowing when to "stop" and consider oocyte donation or other forms of family building is essential. There are several cycle and patient-level variables that may be important when counseling patients regarding cessation of treatment. A 2018 study by Devesa et al. examined the cumulative live birth rates of women ≥38 years old undergoing their first IVF cycle at a single center [48]. As expected, they found that live birth rates decrease with increasing age,

with the most prominent decline occurring in the 42–43 year old age group (7%) and progressing to 1.2% from 44 years onwards. For patients over 40 years completing their IVF cycle and undergoing fresh transfer, the lack of success with their first embryo transfer was not shown to portend a poor future prognosis [49]. In their study, approximately one in every five patients who experienced either a pregnancy loss or negative beta-human chorionic gonadotropin in their initial IVF cycle went on to have a successful delivery in a future cycle. Importantly, the same study showed that future pregnancies are typically achieved within four to six treatment cycles, with no further pregnancies leading to delivery identified beyond that.

A study by Klipstein et al. analyzed 2,705 ART cycles in over 1,200 women age 40 or above to describe live birth rates and predictors of ART success (Figure 6.2) [6]. One-hundred and forty-eight (87.1%) women who had a live birth conceived within the first three IVF cycles. The cumulative live birth rate was not significantly different for women starting ART at ages 40, 41, and 42 but was significantly lower for that subgroup of women undergoing their first ART cycle at age 43 or 44 compared with the lower ages at first cycle start. Furthermore, the live birth rate increased with each additional embryo transferred in each age group with a mean number of embryos transferred for all women of 3.3 for an overall multiple birth rate of 15.3% (92.5% of which were twins). In this cohort, the women with the best chance of achieving a live birth were those who had excess embryos available for cryopreservation (only 5.7%), those with more embryos

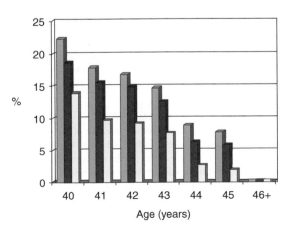

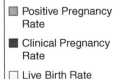

Figure 6.2 Effect of age on positive pregnancy test, clinical pregnancy rate, and live birth rate per cycle start.
Source: Reprinted from Klipstein et al. [6], with permission from Elsevier.

available for transfer (54% had two or fewer embryos transferred), those with low cycle day-3 FSH values (<12 mIU/mL), and women with greater than one fetal heartbeat on initial ultrasound.

When to Stop

There are several important ethical considerations that guide the decision to continue or discontinue treatment when a low likelihood of success is expected. The Ethics Committee of the American Society of Reproductive Medicine (ASRM) defines "futility" as ≤1% chance of live birth and "very poor" prognosis >1% to ≤5% per treatment cycle [50]. The aforementioned study by Klipstein et al. suggests that ART with autologous oocytes has a reasonable chance for success (>5%) up until the end of the 43rd year [6]. While our center does not have a strict number of cycles a patient can attempt before being counseled against further attempts, we take into account various parameters such as previous cycle outcomes, ovarian reserve, and tolerance for low likelihood of cycle success into account. We also discuss other alternatives to family-building such as gestational surrogacy for those with repeated implantation failures or recurrent miscarriage and oocyte donation for poor-responding patients. While oocyte donation does provide a substantially improved chance of live birth over 40, the decision to cease attempts with autologous oocytes and convert to donor oocytes is complex. Beyond the financial considerations of utilizing donor oocytes, there are several societal, ethical, and personal issues that a woman faces when choosing this route. We routinely recommend patients meet with a reproductive psychologist to discuss the complexities of these decisions.

References

1. Martin JA, Hamilton BE, Osterman MJ, Curtin SC, Matthews TJ. Births: final data for 2013. Natl Vital Stat Rep 2015;64(1):1–65.

2. Seifer DB, Baker VL, Leader B. Age-specific serum anti-Müllerian hormone values for 17,120 women presenting to fertility centers within the United States. Fertil Steril 2011;95(2):747–50.

3. Reichman DE, Goldschlag D, Rosenwaks Z. Value of antimüllerian hormone as a prognostic indicator of in vitro fertilization outcome. Fertil Steril 2014;101(4):1012–18.e1.

4. Tokura Y, Yoshino O, Ogura-Nose S, Motoyama H, Harada M, Osuga Y, et al. The significance of serum anti-Müllerian hormone (AMH) levels in patients over age 40 in first IVF treatment. J Assist Reprod Genet 2013;30(6):821–5.

5. Scott RT, Toner JP, Muasher SJ, Oehninger S, Robinson S, Rosenwaks Z. Follicle-stimulating hormone levels on cycle day 3 are predictive of in vitro fertilization outcome. Fertil Steril 1989;51(4):651–4.

6. Klipstein S, Regan M, Ryley DA, Goldman MB, Alper MM, Reindollar RH. One last chance for pregnancy: a review of 2,705 in vitro fertilization cycles initiated in women age 40 years and above. Fertil Steril 2005;84(2):435–45.

7. Rooij van IAJ, Bancsi LFJMM, Broekmans FJM, Looman CWN, Habbema JDF, Velde te ER. Women older than 40 years of age and those with elevated follicle-stimulating hormone levels differ in poor response rate and embryo quality in in vitro fertilization. Fertil Steril 2003;79(3):482–8.

8. Yih MC, Spandorfer SD, Rosenwaks Z. Egg production predicts a doubling of in vitro fertilization pregnancy rates even within defined age and ovarian reserve categories. Fertil Steril 2005;83(1):24–9.

9. Nelson SM, Klein BM, Arce J-C. Comparison of antimüllerian hormone levels and antral follicle count as predictor of ovarian response to controlled ovarian stimulation in good-prognosis patients at individual fertility clinics in two multicenter trials. Fertil Steril 2015;103(4):923–30.e1.

10. Khan HL, Bhatti S, Suhail S, Gul R, Awais A, Hamayun H, et al. Antral follicle count (AFC) and serum anti-Müllerian hormone (AMH) are the predictors of natural fecundability have similar trends irrespective of fertility status and menstrual characteristics among fertile and infertile women below the age of 40 years. Reprod Biol Endocrinol 2019;17(1):20.

11. Hendriks DJ, Mol B-WJ, Bancsi LFJMM, Te Velde ER, Broekmans FJM. Antral follicle count in the prediction of poor ovarian response and pregnancy after in vitro fertilization: a meta-analysis and comparison with basal follicle-stimulating hormone level. Fertil Steril 2005;83(2):291–301.

12. Tsakos E, Tolikas A, Daniilidis A, Asimakopoulos B. Predictive value of anti-müllerian hormone, follicle-stimulating hormone and antral follicle count on the outcome of ovarian stimulation in women following GnRH-antagonist protocol for IVF/ET. Arch Gynecol Obstet 2014;290(6):1249–53.

13. Creanga AA, Syverson C, Seed K, Callaghan WM. Pregnancy-related mortality in the United States, 2011–2013. Obstet Gynecol 2017;**130**(2):366–73.

14. Sheen J-J, Wright JD, Goffman D, Kern-Goldberger AR, Booker W, Siddiq Z, et al. Maternal age and risk for adverse outcomes. Am J Obstet Gynecol 2018;**219**(4):390.e1–390.e15.

15. Wennberg AL, Opdahl S, Bergh C, Aaris Henningsen A-K, Gissler M, Romundstad LB, et al. Effect of maternal age on maternal and neonatal outcomes after assisted reproductive technology. Fertil Steril 2016;**106**(5):1142–9.e14.

16. Sullivan-Pyke CS, Senapati S, Mainigi MA, Barnhart KT. In vitro fertilization and adverse obstetric and perinatal outcomes. Semin Perinatol 2017;**41**(6):345–53.

17. du Fossé NA, van der Hoorn M-LP, van Lith JMM, le Cessie S, Lashley EELO. Advanced paternal age is associated with an increased risk of spontaneous miscarriage: a systematic review and meta-analysis. Hum Reprod Update 2020;**26** (5):650–69.

18. Sharma R, Agarwal A, Rohra VK, Assidi M, Abu-Elmagd M, Turki RF. Effects of increased paternal age on sperm quality, reproductive outcome and associated epigenetic risks to offspring. Reprod Biol Endocrinol 2015;**13**:35.

19. Tsafrir A, Simon A, Revel A, Reubinoff B, Lewin A, Laufer N. Retrospective analysis of 1217 IVF cycles in women aged 40 years and older. Reprod Biomed Online 2007;**14**(3):348–55.

20. Corsan G, Trias A, Trout S, Kemmann E. Ovulation induction combined with intrauterine insemination in women 40 years of age and older: is it worthwhile? Hum Reprod 1996;**11**(5):1109–12.

21. Evans MB, Stentz NC, Richter KS, Schexnayder B, Connell M, Healy MW, et al. Mature follicle count and multiple gestation risk based on patient age in intrauterine insemination cycles with ovarian stimulation. Obstet Gynecol 2020;**135**(5):1005–14.

22. Gunnala V, Irani M, Melnick A, Rosenwaks Z, Spandorfer S. One thousand seventy-eight autologous IVF cycles in women 45 years and older: the largest single-center cohort to date. J Assist Reprod Genet 2018;**35**(3):435–40.

23. van Tilborg TC, Torrance HL, Oudshoorn SC, Eijkemans MJC, Koks CAM, Verhoeve HR, et al. Individualized versus standard FSH dosing in women starting IVF/ICSI: an RCT. Part 1: The predicted poor responder. Hum Reprod 2017;**32** (12):2496–505.

24. Stimpfel M, Vrtačnik-Bokal E, Pozlep B, Kmecl J, Virant-Klun I. Gonadotrophin-releasing hormone agonist protocol of controlled ovarian hyperstimulation as an efficient treatment in Bologna-defined poor ovarian responders. Syst Biol Reprod Med 2016;**62**(4):290–6.

25. Boza A, Cakar E, Boza B, Api M, Kayatas S, Sofuoglu K. Microdose flare-up gonadotropin-releasing hormone (GnRH) agonist versus GnRH antagonist protocols in poor ovarian responders undergoing intracytoplasmic sperm injection. J Reprod Infertil 2016;**17**(3):163–8.

26. Orvieto R, Kruchkovich J, Rabinson J, Zohav E, Anteby EY, Meltcer S. Ultrashort gonadotropin-releasing hormone agonist combined with flexible multidose gonadotropin-releasing hormone antagonist for poor responders in in vitro fertilization/embryo transfer programs. Fertil Steril 2008;**90**(1):228–30.

27. Reichman DE, Zakarin L, Chao K, Meyer L, Davis OK, Rosenwaks Z. Diminished ovarian reserve is the predominant risk factor for gonadotropin-releasing hormone antagonist failure resulting in breakthrough luteinizing hormone surges in in vitro fertilization cycles. Fertil Steril 2014;**102**(1):99–102.

28. Dragisic KG, Davis OK, Fasouliotis SJ, Rosenwaks Z. Use of a luteal estradiol patch and a gonadotropin-releasing hormone antagonist suppression protocol before gonadotropin stimulation for in vitro fertilization in poor responders. Fertil Steril 2005;**84**(4):1023–6.

29. Elassar A, Engmann L, Nulsen J, Benadiva C. Letrozole and gonadotropins versus luteal estradiol and gonadotropin-releasing hormone antagonist protocol in women with a prior low response to ovarian stimulation. Fertil Steril 2011;**95**(7):2330–4.

30. Rubio C, Bellver J, Rodrigo L, Castillón G, Guillén A, Vidal C, et al. In vitro fertilization with preimplantation genetic diagnosis for aneuploidies in advanced maternal age: a randomized, controlled study. Fertil Steril 2017;**107**(5):1122–9.

31. Deng J, Hong HY, Zhao Q, Nadgauda A, Ashrafian S, Behr B, et al. Preimplantation genetic testing for aneuploidy in poor ovarian responders with four or fewer oocytes retrieved. J Assist Reprod Genet 2020;**37**(5):1147–54.

32. Zhou P, Baumgarten SC, Wu Y, Bennett J, Winston N, Hirshfeld-Cytron J, et al. IGF-I signaling is essential for FSH stimulation of AKT and steroidogenic genes in granulosa cells. Mol Endocrinol 2013;**27** (3):511–23.

33. Duffy JM, Ahmad G, Mohiyiddeen L, Nardo LG, Watson A. Growth hormone for in vitro fertilization. Cochrane Database Syst Rev 2010;**1**: CD000099.

34. Garcia-Velasco JA, Moreno L, Pacheco A, Guillén A, Duque L, Requena A, et al. The aromatase inhibitor letrozole increases the concentration of intraovarian androgens and improves in vitro fertilization outcome in low responder patients: a pilot study. Fertil Steril 2005;**84**(1):82–7.

35. Nagels HE, Rishworth JR, Siristatidis CS, Kroon B. Androgens (dehydroepiandrosterone or testosterone) for women undergoing assisted reproduction. Cochrane Database Syst Rev 2015;**11**:CD009749.

36. Özcan P, Fıçıcıoğlu C, Kizilkale O, Yesiladali M, Tok OE, Ozkan F, et al. Can coenzyme Q10 supplementation protect the ovarian reserve against oxidative damage? J Assist Reprod Genet 2016;**33**(9):1223–30.

37. Fragouli E, Wells D. Mitochondrial DNA assessment to determine oocyte and embryo viability. Semin Reprod Med 2015;**33**(6):401–9.

38. Xu Y, Nisenblat V, Lu C, Li R, Qiao J, Zhen X, et al. Pretreatment with coenzyme Q10 improves ovarian response and embryo quality in low-prognosis young women with decreased ovarian reserve: a randomized controlled trial. Reprod Biol Endocrinol 2018;**16**(1):29.

39. Khosravi P, Kazemi E, Zhan Q, Malmsten JE, Toschi M, Zisimopoulos P, et al. Deep learning enables robust assessment and selection of human blastocysts after in vitro fertilization. NPJ Digit Med 2019;**2**:21.

40. Farquhar CM, Wang YA, Sullivan EA. A comparative analysis of assisted reproductive technology cycles in Australia and New Zealand 2004–2007. Hum Reprod 2010;**25**(9):2281–9.

41. Smith ADAC, Tilling K, Lawlor DA, Nelson SM. Live birth rates and perinatal outcomes when all embryos are frozen compared with conventional fresh and frozen embryo transfer: a cohort study of 337,148 in vitro fertilisation cycles. BMC Med 2019;**17**(1):202.

42. Maheshwari A, Pandey S, Amalraj Raja E, Shetty A, Hamilton M, Bhattacharya S. Is frozen embryo transfer better for mothers and babies? Can cumulative meta-analysis provide a definitive answer? Hum Reprod Update 2018;**24**(1):35–58.

43. Roque M, Haahr T, Geber S, Esteves SC, Humaidan P. Fresh versus elective frozen embryo transfer in IVF/ICSI cycles: a systematic review and meta-analysis of reproductive outcomes. Hum Reprod Update 2019;**25**(1):2–14.

44. Marozio L, Picardo E, Filippini C, Mainolfi E, Berchialla P, Cavallo F, et al. Maternal age over 40 years and pregnancy outcome: a hospital-based survey. J Matern Fetal Neonatal Med 2019;**32**(10):1602–8.

45. Penzias A, Bendikson K, Butts S, Coutifaris C, Fossum G, Falcone T, et al. Guidance on the limits to the number of embryos to transfer: a committee opinion. Fertil Steril 2017;**107**(4):901–3.

46. Gunnala V, Reichman DE, Meyer L, Davis OK, Rosenwaks Z. Beyond the American Society for Reproductive Medicine transfer guidelines: How many cleavage-stage embryos are safe to transfer in women ≥43 years old? Fertil Steril 2014;**102**(6):1626–32.e1.

47. Singh B, Reschke L, Segars J, Baker VL. Frozen-thawed embryo transfer: the potential importance of the corpus luteum in preventing obstetrical complications. Fertil Steril 2020;**113**(2):252–7.

48. Devesa M, Tur R, Rodríguez I, Coroleu B, Martínez F, Polyzos NP. Cumulative live birth rates and number of oocytes retrieved in women of advanced age. A single centre analysis including 4500 women ≥38 years old. Hum Reprod 2018;**33**(11):2010–7.

49. Sneeringer R, Klipstein S, Ryley DA, Alper MM, Reindollar RH. Pregnancy loss in the first in vitro fertilization cycle is not predictive of subsequent delivery in women over 40 years. Fertil Steril 2008;**89**(2):364–7.

50. Ethics Committee of American Society for Reproductive Medicine. Fertility treatment when the prognosis is very poor or futile: a committee opinion. Fertil Steril 2012;**98**(1):e6–9.

Optimal IVF Protocols for Women over 40 and Low Functional Ovarian Reserve

David H. Barad and Norbert Gleicher

Introduction

A woman's fertility and fecundity both decrease with age. Until the mid-twentieth century most women achieved childbearing in their peak reproductive years, before their mid-30s. Recent cultural changes created opportunities for women that led to a delay in the first childbirth. Because of this delay more women are trying to conceive at ages once considered to be postreproductive. As a result, the population seeking fertility treatment has become progressively older, especially in developed countries. In the United States, the "graying" of patients in fertility centers is driven by two factors: high in vitro fertilization (IVF) success rates in younger women leads to a quick exit from fertility services after a successful cycle of treatment, and many women over age 40 are now newly seeking care for infertility [1].

This chapter will address approaches recommended by the Center for Human Reproduction in NYC (CHR) on how to treat poor prognosis patients who to try to achieve best possible results, given their reduced reproductive potential.

Expectations for Treatment

When considering fertility treatment for women over 40 years of age, one of the first questions to address is utility versus futility of treatment. The dictionary defines futility as "the quality of having no useful result." However, the definition of a "useful result" is relative. The American Society for Reproductive Medicine (ASRM) has defined futility as treatment that has " a ≤1% chance of achieving a live birth," a live birth rate of 1 to 5% is defined as a "very poor prognosis" [2]. Among our own patients, women of ages 41–42 years achieved a live birth rate of approximately 6%. Over 42 years only women who can produce at least three embryos continue to have reasonable live birth rates [3]. Patients considering treatment at these

ages must be made aware of the much higher live birth rates with using donor eggs and be given the opportunity to reflect on whether a live birth rate of approximately 6% represents a chance worthy of investing their hopes. Many patients will feel angry when denied the possibility of trying to conceive with their own eggs. Such patients often feel the need to try at least one autologous cycle if only to provide a sense of closure. Poor prognosis patients are too rarely given access to IVF. Both in the United States and Europe, most poor prognosis patients are only offered treatment using donor eggs [3]. Our practice has strongly advocated for a patient's right to self-determination when choosing autologous IVF over donor eggs.

A decision to proceed with fertility treatment for poor prognosis patients should be made with full and transparent disclosure of all costs and quantification of risks of failure. Poor prognosis patients also may benefit from consultation with a mental health professional. The struggle to achieve genetic progeny is an ancient human drive and unhappiness over the loss of that connection is a daily experience in most fertility practices. Well-informed patients should have their autonomy respected.

Age and Fertility

Ovarian development proceeds in the first few weeks of gestation, reaching peak concentration of primordial follicles by five months. The follicles then enter a stage of meiotic arrest in which they will remain until puberty. Many follicles will arrest and become atretic during this time, rapidly lowering the population of primordial follicles from the original 6 million to only around 1–2 million at birth. By menarche, follicle counts have further decreased to only 200,000–300,000. The numbers of oocytes will continue to decline as women age, reaching about 25,000 at age 37 and only 1,000 at age 40 years (Figure 7.1).

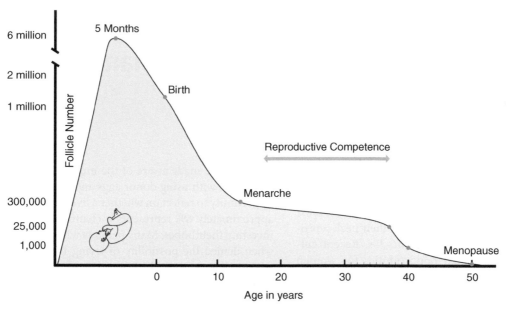

Figure 7.1 Primordial follicles peak at 6 million by five months' gestation as they enter meiotic arrest. In the following months and years many follicles become atretic lowering the population of primordial follicles to only around 1–2 million at birth, only 200,000–300,000 by menarche, 25,000 at age 37 and only 1,000 at age 40.

Natural follicle loss means that ovarian reserve (OR) and normal fertility decline slowly until age 35 and then begin to decline more rapidly, reaching a functional nadir at age 44 years, by which time spontaneous conception usually ends (i.e., "functional menopause").

Ovarian reserve is made up of two distinct components: the resting pool of primordial follicles, which cannot be directly assessed, and the growing follicle pool, represented by all follicles after recruitment between primary follicle stage and the small preantral stages. We can assess the size of the growing pool by measuring cycle day-2 follicle stimulating hormone (FSH), antimüllerian hormone (AMH) and the antral follicle count (AFC). We refer to these estimates of the size of the growing follicle pool as "functional ovarian reserve" (FOR). As most women over the age of 40 years have a significantly reduced population of oocytes, we may consider them all to have diminished "low functional ovarian reserve" (LFOR). Yet, even at age 40, natural conception can occur, with up to 44% of 40-year-old women conceiving within one year and 66% achieving a live birth within four years [4].

Ovarian aging has been characterized by steadily declining follicle and oocyte numbers due to constant active recruitment of follicles out of a finite resting pool of follicles and, secondly, by declining oocyte quality, mostly the consequence of aging mitochondrial and nuclear DNA. Although both mechanisms play significant roles, this traditional view of ovarian aging overlooks a particularly important third component, namely the ovarian microenvironment in which follicles undergo ovarian maturation.

Physiologic microenvironments play crucial roles in many biological processes. Our understanding of the ovarian microenvironment that supports follicle and oocyte maturation has improved. Yet, much is still to be explained, especially as the ovarian microenvironment is not static but changes significantly with advancing age. Changes in the aging ovarian microenvironment represent an overlooked, yet important, third contribution to ovarian aging.

The importance of the role of the ovarian microenvironment lies in the fact that neither loss of follicles and eggs nor time-linked degradation of mitochondrial and nuclear DNA currently can be prevented and/or treated. Yet, assuming changes in the ovarian microenvironment are contributing factors in ovarian aging, some of these changes should be remediable by pharmacologic intervention [5].

Understanding the Physiology of the Ovary after 40

Normal Menstrual Cycle

Most women of reproductive age have a menstrual cycle averaging 28 days. There is an orderly progression of follicles until one follicle assumes dominance and becomes a mature Graafian follicle that will spontaneously ovulate after about 14 days of development. Once ovulation is complete, the follicle will luteinize and become a corpus luteum producing progesterone as its primary steroid hormone together with inhibins that limit the emergence of new Graafian follicles until about two weeks later with the involution of the corpus luteum and subsequent menses, when a cycle begins anew. However, the developmental life of a follicle begins much before these 28 days.

Follicle Development

Most oocytes exist in ovaries from birth within primordial follicles. Primordial follicles are non-growing or "resting" follicles made up of a single oocyte surrounded by a single layer of flat granulosa cells. The DNA of oocytes in primordial follicles arrests in the meiotic prophase I until the time of future ovulation. Although in meiotic arrest, primordial follicles still have minimal ongoing metabolic activity and important active mechanisms for DNA repair [6].

Throughout a women's reproductive lifetime primordial follicles are randomly recruited to begin the process of maturation that will result in production of a mature Graafian follicle. The 200,000–300,000 follicles that are present at puberty are slowly depleted (Figure 7.2).

Activation of primordial follicles to begin maturation depends on a balance of factors: PI3 K/AKT and mTOR signaling within the oocyte control emergence from the resting state, while AMH, produced by more mature growing follicles, provides negative feedback, thereby inhibiting activation [7]. Loss of AMH feedback following chemotherapy can result in unregulated activation and loss of many follicles [8,9].

Upon follicle activation and recruitment, some granulosa cells become cuboidal. After

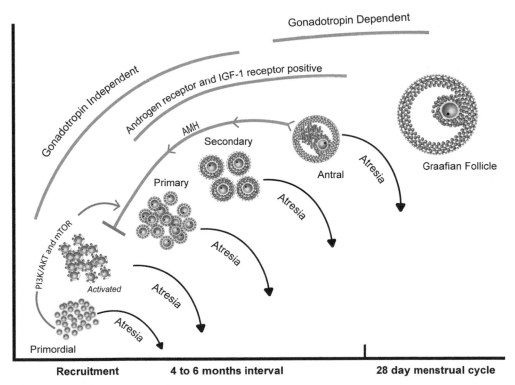

Figure 7.2 Activation of recruitment of primordial follicles by phosphoinositide 3-kinase (PI3 K)/the cascade of PI3K/protein kinase B (AKT) and the mammalian target of rapamycin (mTOR) oocyte signaling. Inhibition of recruitment by antimüllerian hormone (AMH). Gonadotropin independent small follicles have receptors for both androgen and insulin-like growth factor (IGF)-1.

formation of a primary follicle all the granulosa cells become cuboidal, a basement membrane forms around the granulosa cells and the oocyte becomes encased in a zona pellucida. Later, with further proliferation of the granulosa cells, formation of a thecal layer and antrum, the follicle passes from secondary to early antral and antral stages. Next the follicle transitions into a mature Graafian follicle with expansion of the antrum, as granulosa cells differentiate into cumulus cells surrounding the oocyte and mural granulosa cells that line the basement membrane. Whereas mural granulosa cells produce female sex steroids and inhibins, cumulus granulosa cells primarily support the developing oocyte. Together, cumulus cells and oocytes form the cumulus-oocyte complex (COC) with connections that allow bidirectional communication between them. Formation of the COC is dependent on the oocyte's secretion of paracrine growth factors GDF9, BMP15 and fibroblast growth factors [6].

The interval from formation of a primary follicle to ovulation can take several months to even as much as a year. The developing follicle will spend much of this transition in preantral stages and only a few weeks in antral stages before reaching ovulation. Most follicle deaths, known as atresia, occur in the preantral stages of development. Preantral follicle growth is mostly independent of gonadotropins, while postantral follicle growth depends on the gonadotropins FSH and luteinizing hormone (LH). Follicle atresia occurs throughout life, although most atresia occurs shortly after formation of the primordial follicle pool and again shortly after puberty. Follicle atresia will also occur because of exposure to cancer treatments or other toxins. Follicle atresia eliminates follicles with damaged oocytes and those with few granulosa cells but preserves the best follicles. As women age, the primordial follicle pool depletes. Loss of OR, in turn, leads to loss of ability to sustain cyclic promotion of mature Graafian follicles to ovulatory status.

Normal oocyte development depends on interaction between an oocyte and its surrounding cumulus-granulosa cells via gap junctions and cytoplasmic bridges. Granulosa cells produce adenosine diphosphate (ADP) and signals that help regulate oocyte maturation and suppress completion of meiosis until the oocyte has achieved a degree of competence. As women age, cumulus and granulosa cells become less able to suppress luteinization and atresia. Once the oocyte is removed from the COC, meiosis resumes. Maintenance of meiotic arrest is regulated by both granulosa cells and by signals from the oocyte itself [6].

Success of a follicle is, thus, dependent upon competent granulosa cells which, in turn, depend on local growth factors and steroids that allow the follicle to avoid atresia. Successful interaction between the oocyte and its surrounding cumulus granulosa cells is, therefore, central to this process. Supporting mural and cumulus granulosa cells may offer a potential mechanism to improve early follicle development and thereby improve oocyte quality and decrease early follicle atresia. Our center's approach to treating poor prognosis women is focused on trying to decrease atresia through pharmacologic support of the ovarian microenvironment, thereby improving development of early antral follicles.

The Menstrual Cycle over 40

In later reproductive years follicles begin to lose competence. The follicular granulosa cell count decreases, and follicles become less competent to support egg maturation. Most follicles will have evidence of atresia before achieving oocyte competence.

Loss of Luteal Inhibition of Advanced Follicular Recruitment

Such follicles will also produce a poorly functional corpus luteum, unable to restrain the emergence of new Graafian follicles. A net result is the telescoping of the normal menstrual cycle, with follicular development falling back into the previous luteal phase. A hallmark of this telescoping is the common finding of maturing Graafian follicles that have already achieved dominance as early as on the second day of menses in association with rising estradiol (Figure 7.3). This can lead to "early ovulation" and a shortened or irregular menstrual cycle. As ovulation may occur within the first week of the menstrual cycle, there is often inadequate endometrial development to support conception [10]. When recognized at a baseline scan, such follicles are often mistakenly called "cysts." For very poor prognosis patients who often even have difficulty in producing a single follicle, we trigger ovulation in such cases and perform a "cyst aspiration" up to 34 hours later and often retrieve mature oocytes.

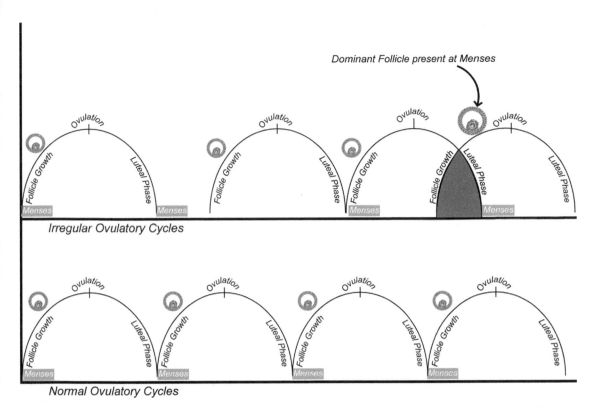

Dominant Follicle present at Menses

Irregular Ovulatory Cycles

Normal Ovulatory Cycles

Figure 7.3 As women age, cycles may become irregular. Cycles collapse into each other as the corpus luteum is not able to suppress emerging new follicular growth. Resulting Graafian follicles may produce mature oocytes.

Luteal phase ovulation induction may be continued if there are remaining antral follicles.

Pretreatment to Try to Improve Functional Ovarian Reserve

The earlier discussion should have demonstrated that a normal development of the Graafian follicle will depend on a healthy pool of antral follicles. A first step in improving follicular recruitment should, therefore, be improvement of the antral follicle pool. We have taken several different approaches to achieving this task.

Hormonal

Androgens

Androgen production is critically important to achieve normal ovarian function [11–13]. Dehydroepiandrosterone (DHEA) is a hormone produced in the adrenals, the gonads [14] and found in the brain [15]. In humans, DHEA, a weak androgen, is produced in abundance and is

primarily a precursor for the synthesis of other androgens and of estrogens. Its production increases with adrenarche, leading to increased testosterone and growth of pubic and axillary hair as well as more oily skin, and adult body odor. Because of its weak affinity for the androgen receptor (AR), DHEA has basically no androgen effect and can, to some degree, act as an androgen antagonist by displacing other more active sex steroids such as testosterone [16].

As women age or are afflicted with other forms of diminished OR, their androgen production progressively decreases [17]. Low androgen levels, however, can negatively affect the growth of small-growing follicles [11–13]. Supplementation with either DHEA or testosterone can improve egg quality and quantity [18], leading to improved embryo quality and increasing rates successful IVF pregnancy and live birth [19].

Sex hormone-binding globulin (SHBG) is a glycoprotein that binds to androgens and estrogens. In the bloodstream testosterone and estradiol are loosely bound to albumin and tightly bound to SHBG. Normally only 1–2% of testosterone is free and biologically active. In the presence of high SHBG, total testosterone values may appear to be elevated but free testosterone levels can be quite low. Hepatic production of SHBG may be increased by other hormones such as estradiol and thyroxine and can be decreased in the presence of hepatic disease, insulin resistance, cachexia and, of course, other hyperandrogenic states such as polycystic ovarian syndrome.

Although adequately powered prospectively randomized studies on the subject have not been performed, studies with lower levels of evidence and animal data are in agreement that LFOR is usually associated with hypoandrogenism [17], and that androgen supplementation can improve markers of OR [11,13].

Normal androgen levels are important for normal follicle maturation and growth. Androgens work on early developing follicles synergistically with FSH in promoting growth. An androgen receptor (AR) knockout model in the mouse demonstrated severe impairment in follicle numbers and growth if the AR on granulosa cells was eliminated but hardly any effects if the AR on oocytes was knocked out [20]. Androgens regulate follicle growth by increasing FSH-receptor and microRNA-125b expression [13]. Reconstitution of androgen levels in hypoandrogenic women with LFOR in ovarian microenvironments, whether with DHEA or testosterone directly has been convincingly demonstrated to improve oocyte numbers and oocyte quality and, ultimately, IVF pregnancy and live birth rates [11].

Our practice introduced androgen supplementation as a treatment for LFOR almost 15 years ago. Investigators at our center were awarded several US patents that claim clinical benefits from androgen supplementation. Currently two companies have been licensed under those patents to make representations regarding micronized DHEA and female fertility, a product named Fertinatal™ (Fertility Nutraceuticals, LLC, New York, N.Y., USA) and a DHEA product produced by Theralogix, LLC (Rockville, MD, USA).

In the United States, DHEA is considered to be a food supplement and is produced by many companies in varying quality. Some of these products have little active DHEA and others have much higher doses than represented by the manufacturers. In the United States, we recommend that only the two abovementioned licensed products be used by women with LFOR. Outside the United States, DHEA is usually considered to be a controlled substance and, therefore, is manufactured under much better quality control. Testosterone products all over the world are controlled substances usually available only by prescription and, therefore, can be trusted.

Patients absorb and metabolize androgens differently. We, therefore, follow androgen levels. Before patients begin androgen supplementation, we obtain a baseline that includes free and total testosterone, DHEA, dehydroepiandrosterone sulfate (DHEAS) and SHBG. Androgen levels reported by liquid chromatography mass spectrometry systems are more accurate and may differ significantly from those reported by immunoassay [21]. The normal age-specific androgen levels in women have not been determined. Normal ranges reported by commercial laboratories reflect women of all ages, including postmenopausal women. In younger women we consider androgen levels in the lower one-third of normal range as low, and the goal of supplementation is to reach at least the middle-third of the range. In general, our target range for total testosterone is between 30 and 60 ng/dL (1–2 nmol/L), free testosterone between 2 and 4 pg/mL and SHBG <80 nmol/L.

Because of fewer side effects and less risk of overdosing patients, at CHR we prefer DHEA over direct testosterone supplementation. Some women are, however, poor metabolizers of DHEA to testosterone [22]. This phenomenon has a genetic basis, mostly occurring only in women of African descent. When testosterone levels remain low despite DHEA supplementation (with a good product), we use direct testosterone supplementation. Side effects observed with DHEA use are minimal, usually restricted to oily skin and acne. Although hair loss has been reported as a side effect of androgen supplementation, in our experience hair loss is usually a temporary telogen effluvium that paradoxically often occurs after a patient ceases DHEA supplementation. Once a patient has begun taking DHEA, we encourage her to continue supplementation uninterrupted until she conceives or until she stops trying to conceive with her own oocytes.

Inositol

Inositols are natural sugars found in fruits, beans, grains and nuts. They are involved in many cellular processes including signal transduction, osmoregulation and ion channel regulation. Inositol has nine stereoisomers. Myoinositol, one of the stereoisomers, is found in all eukaryotic cells. In humans myoinositol synthesis mostly occurs in the kidneys. A metabolic product of myoinositol is d-chiro-inositol. Conversion of myoinositol to d-chiro-inositol is insulin dependent. Insulin resistance results in an imbalance of myoinositol/d-chiro-inositol, which, in turn, promotes insulin mediated androgen metabolism [23]. Combinations of myoinositol and d-chiro-inositol administered to hyperandrogenic women with polycystic ovary syndrome (PCOS) have lowered their androgen levels and improved ovulatory response. However, a recent Cochrane review was unable to substantiate that pretreatment with myoinositol had any beneficial effect for women with PCOS undergoing IVF [24].

Many of our patients come to us already using myo- and d-chiro-inositol among their supplements because they have read on Internet pages that these improve ovulation for women with PCOS. For women with evidence of diminished OR, the hypoandrogenic effects of inositol treatment will be counterproductive. These women are naturally hypoandrogenic and for them inositol treatment is not helpful and may indeed be harmful. There is no benefit to taking inositol when we are trying to raise a women's androgen profile.

Luteal Prime

Luteal Oral Contraceptives

For many years long agonist suppression was the standard approach to ovulation induction. However, it was soon recognized that long agonist suppression was not appropriate for poor responders [25]. Hormonal contraceptives were used instead to prepare patients for ovulation induction, reduce cyst formation and allow scheduling of cycles. We and others have, however, reported that use of oral contraceptives actually reduced oocyte yields [26] and reduces IVF success [27–29]. For these reasons, we do not use oral contraceptives for cycle preparation in women with LFOR.

Progesterone Prime

There have been only few studies on the role of luteal phase progesterone or progestin supplementation prior to ovulation induction [29].

Evidence for an effect of luteal phase progestins on pregnancy or live birth is therefore sparse, although there may be a lower rate of ovarian cyst formation. We have used 200 mg of micronized progesterone administered vaginally along with estradiol priming for women who repeatedly have follicle asynchrony at baseline.

Estradiol Prime

Estradiol, sometimes in combination with a GnRH antagonist, has been used in the luteal phase before the start of ovulation induction for IVF. Luteal estradiol is intended to limit the luteal phase rise of FSH to allow better synchronization of follicles. Women with luteal estradiol priming were shown to have a lower risk of cycle cancelation and an improved chance of clinical pregnancy compared to women without priming [30,31]. We use a transdermal estradiol patch to keep estradiol serum levels of around 100 pg/mL or estradiol valerate 2 mg either orally or vaginally.

Human Growth Hormone

Human growth hormone (HGH) is a peptide hormone produced by the anterior pituitary, which has been shown to induce cell growth, division and regeneration in studies in both humans and animals. In tissues, HGH stimulates production of insulin like growth factor (IGF-1). Secretion of HGH from the anterior pituitary is regulated by growth hormone releasing hormone and growth hormone-inhibiting hormone, with HGH secretion dependent on the balance of these two peptides. Growth hormone secretion decreases with age, with the highest production present in adolescents. Sleep deprivation is known to suppress HGH. Arginine, niacin, sex steroids (estrogen, testosterone and DHEA), exercise and sleep are all known to increase HGH secretion. Although in the past HGH was recovered from cadavers, today all pharmacologic HGH is produced synthetically. In the United States, HGH is approved to treat childhood conditions that produce short stature but is also approved for use in cases of growth hormone deficiency as diagnosed by circulating low values of IGF-1.

Human growth hormone has been used off-label for many years as an antiaging treatment [32], although there is no evidence that it is effective in this regard [33]. The US Congress passed a bill in 1990 that made it illegal to prescribe or distribute HGH for any use in "…in humans other than the treatment of a disease or other recognized medical condition . . . ."

Human growth hormone has been used in IVF for decades but outcome reports have varied. A Cochrane review found no evidence that HGH helps improve birth rates in women who are undergoing ovulation induction prior to IVF and limited evidence of positive effects among women who were considered poor responders [34,35]. The evidence supporting the use of HGH in poor responders is of low quality [36]. Because of limited evidence of effectiveness and prohibitive cost, for many years HGH was not widely used in IVF. However, in more recent times HGH has again gained popularity for patients with a history of poor response to ovulation induction.

At CHR we are currently conducting a registered clinical trial in which HGH treatment is prospectively randomized against our center's standard treatment of women with LFOR. Our practice sees mostly extremely poor prognosis patients with extremely limited responses. As a previous meta-analysis supported the use of HGH for poor responders but the evidence of support was not strong, rather than simply prescribing HGH, we chose to study its possible effectiveness in this highly selected group.

In all past studies of HGH it was given simultaneously within a few days of the beginning of ovulation induction to augment the effects of gonadotropins. We reasoned, as IGF-1 receptors are present on granulosa cells of early antral follicles, that HGH might have greater effectiveness if given before starting an IVF cycle. In our trial HGH is administered at low dose for six to eight weeks before the start of an ovulation induction cycle. All patients in the trial are also given DHEA and CoQ_{10}. The trial is not blinded, and patients pay for their HGH. We, however, do not prescribe HGH to patients outside this trial. As the clinical trial is limited to patients under the age of 45 years, and our center sees a large number of women above this age, an observational study allows HGH use over age 45 outside of trial. Paradoxically, enrolment over age 45 has been more active than under 45. It is too early in both studies to comment on the efficacy of HGH treatments.

Some investigators have recently suggested that HGH may also beneficially affect embryo implantation. Should implantation effects be confirmed, then this could explain why some studies suggested potential outcome benefits from HGH supplementation in IVF, even if given only during ovarian stimulation. Endometrial effects, of course, would not require prolonged presupplementation. When supplementing with HGH, we, therefore, carry our supplementations through cycle simulation until pregnancy test.

Coenzyme Q_{10}

Coenzyme Q_{10} (CoQ_{10}) is commonly found in the mitochondria of animals and bacteria where its primary function is in aerobic cellular respiration resulting in the production of ATP. Organs with the greatest need for energy, such as the heart, liver and kidney, have the highest concentration of CoQ_{10}.

Mitochondrial dysfunction has been implicated as a factor in ovarian aging [37,38]. Mitochondrial nutrients, such as CoQ_{10}, have been used to increase mitochondrial production of energy in an attempt to decrease the effects of reproductive aging [39]. Decreased levels of CoQ_{10} have been found in senescent tissues [40], and supplementation with CoQ_{10} restored mitochondrial function and delayed ovarian aging in mice [41,42]. There are, however, no clinical studies in humans of the effects of CoQ_{10} on LFOR. A combination of DHEA and CoQ_{10} was reported to improve AFC and numbers of mature follicles in an IVF cycle but did not result in significant difference in pregnancy or live birth rates [43]. In spite of a scarcity of evidence, CoQ_{10} is now widely prescribed to women with decreased OR.

As costs of this antioxidant are minor, and there are no known side effects, we consider this treatment to be of potential value. In contrast to DHEA, CoQ_{10} preparations in the marketplace are usually of adequate quality. Because they deliver 999 mg in only three capsules, our preferred products are Ovoenergen™ for women and Androenergen™ for males (both Fertility Nutraceuticals, LLC, New York, NY, USA),

Growth Factors

Platelet-Rich Plasma

Platelet-rich plasma (PRP) has been proposed as a strategy to improve ovarian function [44]. Other medical fields have used PRP to regenerate skin [45] and cartilage [46]. Platelet-rich plasma contains growth factors which can stimulate cellular anabolism, fibrinogen which acts as a scaffold for regenerating tissue and inflammatory modulators that create an anti-inflammatory effect [47–49].

Platelet-rich plasma has been hypothesized to induce the transformation of germline stem cells into primordial follicles, resulting in an increase in the primordial follicle pool [50]. There is only limited evidence in support of this hypothesis [44,51–53].

It is well known that women with premature ovarian insufficiency (POI) may still have occasional irregular periods and may even occasionally achieve a pregnancy [54]. Consequently, it is clear that case reports of pregnancy following any treatment cannot prove efficacy, unless there is a control group for comparison. We are currently sponsoring two randomized controlled trials at CHR testing the efficacy of PRP treatment in women with ovarian failure (NCT03542708) or diminished OR (NCT04278313).

Stem Cells

A bone marrow transplant, also known as a stem cell transplant, may be used to treat leukemia, myeloma and lymphoma and other diseases affecting the bone marrow. Before undergoing bone marrow transplantation, patients receive a combination of chemotherapy and radiation that may result in loss of normal gonadal function. Some patients have, however, been reported to experience restoration of relative normal ovarian function and even pregnancy after apparent iatrogenic menopause [55,56]. These reports have led to a hypothesis that stem cell-based therapies may have a potential regenerative effect on the ovary by driving differentiation of ovarian stem cells into primordial follicles [57]. In mice, bone marrow stem cell infusion was shown to promote ovarian follicle growth and improve ovarian function after induced ovarian failure [58,59]. Regeneration of human ovarian tissue using stem cell therapy is an area of active research with enormous potential but remains unproven at this time [57].

Optimal IVF Stimulation Protocols for Women over 40

Cycle Control

Agonist and Antagonist Cycle Control
When used for women with normal OR, GnRH agonists and antagonists can each supply improved

synchrony of follicle development and prevent premature ovulation leading to better overall cycle control. When these agents are used in poor responding women with evidence of LFOR the apparent benefits often become a significant liability, leading to decreased oocyte production and consequently fewer favorable outcomes [25,60].

Long Agonist
In poor responders long agonist cycles are known to decrease the number of retrieved oocytes [60]. We do not use long agonist protocols when treating poor prognosis patients.

Antagonist
Compared to agonists, GnRH antagonists have fewer hypoestrogenic effects, do not cause flareups and do not require a long time of administration before downregulation [61]. The GnRH antagonists block release of pituitary gonadotropins by competitive binding to the GnRH receptors and can be used effectively at any time during follicle development. Antagonist use is also associated with a lower risk of ovarian hyperstimulation syndrome. In poor responders antagonist protocols were associated with an increased risk of cycle cancelation [61]. We therefore also avoid the use of antagonists for poor prognosis patients.

Microdose Agonist
Microdose GnRH agonist cycles enhance outcomes for poor responders (Figure 7.4). When we feel that cycle control is indicated, we use the so-called microdose agonist flare protocol first reported by Surrey et al. [25]. Our preferred protocol uses 50 mcg subcutaneous injection of leuprolide acetate every 12 hours beginning on the second day of menses. We start gonadotropin injections on the same day. Recently serving ever-increasing increased numbers of patients with severe LFOR, we reserve the microdose agonist protocol for those with AMH >0.5 ng/mL (3.5 pmol/L). For patients who continue to respond poorly when using the microdose agonist protocol, we discontinue the agonist and continue the stimulation for two to three days, after which many patients will have renewed evidence of response.

Clomiphene Citrate and Letrozole
Clomiphene citrate (CC) and letrozole (LTZ) have each been used to induce increased endogenous FSH

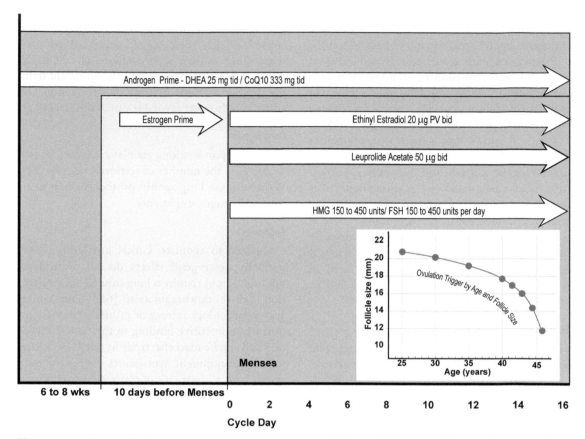

Figure 7.4 Androgen and estrogen priming set up a microdose leuprolide flare cycle. Gonadotropin dose is adjusted according to a patient's estimated ovarian reserve. Ethinyl estradiol allows monitoring of ovarian estrogen response. Timing of the ovulation trigger is based on age and follicle size. HMG, human menopausal gonadotrophin.

production to start ovulation induction. Neither CC nor LTZ has been proven to have any benefit when used in combination with GnRH agonist or antagonist protocols for either the general population of patients undergoing IVF or poor responders [62]. In our practice, we never use long GnRH agonist or antagonist protocols, although recently we have started to use both CC and LTZ in selected poor prognosis patients in addition to gonadotropins and we are seeing progressively positive results.

Clomiphene Citrate

Clomiphene citrate is a is a selective estrogen receptor modulator that functions as a competitive estrogen antagonist in the hypothalamus and pituitary. Administration of CC early in the follicular phase of a menstrual cycle can increase the number of developing follicles by inducing a supraphysiologic level of gonadotropins. Use of CC has an added advantage of helping to suppress the emergence of the midcycle LH surge. One disadvantage of CC is the inhibition of normal endometrial development by blocking estrogen receptors in the endometrium.

We have found CC to be helpful for extreme poor responder patients. We start 100 mg of CC in parallel to gonadotropins on the second day of menses and continue for five days (Figure 7.5). We begin injections of gonadotropins on the same day as CC. If patients were using estradiol priming, we instruct them to stop estradiol with the onset of menses. Following completion of five days of CC, we ask patients to start ethinyl estradiol 20 µg twice a day administered vaginally to counteract the negative effect of CC on the endometrium.

Aromatase Inhibition

Letrozole

Aromatase inhibitors were introduced in 2001 for ovulation induction. Use of aromatase inhibitors

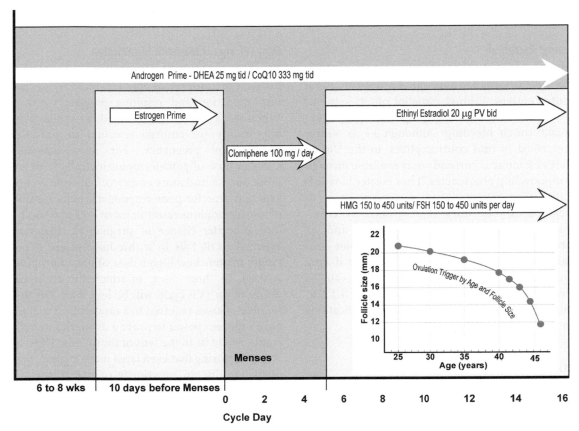

Figure 7.5 Androgen and estrogen priming set up a clomiphene citrate (CC) cycle. Estrogen is stopped when clomiphene is started. Gonadotropin dose is adjusted according to a patient's estimated ovarian reserve. Ethinyl estradiol is started after CC is finished to help build the endometrium. Timing of the ovulation trigger is based on age and follicle size. HMG, human menopausal gonadotrophin.

for ovulation induction has not been approved as an indication by the Food and Drug Administration, making its use "off-label." Letrozole is an aromatase inhibitor that prevents the synthesis of estrogen from androgens by competitive, reversible binding of the enzyme aromatase CYP19. Like CC, LTZ increases endogenous gonadotropin production by reducing the feedback of estradiol on the pituitary and hypothalamus. However, the effect of LTZ is to reduce estradiol production and not as a competitive antagonist.

Patients using LTZ produce only about 10% of the estradiol produced otherwise. This must be remembered when monitoring the response of ovulation induction, as patients using LTZ will have much less evidence of estrogen response despite adequate follicle growth. Oocytes produced in these cycles have the same capacity to produce viable embryos as those produced in traditional cycles. The low estradiol production with

LTZ is seen by some as an advantage when producing oocytes for fertility preservation for patients with breast cancer [63].

As the clinical effect of LTZ depends on decreased estradiol production, using estrogen at the same time as LTZ will preclude benefits. Letrozole's negative effect on estradiol production persists for a few days after the last oral dose as it has a metabolic half-life of two days.

Estrogen Supplementation during Ovulation Induction

Women with poor OR often have poor endometrial development during ovulation induction. Estrogen supplementation can be continued into the ovulation induction cycle to help overcome this problem. However, use of an estradiol patch or of oral estradiol valerate during ovulation induction has the disadvantage of confounding the monitoring of ovarian response by elevating estradiol levels.

Ethinyl Estradiol

Ethinyl estradiol (EE) is the most common estrogen used in combination with a progestin in oral contraceptives. Ethinyl estradiol offsets some of the suppressive effects of progestins, preventing breakthrough bleeding. Although EE is widely prescribed in oral contraceptives, in the United States EE alone is currently only available through compounding pharmacies. It has greater bioavailability than estrogen and is more resistant to metabolism, but does not significantly cross-react with estradiol in immunoassays and, as a result, supplementation with EE will not confound observation of estrogen response during ovulation induction. Ethinyl estradiol can be given following administration of CC or LTZ to balance the negative effects of those medications on the endometrium [64].

Gonadotropins

Human menopausal gonadotropins (HMG) have been used for ovulation induction since the 1960s. Use of exogenous gonadotropins allows recruitment and sustained growth of multiple mature Graafian follicles and their use has been a mainstay in the treatment of infertile couples for many years. While menotropins were originally extracted from urine and had an FSH/LH ration of 1:1, newer recombinant preparations used today often have a much higher ratio of FSH compared to LH activity.

FSH Alone versus FSH Plus LH Activity

Modern ovulation induction protocols using GnRH analogues limit the secretion of endogenous LH. There exists an ongoing controversy over how much LH is needed to produce a competent egg and embryo. A recent meta-analysis [65] examining this question was unable to find clear evidence for a difference between combined recombinant FSH/LH preparations and those with recombinant FSH alone, although moderate evidence supported a finding of more ongoing pregnancies with FSH/LH combinations [65].

In our practice we have always used a combination of FSH and FSH/LH preparations usually in a 2:1 or 3:1 ratio. We have recently begun using only FSH/LH in our poorest

responder population but have not reached final conclusions about efficacy.

Mini IVF versus Maximal Stimulation

There has always been a clear relationship between the number of eggs produced by ovulation induction and resulting pregnancy rates. When more eggs are produced there is a greater opportunity for embryo selection to produce a successful pregnancy. For most patients, a higher dose of gonadotropins logically leads to more oocytes and more embryos. This rule is also generally true for poor responders: higher doses of gonadotrophins result in more eggs and therefore a greater chance of pregnancy. However, eventually OR falls to a threshold where it no longer matters how high a dose of gonadotropins is used. In these cases, in which the expected utility of an IVF cycle will be less than 5%, the number of cases required in a randomized trial to have sufficient power to prove a difference in outcomes would be in the tens of thousands. Thus, it is not surprising that even large meta-analyses are unable to discern superiority of one treatment over another [66]. Still, it is tautological that if no eggs are produced there will be no pregnancy. At CHR, we begin initial ovulation inductions for poor responder patients with dosing as high as 600 units of gonadotropins daily. One result of this approach is a low cancelation rate of 13%, which we consider impressive, especially given the very unfavorable selection of our center's patient population.

In 2014 live births in our center's unfavorable patients represented 1.4% of cycle starts, by 2018 live births represented 5.6% of cycle starts. Concomitantly, the median age of women in this group of patients increased from 41 years in 2014 to 43.0 years in 2018, with median AMH of 0.53 ng/mL (3.78 pmol/L) and baseline FSH of 12 mIU/mL.

If women above age 43 produced three or more transferrable embryos, the live birth rate could reach double digits as many patients in the above noted analysis had only one or two embryos for transfer. We, therefore, do not hesitate to transfer up to five or six embryos, if available, to women of advanced age.

Although live birth rates are still low, they are significantly above what patients are usually advised of by many physicians. If older patients still demonstrate enough OR to produce three or more embryos for transfer, their cumulative live birth chances may be surprisingly high, and they deserve to be advised accordingly.

Back-to-Back Cycles

Most IVF centers require patients to rest for at least one month after a failed cycle of ovulation induction. The rationale for this waiting time is to give the ovaries a chance to return to their normal state after ovulation induction. Follicles are known to develop in waves becoming progressively more responsive to gonadotropins. For poor responders we have noted a carryover effect ("hang-over") when cycles are performed within 100 days of each other [67]. The maximal carryover occurs when cycles are back-to-back. This response is best seen among women preconditioned using androgens, such as DHEA. With back-to-back cycles in combination with androgen supplementation, we have seen some women increase responses from just one or two eggs per cycle to as many as 17 eggs in a single cycle [68]. This effect is dependent on replenishment from the primordial follicle pool. After several cycles, women with severe LFOR can exhaust the ability of the pool to replenish itself and do, indeed, require a few cycles of "rest."

HIER – Highly Individualized Egg Retrieval

Several years ago, we noticed that patients at our center above age 43 experienced a precipitous drop in pregnancy rates, while up to that age the decline had been gradual. We chose to study the differences in our older and younger patients to better understand the reasons. We found that both in vivo and in vitro culture studies of granulosa cells documented progressively excessive premature luteinization of follicles as women aged [69,70]. This finding raised the question, what to do to prevent exposure of oocytes to the toxic microenvironments of prematurely luteinizing follicles? We chose to remove oocytes from those failing follicles earlier, which meant retrieving oocytes earlier. In an initial study, we arbitrarily chose to administer the hCG-trigger to women above age 43 at lead follicle sizes 16 mm. In a small pilot study, that step, alone, improved pregnancy rates [69].

Since then, we have expanded our studies to younger women with premature ovarian aging,

and learned that they, too, prematurely luteinize, although to a lesser degree. In poor prognosis patients early hCG-trigger between 16 and 18 mm lead follicle size not only resulted in greatly improved pregnancy chances in comparison to larger and smaller follicle sizes but also the improvement in clinical pregnancy rates dramatically exceeded improvements we had observed earlier in older women (Figure 7.6). We, in addition, learned that in older women, even at 16 mm lead follicle sizes, an hCG-trigger can be too late. Indeed, the older patients are, the earlier ovulation must be triggered. At our center, hCG-triggers at lead follicle sizes as low as 11–12 mm between ages 45 and 49, therefore, have become routine. We retrieved mature, and sometimes even over-mature eggs, at even smaller lead follicle sizes.

We recently established our center's so-far two "oldest" IVF pregnancies with use of autologous eggs, both only weeks short of their 48th birthday at the time of embryo transfer. One, indeed, delivered a healthy female at 35 weeks' gestational age; the other unfortunately miscarried. The patient who delivered received her hCG-trigger at lead follicle size 12 mm [71].

In poor prognosis patients, we, thus, no longer utilize "standard" protocols. Recognizing that, based on age and/or OR, timing of every patient's egg retrieval must be carefully individualized, we coined the term HIER (Highly Individualized Egg Retrieval) to describe this current practice pattern. Every aspect of a patient's ovarian stimulation is carefully individualized, and this individualization even carries over into the embryology laboratory.

Embryos

Continual improvement in culture media has shifted many IVF practices from cleavage-stage embryo transfer to blastocyst-stage transfer. For young women who can produce many oocytes, and as a result have many embryos, blastocyst culture allows the selection of a single embryo most likely to achieve a healthy singleton pregnancy. However, a recent meta-analysis found only low-quality evidence of improvement of live birth rates with blastocyst transfer and only in good prognosis patients [72]. When few embryos are available for transfer there is little benefit from culture to blastocyst [73]. For women with poor

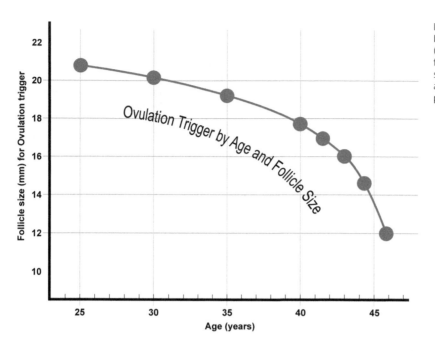

Figure 7.6 Highly Individualized Egg Retrieval (HIER). To compensate for loss of follicular competence, follicle size for the ovulation trigger is adjusted according to the patient's age.

prognosis the risk of multiple pregnancy following multiple embryo transfer is very small as the implantation rate for each embryo is low. Indeed, a Centers for Disease Control and Prevention (CDC) study of over 80,000 IVF cycles found that for poor prognosis women the chance of having a healthy singleton live birth increased directly with the number of embryos transferred [74]. In our practice we discourage all methods of embryo selection, including PGT-A, for our poor prognosis patients, reasoning that the only sure way to deny a chance of live birth is to deny the opportunity for embryo transfer.

Counseling after a Failed Cycle

When treating poor prognosis patients, the unfortunate reality is that most cycles will not result in a successful pregnancy. Patients should be counseled to understand that a successful live birth will be an unusual outcome. They should consider ahead of time how many cycles they would invest their hopes in, always being conscious of the alternative of choosing donor eggs. When we allow patients to be partners in decisions about their care, knowing they have freedom to choose often allows them to choose alternative ways to build their families. If they fail using their own eggs, they at least know they have tried.

Conflict of Interest

NG and DHB are coinventors on several pending and already awarded US patents claiming therapeutic benefits from androgen supplementation in women with LFOR and relating to the FMR1 gene in a diagnostic function in female fertility. Both receive royalties from Fertility Nutraceuticals, LLC, in which NG also holds shares. NG and DHB also are coinventors on three pending AMH-related patent applications. All authors received research grants, travel funds and speaker honoraria from pharma companies, although none in any way related to these presented materials.

References

1. Gleicher N, Kushnir VA, Weghofer A, Barad DH. The "graying" of infertility services: an impending revolution nobody is ready for. *Reprod Biol Endocrinol* 2014; **12**: 63.

2. Ethics Committee of American Society for Reproductive Medicine. Fertility treatment when the prognosis is very poor or futile: a committee opinion. *Fertil Steril* 2012; **98**(1): e6–9.

3. Gleicher N, Vega MV, Darmon SK, et al. Live-birth rates in very poor prognosis patients, who are defined as poor responders under the Bologna criteria, with nonelective single embryo, two-embryo, and three or more embryos transferred. *Fertil Steril* 2015; **104**(6): 1435–41.

4. Leridon H. Can assisted reproduction technology compensate for the natural decline in fertility with age? A model assessment. *Hum Reprod* 2004; **19** (7): 1548–53.

5. Gleicher N, Weghofer A, Barad DH. Defining ovarian reserve to better understand ovarian aging. *Reprod Biol Endocrinol* 2011; **9**: 23.

6. Findlay JK, Dunning KR, Gilchrist RB, Hutt KJ, Russell DL, Walters KA. Chapter 1 - Follicle selection in mammalian ovaries. In: Leung PCK, Adashi EY, eds. The Ovary (Third Edition): Academic Press; 2019: 3–21.

7. Prasasya RD, Mayo KE. Chapter 2 - Regulation of follicle formation and development by ovarian signaling pathways. In: Leung PCK, Adashi EY, eds. The Ovary (Third Edition): Academic Press; 2019: 23–49.

8. Kushnir VA, Seifer DB, Barad DH, Sen A, Gleicher N. Potential therapeutic applications of human anti-Müllerian hormone (AMH) analogues in reproductive medicine. *J Assist Reprod Genet* 2017; **34**(9): 1105–13.

9. Kim H-A, Choi J, Park CS, et al. Post-chemotherapy serum anti-Müllerian hormone level predicts ovarian function recovery. *Endocr Connect* 2018; **7**(8): 949–56.

10. van Zonneveld P, Scheffer GJ, Broekmans FJ, et al. Do cycle disturbances explain the age-related decline of female fertility? Cycle characteristics of women aged over 40 years compared with a reference population of young women. *Hum Reprod* 2003; **18**(3): 495–501.

11. Prizant H, Gleicher N, Sen A. Androgen actions in the ovary: balance is key. *J Endocrinol* 2014; **222**(3): R141–51.

12. Sen A, Prizant H, Hammes SR. Understanding extranuclear (nongenomic) androgen signaling: what a frog oocyte can tell us about human biology. *Steroids* 2011; **76**(9): 822–8.

13. Sen A, Prizant H, Light A, et al. Androgens regulate ovarian follicular development by increasing follicle stimulating hormone receptor and microRNA-125b expression. *Proc Natl Acad Sci U S A* 2014; **111**(8): 3008–13.

14. Schulman RA, Dean C. Solve it with supplements : the best herbal and nutritional supplements to prevent and heal more than 100 common health problems. Emmaus, Pa.: Rodale; 2007.

15. Zwain IH, Yen SSC. Dehydroepiandrosterone: biosynthesis and metabolism in the brain. *Endocrinology* 1999; **140**(2): 880–7.

16. Chen F, Knecht K, Birzin E, et al. Direct agonist/antagonist functions of dehydroepiandrosterone. *Endocrinology* 2005; **146**(11): 4568–76.

17. Gleicher N, Kim A, Weghofer A, et al. Hypoandrogenism in association with diminished functional ovarian reserve. *Hum Reprod* 2013; **28** (4): 1084–91.

18. Gleicher N, Barad DH. Dehydroepiandrosterone (DHEA) supplementation in diminished ovarian reserve (DOR). *Reprod Biol Endocrinol* 2011; **9**: 67.

19. Gleicher N, Kushnir VA, Barad DH. Chapter 24 - The ovarian factor in assisted reproductive technology. In: Leung PCK, Adashi EY, eds. The Ovary (Third Edition): Academic Press; 2019: 379–401.

20. Sen A, Hammes SR. Granulosa cell-specific androgen receptors are critical regulators of ovarian development and function. *Mol Endocrinol* 2010; **24**(7): 1393–403.

21. Gallagher LM, Owen LJ, Keevil BG. Simultaneous determination of androstenedione and testosterone in human serum by liquid chromatography-tandem mass spectrometry. *Ann Clin Biochem* 2007; **44**(Pt 1): 48–56.

22. Shohat-Tal A, Sen A, Barad DH, Kushnir V, Gleicher N. Genetics of androgen metabolism in women with infertility and hypoandrogenism. *Nat Rev Endocrinol* 2015; **11**(7): 429–41.

23. Wojciechowska A, Osowski A, Jóźwik M, Górecki R, Rynkiewicz A, Wojtkiewicz J. Inositols' importance in the improvement of the endocrine-metabolic profile in PCOS. *Int J Mol Sci* 2019; **20** (22): 5787.

24. Showell MG, Mackenzie-Proctor R, Jordan V, Hodgson R, Farquhar C. Inositol for subfertile women with polycystic ovary syndrome. *Cochrane Database Syst Rev* 2018; **12**: CD012378.

25. Surrey ES. Management of the poor responder: the role of GnRH agonists and antagonists. *J Assist Reprod Genet* 2007; **24**(12): 613–19.

26. Barad DH, Kim A, Kubba H, Weghofer A, Gleicher N. Does hormonal contraception prior to in vitro fertilization (IVF) negatively affect oocyte yields? A pilot study. *Reprod Biol Endocrinol* 2013; **11**: 28.

27. Smulders B, van Oirschot SM, Farquhar C, Rombauts L, Kremer JA. Oral contraceptive pill, progestogen or estrogen pre-treatment for ovarian stimulation protocols for women undergoing assisted reproductive techniques. *Cochrane Database Syst Rev* 2010;**1**: CD006109.

28. Farquhar C, Rombauts L, Kremer JA, Lethaby A, Ayeleke RO. Oral contraceptive pill, progestogen or oestrogen pretreatment for ovarian stimulation protocols for women undergoing assisted reproductive techniques. *Cochrane Database Syst Rev* 2017; **5**: CD006109.

29. Farquhar C, Rombauts L, Kremer JA, Lethaby A, Ayeleke RO. Oral contraceptive pill, progestogen or oestrogen pretreatment for ovarian stimulation protocols for women undergoing assisted reproductive techniques. *Cochrane Database Syst Rev* 2017; **5**: CD006109-CD.

30. Fanchin R, Cunha-Filho JS, Schonauer LM, Kadoch IJ, Cohen-Bacri P, Frydman R. Coordination of early antral follicles by luteal estradiol administration provides a basis for alternative controlled ovarian hyperstimulation regimens. *Fertil Steril* 2003; **79**(2): 316–21.

31. Reynolds KA, Omurtag KR, Jimenez PT, Rhee JS, Tuuli MG, Jungheim ES. Cycle cancellation and pregnancy after luteal estradiol priming in women defined as poor responders: a systematic review and meta-analysis. *Human Reprod* 2013; **28**(11): 2981–9.

32. Kuczynski A. Anti-aging potion or poison? *The New York Times* 1998; April 12, Sect. 1.

33. Liu H, Bravata DM, Olkin I, et al. Systematic review: the safety and efficacy of growth hormone in the healthy elderly. *Ann Intern Med* 2007; **146**(2): 104–15.

34. Duffy JM, Ahmad G, Mohiyiddeen L, Nardo LG, Watson A. Growth hormone for in vitro fertilization. *Cochrane Database Syst Rev* 2010; **1**: CD000099.

35. Cozzolino M, Cecchino GN, Troiano G, Romanelli C. Growth hormone cotreatment for poor responders undergoing in vitro fertilization cycles: a systematic review and meta-analysis. *Fertil Steril* 2020; **114**(1): 97–109.

36. Bortoletto P, Spandorfer S. Growth hormone: in search of the Holy Grail for poor responders (or a felony). *Fertil Steril* 2020; **114**(1): 63–4.

37. Kasapoğlu I, Seli E. Mitochondrial dysfunction and ovarian aging. *Endocrinology* 2020; **161**(2).

38. Wang T, Zhang M, Jiang Z, Seli E. Mitochondrial dysfunction and ovarian aging. *Am J Reprod Immunol* 2017; **77**(5): e12651.

39. Bentov Y, Yavorska T, Esfandiari N, Jurisicova A, Casper RF. The contribution of mitochondrial function to reproductive aging. *J Assist Reprod Genet* 2011; **28**(9): 773–83.

40. Kalén A, Appelkvist E-L, Dallner G. Age-related changes in the lipid compositions of rat and human tissues. *Lipids* 1989; **24**(7): 579–84.

41. Ben-Meir A, Burstein E, Borrego-Alvarez A, et al. Coenzyme Q10 restores oocyte mitochondrial function and fertility during reproductive aging. *Aging Cell* 2015; **14**(5): 887–95.

42. Bentov Y, Casper RF. The aging oocyte--can mitochondrial function be improved? *Fertil Steril* 2013; **99**(1): 18–22.

43. Gat I, Blanco Mejia S, Balakier H, Librach CL, Claessens A, Ryan EA. The use of coenzyme Q10 and DHEA during IUI and IVF cycles in patients with decreased ovarian reserve. *Gynecol Endocrinol* 2016; **32**(7): 534–7.

44. Pantos K, Nitsos N, Kokkali G, et al. Ovarian rejuvenation and folliculogenesis reactivation in peri-menopausal women after autologous platelet-rich plasma treatment. Abstracts of the 32nd Annual Meeting of the European Society of Human Reproduction and Embryology, Helsinki, Finland. *Hum Reprod* 2016: i301.

45. Fabi S, Sundaram H. The potential of topical and injectable growth factors and cytokines for skin rejuvenation. *Facial Plast Surg* 2014; **30**(02): 157–71.

46. Xie X, Zhang C, Tuan RS. Biology of platelet-rich plasma and its clinical application in cartilage repair. *Arthritis Res Ther* 2014; **16**(1): 204.

47. Macaulay IC, Carr P, Gusnanto A, Ouwehand WH, Fitzgerald D, Watkins NA. Platelet genomics and proteomics in human health and disease. *J Clin Invest* 2005; **115**: 3370–7.

48. McRedmond JP, Park SD, Reilly DF, et al. Integration of proteomics and genomics in platelets: a profile of platelet proteins and platelet-specific genes. *Mol Cell Proteomics* 2004; **3**: 133–44.

49. Watson SP, Bahou WF, Fitzgerald D, Ouwehand W, Rao AK, Leavitt AD. ISTH platelet physiology subcommittee: mapping the platelet proteome: a report of the ISTH platelet physiology subcommittee. *J Thromb Haemost* 2005; **3**: 2098–101.

50. Sills ES, Wood SH. Autologous activated platelet-rich plasma injection into adult human ovary tissue: molecular mechanism, analysis, and discussion of reproductive response. *Biosci Rep* 2019; **39**(6): BSR20190805.

51. Farimani M, Heshmati S, Poorolajal J, Bahmanzadeh M. A report on three live births in women with poor ovarian response following intra-ovarian injection of platelet-rich plasma (PRP). *Mol Biol Rep* 2019; **46**(2): 1611–16.

52. Hosseini L, Shirazi A, Naderi MM, et al. Platelet-rich plasma promotes the development of isolated human primordial and primary follicles to the preantral stage. *Reprod Biomed Online* 2017; **35**(4): 343–50.

53. Sills ES, Rickers NS, Li X, Palermo GD. First data on in vitro fertilization and blastocyst formation after intraovarian injection of calcium gluconate-activated autologous platelet rich plasma. *Gynecol Endocrinol* 2018; **34**(9): 756–60.

54. Bidet M, Bachelot A, Bissauge E, et al. Resumption of ovarian function and pregnancies in 358 patients with premature ovarian failure. *J Clin Endocrinol Metab* 2011; **96**(12): 3864–72.

55. Gulati SC, Van Poznak C. Pregnancy after bone marrow transplantation. *J Clin Oncol* 1998; **16**(5): 1978–85.

56. Loren AW, Chow E, Jacobsohn DA, et al. Pregnancy after hematopoietic cell transplantation: a report from the late effects working committee of the Center for International Blood and Marrow Transplant Research (CIBMTR). *Biol Blood Marrow Transplant* 2011; **17**(2): 157–66.

57. Akahori T, Woods DC, Tilly JL. Female fertility preservation through stem cell-based ovarian tissue reconstitution in vitro and ovarian regeneration in vivo. *Clin Med Insights Reprod Health* 2019; **13**: 1179558119848007.

58. Herraiz S, Buigues A, Diaz-Garcia C, et al. Fertility rescue and ovarian follicle growth promotion by bone marrow stem cell infusion. *Fertil Steril* 2018; **109**(5): 908–18 e2.

59. Liu R, Zhang X, Fan Z, et al. Human amniotic mesenchymal stem cells improve the follicular microenvironment to recover ovarian function in premature ovarian failure mice. *Stem Cell Res Ther* 2019; **10**(1): 299.

60. Pandian Z, McTavish AR, Aucott L, Hamilton MP, Bhattacharya S. Interventions for 'poor responders' to controlled ovarian hyper stimulation (COH) in in-vitro fertilisation (IVF). *Cochrane Database Syst Rev* 2010; (1): CD004379.

61. Al-Inany HG, Youssef MA, Ayeleke RO, Brown J, Lam WS, Broekmans FJ. Gonadotrophin-releasing hormone antagonists for assisted reproductive technology. *Cochrane Database Syst Rev* 2016; (4): CD001750.

62. Kamath MS, Maheshwari A, Bhattacharya S, Lor KY, Gibreel A. Oral medications including clomiphene citrate or aromatase inhibitors with gonadotropins for controlled ovarian stimulation in women undergoing in vitro fertilisation. *Cochrane Database Syst Rev* 2017; (11): CD008528.

63. Dahhan T, Balkenende E, van Wely M, Linn S, Goddijn M. Tamoxifen or letrozole versus standard methods for women with estrogen-receptor positive breast cancer undergoing oocyte or embryo cryopreservation in assisted reproduction. *Cochrane Database Syst Rev* 2013; (11): CD010240.

64. Check JH. The multiple uses of ethinyl estradiol for treating infertility. *Clin Exp Obstet Gynecol* 2010; **37**(4): 249–51.

65. Mochtar MH, Danhof NA, Ayeleke RO, Van der Veen F, van Wely M. Recombinant luteinizing hormone (rLH) and recombinant follicle stimulating hormone (rFSH) for ovarian stimulation in IVF/ICSI cycles. *Cochrane Database Syst Rev* 2017; (5): CD005070.

66. Youssef MA, van Wely M, Mochtar M, et al. Low dosing of gonadotropins in in vitro fertilization cycles for women with poor ovarian reserve: systematic review and meta-analysis. *Fertil Steril* 2018; **109**(2): 289–301.

67. Barad DH, Kushnir VA, Lee HJ, Lazzaroni E, Gleicher N. Effect of inter-cycle interval on oocyte production in humans in the presence of the weak androgen DHEA and follicle stimulating hormone: a case-control study. *Reprod Biol Endocrinol* 2014; **12**: 68.

68. Barad DH, Gleicher N. Increased oocyte production after treatment with dehydroepiandrosterone. *Fertil Steril* 2005; **84**(3): 756.

69. Wu YG, Barad DH, Kushnir VA, et al. Aging-related premature luteinization of granulosa cells is avoided by early oocyte retrieval. *J Endocrinol* 2015; **226** (3): 167–80.

70. Wu YG, Barad DH, Kushnir VA, et al. With low ovarian reserve, Highly Individualized Egg Retrieval (HIER) improves IVF results by avoiding premature luteinization. *J Ovarian Res* 2018; **11**(1): 23.

71. Gleicher N, Kushnir VA, Darmon S, Albertini DF, Barad DH. Older women using their own eggs? Issue framed with two oldest reported IVF pregnancies and a live birth. *Reprod Biomed Online* 2018; **37**(2): 172–7.

72. Glujovsky D, Farquhar C, Quinteiro Retamar AM, Alvarez Sedo CR, Blake D. Cleavage stage versus blastocyst stage embryo transfer in assisted reproductive technology. *Cochrane Database Syst Rev* 2016; (6): CD002118.

73. Xiao JS, Healey M, Talmor A, Vollenhoven B. When only one embryo is available, is it better to transfer on Day 3 or to grow on? *Reprod Biomed Online* 2019; **39**(6): 916–23.

74. Kissin DM, Kulkarni AD, Kushnir VA, Jamieson DJ, National ARTSSG. Number of embryos transferred after in vitro fertilization and good perinatal outcome. *Obstet Gynecol* 2014; **123** (2 Pt 1): 239–47.

Fertility Counseling beyond 40

Amir Mor and David B. Seifer

Introduction

Throughout the past decades, in developed countries, there is a trend of long-term decline in the overall birth and fertility rates. The trend has been driven mostly by delayed childbearing. Childbearing at a later age is attributed to the following changes in social trends:

- higher rates of pursuing advanced education among women,
- increasing proportion of women in the workforce,
- improved and wider use of contraception,
- marriage at a later age,
- more frequent divorce followed by remarriage,
- planning a smaller family size.

These major social trends have led women to attempt conception at a time when they are experiencing a physiological decline in their fertility potential. Maximum fertility potential is between the ages of 20 and 24. There is a modest progressive decrease in this potential by the age of 30–32, with a relatively steep decline between the ages of 35 and 40 [1]. Furthermore, as the fertility potential diminishes the miscarriage rate increases. Natural conception miscarriage rates, which are low before the age of 30 (7–15%), gradually rise to 34–52% after the age of 40 [2,3].

Reproductive Challenges over the Age of 40

Follicular Pool Depletion of Egg Number

In utero the female fetus is endowed through mitosis with the greatest number of follicles. By 20 weeks' gestation the female fetus has completed creating all her ovarian follicles. Each follicle surrounds and protects a single oocyte. By 20 weeks the female fetus has on average, 6–7 million follicles [4]. From this moment to the time of puberty the number of follicles (with their accompanied oocytes) is decreasing exclusively through programmed cell death (apoptosis) [5] with 1–2 million at birth and 300,000–400,000 by puberty [6,7]. From these few hundreds of thousands of follicles at puberty, only about 400 will ovulate (a gonadotrophin dependent process) during the reproductive years till menopause. Atresia/apoptosis (a gonadotrophin independent process) occurs regardless of pregnancies or use of birth control. Smokers appear to experience menopause about 1–4 years earlier than non-smokers. By the age of 37–38 about 25,000 follicles survive. These 25,000 follicles are still capable of maintaining the ovarian endocrine function for about a decade, but their ability to ovulate a genetically well-balanced oocyte is severely compromised (good endocrine function but poor fertilization potential). By menopause (age 51 on average in the US) about 1000 follicles remain. These follicles have already lost both their endocrine and fertilization potential [8–11].

At several years before menopause, women may ovulate more frequently than younger women. This is due to the shortening of the follicular phase. Higher levels of follicle stimulating hormone (FSH) compensate for the decrease in follicular pool [12]. The lead follicle has an earlier start in the menstrual cycle but grows at a normal pace. Shorter menstrual cycles are a sign for depleted follicular pool but are not a direct cause for decreased fertility. Young women may have a depleted follicular pool due to smoking, prior ovarian surgery and family history of premature ovarian insufficiency due to genetic related causes such as the presence of the FMR-1 or BRCA genes. Young women may have diminished ovarian reserve even if they have no known risk factors. To date, there is no good model that can reliably predict the female reproductive life span nor is there a proven reliable clinical intervention that can delay or stop follicular atresia.

Decrease in Oocyte Quality

With age, as the number of follicles decreases, oocyte quality also declines. The major cause is genetic imbalances. It is believed that in utero all 6–7 million oocytes have started their first meiotic division and that they are all arrested at the prophase of meiosis I [4,13]. It is worth mentioning that each one of these immature oocytes contains four copies of each maternal gene. When some of these oocytes are selected for ovulation, only then will they continue development into the second meiotic division expelling two out of the four copies of the maternal genes (the first polar body that may divide later). The first meiotic division is dependent on the normal functioning of the microtubules which make up the meiotic spindle that is critically responsible for normal alignment of the chromosomes on the metaphase plate prior to cell division. The meiotic spindle is at least 40 years old if natural conception is attempted at 40 years of age. Therefore, it is not a surprise that meiotic errors become common as women age and that the global rate of oocyte aneuploidy increases with advancing maternal age as the microtubules of the meiotic spindle become disorganized concomitantly with advancing age [14–17]. Aging mitochondria may contribute to the disorganization of microtubules through their inability to supply sufficient energy to accommodate the function of the meiotic spindle. Oocyte aneuploidy results primarily from premature separation of sister chromatids during meiosis I or from whole chromosome nondisjunction during meiosis II resulting in the abnormal absence (i.e., Turner's) or addition of a chromosome (i.e., Down's Syndrome) [17]. About half of all clinical miscarriages show chromosomal abnormality. The probability of chromosomal abnormality increases with age, from as low as 35% at age 20 to about 80% over the age of 42 [18]. Trisomies are by far the most common abnormality, followed by polyploidies and monosomy X (45,X).

Unfortunately, to date, there is no reliable technology to assess oocyte euploidy prior to fertilization with sperm. This is in part due to the fact that the second polar body is expelled only after fertilization. Furthermore, follicular pool studies (i.e., ovarian reserve tests) such as antimüllerian hormone (AMH), cycle day 2–4 FSH and antral follicle count (AFC) are our best estimation of the number of remaining follicles and provide limited reliable data about the oocytes' quality or their ability to complete the meiotic divisions correctly. The strongest predictor for oocyte quality is maternal age.

The Uterus

The uterus does not appear to be significantly affected by age. Uterine receptivity and its ability to support pregnancy are not thought to be significantly decreased by age [19,20]. This can be explained, at least partially, by good success rates when transferring embryos created from a young donor's oocytes into uteri of aging women (including women in their menopause) [21,22].

Aging and Male Fertility

Semen volume, sperm motility, sperm concentration, and percentage of sperm cells with normal morphology all decrease with age [23,24]. However, neither semen parameters nor luteinizing hormone, FSH, or testosterone faithfully predict fertilizing potential [25]. Overall, there is little or no decline in male fertility before the age of 45–50. After age 50 random mutations within sperm increase. Therefore, male factor contributes relatively little to the overall age-related decline in fertility unless the male is older than 50 when it may have some impact [26]. However, congenital syndromes and abnormalities (such as achondroplasia and neurofibromatosis), acute lymphocytic leukemia, autism, and schizophrenia are strongly associated with advanced paternal age [27].

Infertility Evaluation and Counseling Women over 40 Years of Age

Follicular pool depletion and declining oocyte quality are the two major factors affecting female fertility over 40 years of age. To date, there is no reliable test to evaluate oocyte quality. Therefore, we will elaborate on the available testing for assessing the size of the follicular pool (i.e., ovarian reserve). For the sake of clarity ovarian reserve and follicular pool are used interchangeably throughout this chapter.

Due to the reasons above, when a 40-year-old (or older) woman wishes to conceive, infertility evaluation is indicated without delay. The recommendation is to initiate a complete evaluation immediately without consideration of any time period of unprotected intercourse attempts [1]. This is in contrast to evaluation of younger women, who must demonstrate failure of attempts to conceive spontaneously over a certain period of time: 12 months for women younger than 35 and 6 months for women who are 35–40 years of age [1].

The complete evaluation includes lab work, imaging studies, and semen analysis. These studies are described elsewhere in this book. In this chapter, we elaborate on the various tests for follicular pool depletion as this is one of the major factors affecting women over 40 years of age. Although assessment of the follicular pool provides little information about oocyte quality, it does assist in predicting fecundity and successful ovarian response to hormonal stimulation. Additionally, one should bear in mind that all ovarian reserve testing has limited sensitivity and specificity rates (dependent on preselected cut-off values) with inherent false positive and false negative results. Furthermore, not infrequently there may be discordance among the different ovarian reserve testing results. Therefore, results should be interpreted with caution. Women should not be told that they cannot conceive spontaneously or denied fertility treatments based solely on any single test consistent with decreased ovarian reserve.

Basal FSH and Estradiol Levels

Cycle day 2–4 ("baseline") FSH levels increase as the follicular pool diminishes. The loss of follicles with their granulosa cells leads to decreased levels of Inhibin B (secreted by the granulosa cells). Lower levels of Inhibin B in the early follicular phase lead to reduced inhibition of FSH secretion during cycle days 2–4 [28,29]. There are several commercial assays available for quantifying serum FSH. These assays have different reference values and therefore, comparison of FSH levels between assays is not advised. Another significant challenge is same patient cycle-to-cycle baseline FSH variability. As cycle day 2–4 FSH values increase, the number of oocytes retrieved from an in vitro fertilization (IVF) cycle would

decrease. Obtaining fewer oocytes will result in a lower probability for pregnancy and live birth [30].

Consistently high day 2–4 FSH values are associated with poor prognosis but a single FSH level that is around 10–15 IU/L does not necessarily provide high specificity for a poor outcome [31]. As previously mentioned, FSH levels may vary significantly between consecutive cycles of the same woman. Therefore, when FSH levels are borderline elevated (10–15 IU/L), many clinicians prefer to repeat the test and choose to initiate a treatment cycle when the FSH level is relatively low. However, this approach has not been shown to improve treatment outcomes [32]. There is a natural aging progression over time from consistently low FSH to sometimes low accompanied by sometimes elevated FSH to consistently elevated FSH.

Cycle day 2–4 serum estradiol concentration may provide additional data in conjugation with basal FSH levels. As previously mentioned, aging women experience shortening of their menstrual cycles due to shortening of the follicular phase. This involves an earlier selection of a lead follicle and a resulting earlier ovulation. Earlier selection of a lead follicle can be followed by an early rise of estradiol level (secreted by this follicle) on cycle days 2–4. This early rise of estradiol can suppress the cycle day 2–4 basal FSH level. Therefore, relatively low basal FSH with a relatively high estradiol level are also suggestive of diminished ovarian reserve. When day 2–4 FSH is normal but day 2–4 estradiol is elevated (>60–80 pg/mL), the ovaries are less likely to respond well to exogenous gonadotropins and the chances for pregnancy are decreased [33]. When both FSH and estradiol are elevated, the success rates are even lower. Day 2–4 FSH and estradiol measurements are cycle dependent with greater intercycle variability in contrast to measurements of AFC and AMH (see below).

Antral Follicle Count

During the reproductive years about 20–150 follicles are growing at any given time. However, only a minority are in their antral stage (containing fluid) and are large enough (>1–2 mm in diameter) to be visualized by transvaginal ultrasound [34]. Studies have shown that the visualized number of antral follicles is not only a good representation of growing follicles but also proportional to the size of the resting (primordial) follicular pool [35]. Antral follicle count can be, therefore, a useful indirect measure of the ovarian reserve. Low AFC also correlates with the onset of menopause. Antral follicle count correlates well with oocyte yield in IVF cycles [35]. Assessment of AFC can be impaired by high body mass index (BMI) of a patient and/or assessment by multiple sonographers which introduces interobserver variation. However, it should be noted that during an IVF cycle, one should not expect all antral follicles to grow following FSH stimulation. This is because a significant portion of these sonographically visible antral follicles are already in an ongoing natural process of atresia. A low total AFC threshold of three to four follicles has an acceptable specificity (73–100%) for predicting poor ovarian response in IVF cycles and failure to conceive (64–100%) [36,37].

Antimüllerian Hormone

Antimüllerian hormone plays a fundamental role in early folliculogenesis by regulating follicular recruitment and cyclic selection. It is produced by the granulosa cells of small and large preantral as well as small antral growing follicles. It is initially secreted by primary follicles (immediately after recruitment) and ceases in the antral follicles that reach 6 mm. Antimüllerian hormone also suppresses additional recruitment of primordial follicles into the growing pool (a protective effect against premature exhaustion of the follicular pool) [38]. Small antral follicles contain a large number of granulosa cells, which are likely to be the main source of AMH. Therefore, AMH, as AFC, is an excellent marker for ovarian reserve. Cycle-to-cycle variability is less for AMH compared to AFC and therefore AMH is the preferable ovarian reserve test [39].

In contrast to day 2–4 FSH, AMH level does not fluctuate significantly throughout the menstrual cycle [40]. Because AMH derives mainly from small antral follicles, it is not surprising that gonadotropin-releasing hormone agonists and oral contraceptives suppress its level after 3 months of use (through suppression of pituitary FSH) [41]. Prolonged use (>3 months) of oral contraceptives leads to a transient decrease in AMH levels and AFC. By contrast, polycystic ovaries often present with very high levels of AMH (≥5 ng/mL). This is due to a high number of arrested small antral follicles constantly secreting large amounts of AMH.

Overall, low AMH level is associated with decreased ovarian reserve, poor response to ovarian stimulation, and low oocyte yield in IVF cycles [42]. In older women AMH may be more important in predicting livebirth than in young women [43,44]. In women 40 or older with AMH <1 ng/mL, workup and treatment options should be pursued in an expeditious focused fashion to avoid further age-related loss of egg quantity and quality.

Clomiphene Citrate Challenge Test

The Clomiphene Citrate Challenge Test (CCCT) is a provocative test that is supposed, in theory, to reveal diminished ovarian reserve while basal FSH levels are still in the normal range. Cycle day 3 FSH is measured, then 100 mg of clomiphene citrate is taken daily on cycle days 5–9. The FSH is measured again on cycle day 10 [45]. Physiologically, clomiphene citrate increases endogenous FSH levels in all women and the responding follicular cohort (to the supraphysiological FSH levels) secretes in return inhibin B and estradiol that suppress additional FSH secretion. In aging women, a smaller follicular cohort is expected to respond to this initial supraphysiological FSH level and therefore, exerts less negative feedback on FSH secretion. The expected result is a higher FSH level on day 10 [46]. In theory, a frankly elevated cycle day 10 FSH concentration can identify women with diminished ovarian reserve who might otherwise go unrecognized if evaluated with basal cycle day 2–4 FSH and estradiol levels alone [47]. However, studies have shown that this test has a limited clinical value and no benefit over AMH, AFC, or basal FSH [48]. CCCT is being used less often in clinical practice.

General Considerations When Counseling Women over 40

The age of a woman's mother at menopause and reproductive history of any older sisters may provide important predictive information. Family history of premature menopause may indicate the expedited workup of possible premature ovarian insufficiency.

Testing for FMR-1 and/or BRCA genes in the background of a family history for breast and/or ovarian cancer or in the case of unexpectedly diminished ovarian reserve may be indicated. Family history of multiple miscarriages, birth defects, and developmental abnormalities may suggest inherited genetic abnormalities that warrant specific evaluation and treatment.

Smoking is associated with impaired fecundity and increased risks of spontaneous miscarriage and ectopic pregnancy. It appears to accelerate the loss of reproductive function and may advance the time of menopause by 1–4 years. Regarding fertility treatments, smoking is associated with almost doubling the number of IVF attempts to conceive. Nonsmokers with excessive exposure to tobacco smoke (passive smoking) may have reproductive consequences as great as those observed in smokers. Medications such as varenicline, bupropion, and nicotine (gums, patches, etc.) should be offered for smoking cessation. These approaches have been shown to be twice as effective as placebo [49].

Women with a history of cancer treated by chemotherapy and/or radiation therapy are at increased risk of premature ovarian insufficiency or may already be in iatrogenic menopause. These women should be appropriately counseled about their possibly limited reproductive potential [50].

Oral contraceptives have not been shown to interfere with fertility potential once they are discontinued [51,52]. There is some evidence that combined oral contraceptive use just before IVF may decrease the success rates (in some ovarian stimulation protocols) but this effect was not seen when progesterone only was used [53,54].

Personal obstetric and gynecologic histories may include miscarriages, preterm births, change in menstrual frequency and flow, anatomical abnormalities (e.g., fibroids, polyps, uterine septum), as well as uterine, ovarian, and tubal surgeries (e.g., dilation and curettage, bilateral tubal ligation, salpingectomy, ovarian cyst removal, and endometriosis resection). These histories should be carefully documented to select the most appropriate intervention before any fertility treatment.

High BMI is a major risk factor when considering fertility treatments under general anesthesia (e.g., oocyte retrieval and hysteroscopic polypectomy). As time is of the essence for all mature women, weight loss and achievement of a BMI < 35 as soon as possible should be encouraged. Daily exercise, balanced diet, and proper vitamin intake should be rapidly optimized. Consideration may be given to supplementing women with low AMH with coenzyme Q 10, DHEA, and vitamin D3 when vitamin D levels are <30 ng/mL. Normal vitamin D levels are believed to be of importance in optimizing AMH levels and particularly in treatment outcomes of women with polycystic ovarian syndrome. Additionally, all recommended vaccinations should be administered in anticipation of pregnancy.

Lastly, lifestyle choices, stress, and sleep disturbances may negatively affect fertility potential through altering the functions of the hypothalamus, pituitary, and gonads. The exact mechanisms are yet to be fully understood; however, it is clear that stress reduction techniques are an important part of the multidisciplinary fertility treatments [55–57].

Special Considerations When Counseling Women over 40

Personal timeline and meeting realistic expectations are a priority in fertility counseling especially for women over 40 [58,59]. It is advised that no more than four cycles of oral ovulation induction cycles with intrauterine insemination be pursued before proceeding to IVF [58,59]. If the goal is to have one or more children, IVF with or without embryo banking should be discussed. If a male partner is not available and donor sperm is not an option, oocyte freezing is a reasonable alternative for fertility preservation. Nowadays, oocyte vitrification and thawing are considered to yield the same results as using fresh oocytes [50]. However, one should note that not all thawed oocytes will be fertilized following sperm injection. Therefore, in general, good-quality embryo banking is considered more reliable than oocyte freezing.

As the window of opportunity is narrower, expanded genetic diseases carrier screening should be offered and expedited for women over 40 and their partners to identify potential genetic problems that may be overcome with IVF and preimplantation genetic testing (PGT) directed to the known single gene mutations (PGT-M) or to the known structural chromosomal rearrangements (PGT-SR) carried by either of the partners if recurrent pregnancy loss has been an issue. Both PGT-M and PGT-SR are robust approaches to detect and perhaps treat specific conditions in the embryonic genome prior to embryo transfer. This is in contrast to the less accurate general approach to detect imbalances in the embryonic genetic material: PGT for aneuploidy (PGT-A) [60]. An additional point worthy of mention during the workup is, if any uterine pathology is noted on the hysterosalpingogram or sono-hysterogram which is consistent with uterine pathology (i.e., polyp, fibroid, adhesions), consideration should be given to first proceeding with egg retrieval and banking to obtain the desired number of cryopreserved items then proceeding with the appropriate surgery to normalize uterine anatomy in preparation for eventual transfer. In summary, before proceeding to donor oocytes, decisiveness and tailoring the optimal treatment with which the woman (or couple) is most comfortable deserves important consideration in the timeliest fashion. The tailored treatment plan should take into consideration the increased risks in pregnancy and may include preconception counseling with an obstetrician, a geneticist, and a psychologist.

Summary

The two main fertility challenges faced by women over 40 are decreased oocyte quality and quantity. Age is the most significant predictor of oocyte quality. There is no reliable test aimed at evaluating single oocyte quality in vivo or in vitro following oocyte retrieval or just prior to fertilization. On the other hand, there are informative ovarian reserve tests aimed at estimating the residual follicular pool in aging women: AMH, AFC, and cycle day 2–4 FSH [61]. Each has acceptable specificity for detecting diminished ovarian reserve. The majority of clinicians prefer AMH over AFC and FSH due to its technical simplicity, lower intra- and intercycle variability and increased prognostic value in the context of older women [43,44]. Once stating a desire to conceive, women who are 40 or older should have an immediate comprehensive infertility evaluation that must include prompt ovarian reserve testing. Lifestyle changes including nutrition, vitamins, exercise, stress reduction, and adequate sleep [62] can only assist in the goal. Lastly, preparation, engagement, and support from a team of professionals are essential to approach conceiving over the age of 40.

References

1. American College of Obstetricians and Gynecologists Committee on Gynecologic Practice and Practice Committee. Female age-related fertility decline. Committee Opinion No. 589. *Fertil Steril* 2014;**101**:633–4.

2. Stein ZA. A woman's age: childbearing and child rearing. *Am J Epidemiol* 1985;**121**:327–42.

3. Gosden RG. Maternal age: a major factor affecting the prospects and outcome of pregnancy. *Ann N Y Acad Sci* 1985;**442**:45–57.

4. Baker TG. A Quantitative and Cytological Study of Germ Cells in Human Ovaries. *Proc R Soc Lond B Biol Sci* 1963;**158**:417–33.

5. Vaskivuo TE, Anttonen M, Herva R, et al. Survival of human ovarian follicles from fetal to adult life: apoptosis, apoptosis-related proteins, and transcription factor GATA-4. *J Clin Endocrinol Metab* 2001;**86**:3421–9.

6. Markstrom E, Svensson E, Shao R, Svanberg B, Billig H. Survival factors regulating ovarian apoptosis – dependence on follicle differentiation. *Reproduction* 2002;**123**:23–30.

7. te Velde ER, Pearson PL. The variability of female reproductive ageing. *Hum Reprod Update* 2002;**8**:141–54.

8. Richardson SJ, Senikas V, Nelson JF. Follicular depletion during the menopausal transition: evidence for accelerated loss and ultimate exhaustion. *J Clin Endocrinol Metab* 1987;**65**:1231–7.

9. Faddy MJ, Gosden RG. A model conforming the decline in follicle numbers to the age of menopause in women. *Hum Reprod* 1996;**11**:1484–6.

10. Battaglia DE, Goodwin P, Klein NA, Soules MR. Influence of maternal age on meiotic spindle assembly in oocytes from naturally cycling women. *Hum Reprod* 1996;**11**:2217–22.

11. Gougeon A, Ecochard R, Thalabard JC. Age-related changes of the population of human ovarian follicles: increase in the disappearance rate of non-growing and early-growing follicles in aging women. *Biol Reprod* 1994;**50**:653–63.

12. Jacobs SL, Metzger DA, Dodson WC, Haney AF. Effect of age on response to human menopausal gonadotropin stimulation. *J Clin Endocrinol Metab* 1990;**71**:1525–30.

13. Block E. A quantitative morphological investigation of the follicular system in newborn female infants. *Acta Anat (Basel)* 1953;**17**:201–6.

14. Nasmyth K. Disseminating the genome: joining, resolving, and separating sister chromatids during mitosis and meiosis. *Annu Rev Genet* 2001;**35**:673–745.

15. Pellestor F, Anahory T, Hamamah S. Effect of maternal age on the frequency of cytogenetic abnormalities in human oocytes. *Cytogenet Genome Res* 2005;**111**:206–12.

16. Pellestor F, Andreo B, Arnal F, Humeau C, Demaille J. Maternal aging and chromosomal abnormalities: new data drawn from in vitro unfertilized human oocytes. *Hum Genet* 2003;**112**:195–203.

17. Pellestor F, Andreo B, Anahory T, Hamamah S. The occurrence of aneuploidy in human: lessons from the cytogenetic studies of human oocytes. *Eur J Med Genet* 2006;**49**:103–16.

18. Hassold T, Chiu D. Maternal age-specific rates of numerical chromosome abnormalities with special reference to trisomy. *Hum Genet* 1985;**70**:11–17.

19. Noci I, Borri P, Chieffi O, et al.I. Aging of the human endometrium: a basic morphological and immunohistochemical study. *Eur J Obstet Gynecol Reprod Biol* 1995;**63**:181–5.

20. Abdalla HI, Burton G, Kirkland A, et al. Age, pregnancy and miscarriage: uterine versus ovarian factors. *Hum Reprod* 1993;**8**:1512–7.

21. Borini A, Bafaro G, Violini F, Bianchi L, Casadio V, Flamigni C. Pregnancies in postmenopausal women over 50 years old in an oocyte donation program. *Fertil Steril* 1995;**63**:258–61.

22. Melnick AP, Rosenwaks Z. Oocyte donation: insights gleaned and future challenges. *Fertil Steril* 2018;**110**:988–93.

23. Kidd SA, Eskenazi B, Wyrobek AJ. Effects of male age on semen quality and fertility: a review of the literature. *Fertil Steril* 2001;**75**:237–48.

24. Eskenazi B, Wyrobek AJ, Sloter E, et al. The association of age and semen quality in healthy men. *Hum Reprod* 2003;**18**:447–54.

25. Vermeulen A, Kaufman JM. Ageing of the hypothalamo-pituitary-testicular axis in men. *Horm Res* 1995;**43**:25–8.

26. Almeida S, Rato L, Sousa M, Alves MG, Oliveira PF. Fertility and sperm quality in the aging male. *Curr Pharm Des* 2017;**23**:4429–37.

27. Nybo Andersen AM, Urhoj SK. Is advanced paternal age a health risk for the offspring? *Fertil Steril* 2017;**107**:312–8.

28. Mihm M, Gangooly S, Muttukrishna S. The normal menstrual cycle in women. *Anim Reprod Sci* 2011;**124**:229–36.

29. Sowers MR, Eyvazzadeh AD, McConnell D, et al. Anti-mullerian hormone and inhibin B in the definition of ovarian aging and the menopause transition. *J Clin Endocrinol Metab* 2008;**93**:3478–83.

30. Bukman A, Heineman MJ. Ovarian reserve testing and the use of prognostic models in patients with subfertility. *Hum Reprod Update* 2001;**7**:581–90.

31. Roberts JE, Spandorfer S, Fasouliotis SJ, Kashyap S, Rosenwaks Z. Taking a basal follicle-stimulating hormone history is essential before initiating in vitro fertilization. *Fertil Steril* 2005;**83**:37–41.

32. Abdalla H, Thum MY. Repeated testing of basal FSH levels has no predictive value for IVF outcome in women with elevated basal FSH. *Hum Reprod* 2006;**21**:171–4.

33. Buyalos RP, Daneshmand S, Brzechffa PR. Basal estradiol and follicle-stimulating hormone predict fecundity in women of advanced reproductive age undergoing ovulation induction therapy. *Fertil Steril* 1997;**68**:272–7.

34. Pache TD, Wladimiroff JW, de Jong FH, Hop WC, Fauser BC. Growth patterns of nondominant ovarian follicles during the normal menstrual cycle. *Fertil Steril* 1990;**54**:638–42.

35. Scheffer GJ, Broekmans FJ, Dorland M, Habbema JD, Looman CW, te Velde ER. Antral follicle counts by transvaginal ultrasonography are related to age in women with proven natural fertility. *Fertil Steril* 1999;**72**:845–51.

36. Frattarelli JL, Lauria-Costab DF, Miller BT, Bergh PA, Scott RT. Basal antral follicle number and mean ovarian diameter predict cycle cancellation and ovarian responsiveness in assisted reproductive technology cycles. *Fertil Steril* 2000;**74**:512–7.

37. Kupesic S, Kurjak A, Bjelos D, Vujisic S. Three-dimensional ultrasonographic ovarian measurements and in vitro fertilization outcome are related to age. *Fertil Steril* 2003;**79**:190–7.

38. Themmen AP. Anti-Mullerian hormone: its role in follicular growth initiation and survival and as an ovarian reserve marker. *J Natl Cancer Inst Monogr* 2005;**34**:18–21.

39. Fleming R, Seifer DB, Frattarelli JL, Ruman J. Assessing ovarian response: antral follicle count versus anti-Mullerian hormone. *Reprod Biomed Online* 2015;**31**:486–96.

40. Hehenkamp WJ, Looman CW, Themmen AP, de Jong FH, Te Velde ER, Broekmans FJ. Anti-Mullerian hormone levels in the spontaneous menstrual cycle do not show substantial fluctuation. *J Clin Endocrinol Metab* 2006;**91**:4057–63.

41. Broer SL, Broekmans FJ, Laven JS, Fauser BC. Anti-Mullerian hormone: ovarian reserve testing and its potential clinical implications. *Hum Reprod Update* 2014;**20**:688–701.

42. Gnoth C, Schuring AN, Friol K, Tigges J, Mallmann P, Godehardt E. Relevance of anti-Mullerian hormone measurement in a routine IVF program. *Hum Reprod* 2008;**23**:1359–65.

43. Goswami M, Nikolaou D. Is AMH level, independent of age, a predictor of live birth in IVF? *J Hum Reprod Sci* 2017;**10**:24–30.

44. Tal R, Seifer DB, Tal R, Grainger E, Wantman E, Tal O. AMH highly correlates with cumulative live birth rate in women with diminished ovarian reserve independent of age. *J Clin Endocrinol Metab* 2021;**106**:2754–66.

45. Navot D, Rosenwaks Z, Margalioth EJ. Prognostic assessment of female fecundity. *Lancet* 1987;**2**:645–7.

46. Yong PY, Baird DT, Thong KJ, McNeilly AS, Anderson RA. Prospective analysis of the relationships between the ovarian follicle cohort and basal FSH concentration, the inhibin response to exogenous FSH and ovarian follicle number at different stages of the normal menstrual cycle and after pituitary down-regulation. *Hum Reprod* 2003;**18**:35–44.

47. Csemiczky G, Harlin J, Fried G. Predictive power of clomiphene citrate challenge test for failure of in vitro fertilization treatment. *Acta Obstet Gynecol Scand* 2002;**81**:954–61.

48. Hendriks DJ, Broekmans FJ, Bancsi LF, de Jong FH, Looman CW, Te Velde ER. Repeated clomiphene citrate challenge testing in the prediction of outcome in IVF: a comparison with basal markers for ovarian reserve. *Hum Reprod* 2005;**20**:163–9.

49. Practice Committee of the American Society for Reproductive Medicine. Smoking and infertility: a committee opinion. *Fertil Steril* 2018;**110**:611–18.

50. Ladanyi C, Mor A, Christianson MS, Dhillon N, Segars JH. Recent advances in the field of ovarian tissue cryopreservation and opportunities for research. *J Assist Reprod Genet* 2017;**34**:709–22.

51. Girum T, Wasie A. Return of fertility after discontinuation of contraception: a systematic review and meta-analysis. *Contracept Reprod Med* 2018;**3**:9.

52. Barnhart KT, Schreiber CA. Return to fertility following discontinuation of oral contraceptives. *Fertil Steril* 2009;**91**:659–63.

53. Wei D, Shi Y, Li J, et al. Effect of pretreatment with oral contraceptives and progestins on IVF outcomes in women with polycystic ovary syndrome. *Hum Reprod* 2017;**32**:354–61.

54. Farquhar C, Rombauts L, Kremer JA, Lethaby A, Ayeleke RO. Oral contraceptive pill, progestogen or oestrogen pretreatment for ovarian stimulation protocols for women undergoing assisted reproductive techniques. *Cochrane Database Syst Rev* 2017;**5**:CD006109.

55. Kloss JD, Perlis ML, Zamzow JA, Culnan EJ, Gracia CR. Sleep, sleep disturbance, and fertility in women. *Sleep Med Rev* 2015;**22**:78–87.

56. Palomba S, Daolio J, Romeo S, Battaglia FA, Marci R, La Sala GB. Lifestyle and fertility: the influence of stress and quality of life on female fertility. *Reprod Biol Endocrinol* 2018;**16**:113.

57. Joseph DN, Whirledge S. Stress and the HPA axis: balancing homeostasis and fertility. *Int J Mol Sci* 2017;**18**.

58. Kaser DJ, Goldman MB, Fung JL, Alper MM, Reindollar RH. When is clomiphene or gonadotropin intrauterine insemination futile? Results of the Fast Track and Standard Treatment Trial and the Forty and Over Treatment Trial, two prospective randomized controlled trials. *Fertil Steril* 2014;**102**:1331–7 e1.

59. Reindollar RH, Regan MM, Neumann PJ, et al. A randomized clinical trial to evaluate optimal treatment for unexplained infertility: the fast track and standard treatment (FASTT) trial. *Fertil Steril* 2010;**94**:888–99.

60. Mochizuki L, Gleicher N. The PGS/PGT-A controversy in IVF addressed as a formal conflict resolution analysis. *J Assist Reprod Genet* 2020;**37**:677–87.

61. Tal R, Seifer DB. Ovarian reserve testing: a user's guide. *Am J Obstet Gynecol* 2017;**217**:129–40.

62. Beroukhim G, Esencan E, Seifer DB. Impact of sleep patterns upon female neuroendocrinology and reproductive outcomes: a comprehensive review. *Reprod Biol Endocrinol* 2022;**20**:16.

Support Systems and Patient Experience Architecture for Fertility Care of Women over 40 in the 2020s

Dimitrios S. Nikolaou and David B. Seifer

Introduction

This chapter is directed toward optimizing patient support going through a fertility service, with emphasis on women over 40. "Patient support" is a concept far broader than the traditional offer of a phone number for a counselor and handing out a pamphlet. It encompasses optimal clinical management, as well as an organizational structure for the whole service to optimize patient experience. We first summarize supporting women over 40 during the COVID pandemic, followed by providing key steps of an individualized clinical management strategy, and the requirements of patient support structures. However, unlike previous publications, this chapter does not end by simply outlining what is desirable. It proceeds to a number of practical steps that fertility services can follow, using the framework of "patient experience architecture" to build suitable structured pathways. Furthermore, it explores the path of digital transformation in an effort to reduce cost and improve consistency delivering core professional values in every interaction. At the end of the chapter there is a short list of useful reading.

COVID Update

It seems appropriate to emphasize, in this chapter, remarks focusing on supporting patients over 40, specifically, during the COVID pandemic. Over the last year many assisted reproductive technology (ART) programs worldwide were suspended, completely or partly, causing delays in treatments and backlog. This has undoubtedly added to the distress and stress of patients, especially those over 40 or with very poor ovarian reserve, who worry that time is running out for their ability to have a child. The main professional organizations have been issuing guidance and this included advice on patient-support mechanisms during the pandemic [1–7]. For example, the American Society for Reproductive Medicine (ASRM) recommends that clinics should reach out to patients, ask them how they are doing, understand that some patients need to "vent" and "blame," while explaining that "we are all in this together," provide good-quality information and support and stay connected [2].

Fertility Units should be able to continue with fertility preservation for cancer. Age and poor ovarian reserve are time-sensitive, but the ASRM recommended early in the crisis that these should not be included in the definition of "urgent case" during the lockdown. Clinics should have a transparent clinical prioritization policy in place, as part of their service continuity and recommencement strategy. The COVID-19 service continuity strategy needs to include the following elements of transparency and organization (Table 9.1).

Academic work should be encouraged to continue, as it generates new knowledge to help, and develop effective strategies during the pandemic. For example: it has been shown recently that delaying in vitro fertilization (IVF) between 3 and 6 months from the decision to treat does NOT have significant adverse effect on livebirth rates, over starting treatment immediately (0–3 months) for women over 40 with low or extremely low ovarian reserve. If anything, it appears that a small delay (3–6 months) is associated with slightly better success rates [8]. There may be various explanations, but one possible factor is that there is time to optimize physical and mental health, weight, and pre-treat as necessary.

Delaying treatment beyond 6 months likely will have an adverse effect, especially for women over 40 with additional known causes such as tubal or male factor, based on mathematical

Table 9.1 Elements of a service continuity strategy during COVID-19

- Direct patient care: virtual outpatient clinics, answering of messages from patients, early pregnancy and OHSS reviews, issuing repeat prescriptions, virtual multidisciplinary team meetings
- A strategy for minimizing the risk of exposure to COVID-19 for patients and staff: contact tracing, testing, safe distancing, PPE policy, policy of partners accompanying patients for office visits
- Other patient support: counselling sessions, virtual meetings for information, group-support meetings, webinars
- Regular timely website and social media updates regarding the office practice
- Audits, protocol update, mandatory training, and quality management
- Staff training and education. Cross-training staff to be able to effectively cope with absences, development of back-up cover pathways
- Academic work that does not require direct patient contact

OHSS, ovarian hyperstimulation syndrome; PPE, personal protective equipment.

modeling but not yet confirmed with actual data [9]. This model, however, was built on the fact that fertility prognosis is affected adversely by female age and duration of infertility. If 6–12 more months are added to the age and duration of infertility for each patient, then their estimated prognosis will be affected. Information such as the above should be taken into account when discussing the prioritization of cases for recommencement after a lockdown.

An important aspect of this is the added pressure on fertility clinic staff. The patients are more stressed, and need to "vent out." This is superimposed upon a background of globally deteriorating mental health, with huge increases of mental disorders reported in all segments of the population. The medical team is already under pressure as there is a constantly changing environment, demands to change work patterns and content, uncertainty, redeployment, a control and command culture that seeps in and seems to want to settle long term, and various other agendas that are being promoted. There are also pressures at home (health, homeschooling) and financial concerns, in addition to caring for patients who are stressed and angry.

In planning for the future, more robust strategies need to be developed for coping with

similar epidemics. This could be informed by public health modeling. There are various suggestions that, with more flexibility, not all clinical services will need to be suspended every time, but only certain sections of the hospital will be allocated as red zones, while the rest of the hospital can carry on with its normal activity [10].

The Wider Concept of "Patient Support"

In terms of *supporting* women over 40 who want to have a baby, the first step it to actually *want* to support them. This does not necessarily mean offering IVF or similar in every case. It does mean, however, responding positively to their request for medical advice and help. This is the cultural perspective reflected throughout this book. Traditionally, chapters on fertility for women over 40 ended mirroring the rapid natural decline in fertility and the accompanied increases in the rate of miscarriage and fetal abnormalities, as well as the various adverse obstetric and neonatal outcomes. Most would feel that women should be advised to have their babies earlier in life to avoid disappointment. However, there are many women over 40 who want to have a baby or present when they are pregnant already while asking for advice. Thus, begging the following questions: Is the medical community going to engage positively with them? Is there anything at all that can be done, individually and organizationally, to improve their chance of achieving all that is achievable? If they are already pregnant, are there steps that can be taken to manage the risk for their pregnancy and optimize the outcome? And if there is no effective treatment, how should they be supported, otherwise? Here is one example, as a point of reference: a 42-year-old with no prior children and recently separated, who anxiously wants to explore her fertility "options."

Staying on the concept of "support," traditionally this was limited to arrangements for providing "psychological" support for patients who were anxious or upset or otherwise distressed. This might include a kind nurse and possibly a qualified counselor. As crucial and as necessary as these may be, no amount of kindness from a nurse or professional ability of the fertility counsellor can adequately compensate for the distress caused by poor service organization. For example, the fact that there was no sufficient discussion of

the various options, the overall prognosis, and clarity about the total cost, not enough information (to reach a proper understanding) about the treatment, or no effective interactive channel of communication with the clinic during the treatment. In other words, "patient support" has many underlying aspects, beyond psychological counseling including two crucial points which are the development of suitable "patient management strategies" and "clinic organizational structures."

The Scope of "Management" of Infertility in the 40s

Infertility is a complex condition incorporating reproductive, medical, psychological, mental, spiritual, and social concerns. Our patients have to deal with their own body and mind as well as navigate a complex ecosystem that includes their partner, extended family, social cycle, work environment, fertility clinics, various public and private organizations, and support groups. Infertility is also a rapidly growing global business and has attracted various entrepreneurs, each of whom pursues their own marketing strategy. In this environment it is hard for patients to know who to trust.

The National Institute for Health and Care Excellence provides national guidance and advice to improve health and social care. It produces evidence-based guidance and advice. For women over 40 there are no recommendations in the NICE guidelines (National Institute for Clinical Excellence) and there is little or no state funding for IVF. What makes patients happy is difficult to define. The Human Fertilization and Embryology Authority (HFEA) is the government regulator responsible for making sure fertility clinics and research centers comply with the law. It collects data directly from the clinics and carries our regular planned or unannounced inspections. The HFEA asks patients to rate their clinic on the basis of several criteria. It advises patients that "a great fertility clinic isn't just one that can give them effective treatment, it's one with compassionate staff, clear pricing, seamless administrative processes and exceptional emotional support" [11].

The concept of "management," in any setting, implies setting and overseeing a process of transition from the point of origin (point A: current situation) to an agreed destination (point B).

A suitable "patient management strategy" should include the steps outlined in Table 9.2.

Clinic Support Structures

The Requirements of the HFEA Code of Practice

In the ninth edition of its code of practice, in 2019, the HFEA in the UK includes specific requirements for counseling and patient support, which we recommend as essential reading [11]. Specifically, on patient support the code of practice requires that each fertility center develops a "patient support policy" to describe exactly how the patients will be supported before, during, and after treatment. The recommendations include, among others:

- All staff (not just the counselor) should provide psychological and other support to the patients, before, during, and after the treatment.
- Support should be patient-centered.
- Support should be adapted for each patient according to their requirements, preferences, and circumstances.
- The policy should describe each individual staff member's role in supporting patients.
- A list of information resources and how to access them.
- A list of patient-support activities such as support groups and forums.
- A description of the interactive communication channels with the clinic in and out of hours.
- A list of training to be provided to the center staff relating to patient support, such as e-learning courses.
- Feedback mechanisms for collecting data on patient/donor experience.
- Quality indicators for systematically monitoring the center's provision of patient support.

The HFEA Code of Practice also says that treatments should not be initiated unless the patient has been given a suitable opportunity to receive proper counseling about the implications, and information about the treatment. It is a mandatory requirement to offer counselling, among else, if the treatment involves donated gametes, or the creation of embryos in vitro, or embryo storage.

Table 9.2 Essential steps of an individualized clinical management strategy

1. **Defining point A**

   In medicine, point A is when a patient first presents. It includes all the various diagnostic steps: review of previous medical information, clinical history, clinical examination, laboratory and other imaging tests

2. **Mapping the problem:**

   The purpose of all this is to "map" the situation, including all the "issues" that arise from the history and other clinical investigations. For women over 40, AGE is the first and, prognostically, usually the most important "issue," as it directly impacts egg-quality and is the main determinant of the overall prognosis for outcome. Other issues may include:

   • **Reproductive: uterine, tubal, male, endometriosis, anovulation**

   • **General medical: thyroid, comorbidities, i.e., obesity, systemic diseases**

   • **Psychological**

   • **Social: partner, employment, finances**

   • **Ideological, spiritual**

3. **Estimating the overall prognosis:** Based on the above analysis, the next keystone of management is the estimation of prognosis. This will be based on the patient's individual circumstances in the context of the clinic's own success rates as well as national and international success rates

4. **Adjusting point B:** Based on the above, there is often a need to readjust point B. This is called "managing expectations and achieving realism." There needs to be an agreement on what is achievable or what chance of success is acceptable. Unless this crucial point is reached, all subsequent steps are destined to fail, and the patient will not be satisfied

5. Define "success" in operational terms the patient or couple understands. Success has different meanings to different people in different circumstances. For some, it is a healthy baby. For others, it can be having tried what was possible and achieving what was achievable, or even trying and failing but having achieved "peace of mind" that they did whatever was within their power to try

6. Discuss the whole range of options, with own eggs or donor eggs, along with success rates, costs, risks, alternatives, and requirements

7. The role of the doctor includes offering advice at this point, not just a range of options. This advice will be based on the best available evidence and consideration of the patient's/couple's value system

8. Finally, the management strategy, i.e., the path from A to B, will be codesigned with the patient. Any such strategy should have at least three components:

   • **Pretreatment optimization of health and information. Including preconceptional counselling on obstetric risks, dietary advice, and psychological counseling**

   • **If appropriate, a plan of ART treatment(s). After the first treatment cycle there should be a session for reviewing the recent cycle in detail, debriefing and possible therapeutic adjustments discussed**

Table 9.2 (cont.)

   • **Support structures throughout and an initial discussion of options if the first attempted treatment is unsuccessful**

Regarding the provision of counseling in circumstances such as the above, the code of practice is clear that only *qualified* counselors should provide counseling. The provision of counseling should be clearly distinguished from the normal supporting relationship between the clinic staff and patients.

Formal Counseling: British Infertility Counselling Association Guidelines

Counselling is a distinct professional process based on a body of theoretical knowledge and agreed codes of ethics and values. It needs to be distinguished from the normal advice and support that is provided by the doctor and other members of the medical team, or any other support or coaching. Counselling takes place when a counsellor contracts with a client to explore any difficulty, distress, uncertainty, or dissatisfaction that the client may be experiencing. It is confidential within specific boundaries and conducted in private either face-to-face, by telephone or online. According to the British Infertility Counselling Association (BICA) guidelines [12], the counseling service should comply with current professional guidance on good practice in infertility counseling. Only qualified counselors should provide counseling (Table 9.3).

The European Society of Human Reproduction and Embryology Recommendations for Patient Support

In our essential reading recommendations, we include the European Society of Human Reproduction and Embryology (ESHRE) guideline on "Routine psychosocial care in infertility and medically assisted reproduction," which was produced by the Psychology and Counselling Guideline Development Group in March 2015 [13,14]. This guideline is freely available online in the extended form, as well as summary and patient forms. It includes the fact that individual patients have clear preferences about the psychosocial care that they need, and fertility staff should be aware of these preferences and try to address them in each case. Particularly, patients appreciate the provision

Table 9.3 BICA Fourth Edition Version 1, 2019

The purpose of counseling for infertility, involuntary childlessness, and assisted conception is to:
Provide emotional support before, during, and after treatment or donation of sperm, eggs, and embryos or a surrogacy arrangement, particularly if the person is experiencing stress, ambivalence, or distress
Assist people in developing successful coping strategies for dealing with both the short- and longer-term consequences of infertility, involuntary childlessness, and treatment
Help people to try to adjust to, and accommodate, their particular situation
Counseling may be an ongoing process and can be continued, or take place for the first time, after a course of treatment has been completed. The duration of counselling is determined by the individual's needs and wishes. Any referral to alternative sources of counselling should only be made with the agreement of the client. Counselling should be provided by a qualified counsellor who meets the accreditation criteria

of clear and detailed information about the treatment before it starts.

It is important to realize not only that different patients have different needs for support, but also that each patient's needs will evolve during their individual journey. Some patients are particularly vulnerable during treatment and need additional support for "special needs."

For example, at the relational level, some women lack adequate support from significant people in their life and are absent from work. Some women use avoidance coping strategies and some couples have different views about the importance of parenthood. Some patients have passive coping mechanisms, such as withdrawal. Patients with lower educational levels may need more input. There may be language or cultural barriers that need to be addressed. Couples in which there is severe male infertility may need extra support. During treatment, patients need more support if they have a history of vulnerability to mental health disorders.

Emotional needs tend to peak at crucial stages of the treatment, such as before the egg collection, the embryo transfer, and especially after unsuccessful treatment. In pregnancy, women with a history of infertility treatment tend to be more anxious than other women. There are infertility-specific or generic assessment tools that can be used by infertility clinic staff to assess individual patient needs [13]. These need to be part of staff training, treatment protocols, and management strategy.

The HFEA Pilot National Patient Survey

The HFEA Pilot National Fertility Patient Survey [15] is recommended as it provides valuable insight into what patients most highly value in their fertility care. This was the largest and most representative survey of fertility patients in the UK and was carried out by YouGov. It provides an opportunity to understand the experiences of patients and what changes could have the greatest impact. There is a large amount of data to process. Here, we provide our own pick of interesting findings, although we recommend that each reader draws their own conclusions.

- The outcome is a key determinant in overall satisfaction. None of the patients who were successful said they were dissatisfied. For those who were unsuccessful, 30% said that they were dissatisfied. This finding is discussed later in this chapter.
- In key driver analysis, the "interest shown in you as a person" comes out as top driver of overall satisfaction. The ease of accessing fertility treatment through the National Health Service (NHS) is one of the least important drivers.
- The subsequent most important drivers are the respect and courtesy patients are shown and how safe they felt during treatment.
- Other key factors were the quality of counseling and the coordination and administration of treatment.
- 75% of patients remember receiving information about how to access counseling.
- The most popular reasons for choosing a particular clinic were the location (51%), information about success rates (44%), and having a good first impression of the clinic staff (36%).
- Having the option to ask questions after consultations is also key. Many said that it was only after they left the room that they would think of questions to ask.
- Over a quarter (27%) of NHS clinic users disagreed that they had enough time with the healthcare professionals, dropping to one-sixth (16%) of those who most recently used a private clinic.

- Some felt that the healthcare professionals lacked empathy and that the process felt rushed.
- Consultants are seen to play a very specific role in the process: they are delivering factual information, rather than emotional support. Many find their consultants blunt or brusque in interactions, especially when delivering negative news, and often difficult to contact.
- Sometimes the amount of information received in the consultation can be overwhelming, and it would be helpful to have hard-top-access information recorded to take away in some form.
- One in four felt the chances of success were not made clear.
- There was a preference for succinct documents (e.g., PowerPoint format), rather than long Word documents. They are looking for a succinct treatment plan that gives them all the information they need (visually/graphically where possible), in a simple and succinct format.
- Many patients commented on poor internal communication. For example, doctors not reading notes, not knowing what other doctors are doing.
- Just over half (55%) were satisfied they could contact a named person at the clinic.
- A large number felt frustrated with the administrative process.
- 63% of responders said they felt able to provide feedback.
- 62% of those whose most recent treatment was at a private clinic said they paid more than expected.
- Private clinics in general are perceived to be more flexible, with their users more likely to be satisfied than NHS clinic users
- The advice provided by general practitioners (GPs) and the ease of access to fertility treatment are the lowest performing measures for patient satisfaction; however, they are not significant drivers of overall satisfaction.
- Just under half (46%) said they were satisfied with how long it took to begin fertility treatment.
- Online support forums have become a more popular form of support over recent years, with 31% of those that have used a clinic in the past 2 years citing them.

- Shared waiting rooms are often unpleasant and unsettling for patients. Mixing maternity and fertility patients in waiting rooms is insensitive and distasteful, particularly for those that are in hospital for important checks or following miscarriage. Waiting room information materials such as posters of babies and mothers can be seen as insensitive, and a stark reminder for those struggling to conceive.

Practical Elements of a Patient Support Strategy, Focusing of Improved Patient Experience

The feedback from patients and patient groups, as well as the recommendations of ESHRE, HFEA, and other professional bodies provide an understanding of what is desirable in terms of patient support. The challenge is to build systems to meet these requirements in a consistent manner. This will not happen by chance and cannot rely on certain individuals. Organizations need to see "patient experience" as a key strategic objective, along with financial performance, success rates, and complication rates. Even if approached from a purely business perspective, this is good investment in terms of brand development and resilience in a very competitive and dynamic ecosystem. Putting patients first is the guiding principle that should be the common thread throughout the practice.

Reorganization of Outpatient Infertility Clinics in the NHS

Practical steps for the reorganization of NHS outpatient infertility clinics are summarized in Table 9.4.

How Do We Support Staff To Support Patients?

Only healthy and happy staff can provide proper patient support. The role of fertility clinic staff is to support the patients. The role of the senior management (clinical and business) is to support the clinic staff. It needs to be recognized that looking after patients with infertility poses special challenges. There is often a background of mental distress. Fertility treatments are expensive, time-consuming,

Table 9.4 Elements of patient support strategy

Organizational standards of NHS infertility clinics to optimize patient support

- For public organizations such as the NHS, to provide the expertise of a subspecialist consultant to every patient, at each appointment, the most effective model is the "hub and spoke." The various resources (spokes) are booked with a small number of patients each, according to their level of competence, and the subspecialist consultant (the hub) is supernumerary so that they can make all key management decisions and see the patients that need personal input: for example, a difficult decision about open myomectomy versus straight to IVF for a 41-year-old woman with poor ovarian reserve [16–18]

- Time allocation: especially for the follow-up consultation, when all test results are discussed along with "issues identified", prognosis, options, and strategy, most successful programs allocate 1 hour per appointment. This includes welfare of the child assessment, legal parenthood, and assessment of each patient's individual needs for support during treatment

- Number of patients per resource need to be capped to five or six as a maximum per clinic session (usually 3–5 hours)

- A member of the team should be allocated to coordinate patient numbers with available resources per session and develop the schedule for the clinic

- Preclinic triage is a very important function and should be done by an experienced member of the team based on pre-agreed criteria

- Nurse-led clinic appointment, as a first step, to even out the path, is usually associated with higher patient satisfaction

- After each clinic session there should be a clinic meeting for discussion of complex or interesting cases and shared learning

- There should be a clinical management strategy outlining the clinic's policy for all key indications and when to escalate. This should be discussed at regular operational meetings to comply with local and national standards

- There should also be a referral policy outlining referral acceptance criteria

- From the patient's perspective, the clinic "appointment" should be a small trail with several stops, including nurse meeting, doctor meeting, and admin meeting (to organize investigations, book next steps, discuss funding options, provide information material)

- The clinic session should be supported with teaching material, videos

- There should be a help point (specific individual) with telephone number/email/patient portal via electronic medical records for queries and troubleshooting after the appointment

- The clinical team should be proactive in educating the wider community in and out of the hospital (other consultants, general practitioners, patient groups) so that there is uniformity of message

- There should be active communication channels with the general practitioners to discuss queries

painful, and involve supraphysiological levels of hormones that affect the patients physically and mentally. This affects their ability to absorb and retain information and also may contribute to the higher levels of passive aggression, compared to patients in other fields [19]. Furthermore, infertility patients tend to be relatively young and physically well, unlike oncology or cardiology patients, and often do their own research and seek opinion from various doctors. Most patients with infertility have to pay for part or the whole of their treatment and express an expectation to receive concierge service.

The staff working in the ART Units may not receive special training to meet these expectations. Just like most "patient support" policies, most policies on "staff wellbeing" may be limited to a pamphlet, helpline, or perhaps the offer of some mentoring. This is not optimal. Staff happiness should be a key part of the service strategy. This would recognize the special challenges of their jobs and inform the planning of staff rotations, working environment, and workload: quantitative and qualitative. For example, one very difficult consultation with a very upset patient, or investigating and dealing with a complaint, could be enough load for someone's morning session. Many clinics may be crowded with tiny scanning rooms, little room for recuperation, overbooked schedules, where there is little space or time for staff to decompress and recover. The wider context is that only motivated staff will excel and this requires a sense of pride of ownership and a feeling of achievement and meaning. This requires ecological leadership models where the managers support and enable staff to grow, rather than monitoring performance and handing down instructions in a traditional manner [20]. Importantly, clinic staff need to feel appreciated more than they need to be paid.

Dealing with Complaints

In the HFEA National Patient Survey none of the patients who were successful said they were dissatisfied with the service, as opposed to 30% of those who were unsuccessful. This means that, dealing with women over 40, often accompanied by poor prognosis, appears to be a lose–lose scenario. When complaints arise (and they WILL), there should be a psychological buffer to protect clinical staff, so that they do not feel that their professionalism and integrity are being questioned each time. Staff should be supported, as well as patients.

The Crucial Function of IVF Coordination

This is an extremely important part of the service, which is often not acknowledged in staff schedules. This is not an administrative task, to be pushed to the margin of other activities. It is important, direct, patient care. IVF coordination is the function of connecting the dots between consultant review and commencement of treatment, or embryo transfer and next consultant review, or steps of treatment, or clinics and all other parties such as other specialties, the GP, etc. There are usually several loose ends to be sorted to produce a seamless treatment pathway.

IVF coordination sessions should be acknowledged as important clinical – not administrative – sessions and should be carried out by an integrated team of doctors, nurses, and embryologists. There needs to be a system to follow the progress of every patient who is approaching treatment, going through treatment, or finishing treatment, analogous to a control tower watching air traffic at an airport.

The Caveats of "Personalized Care" in Infertility

Most patients express the need to see the same person each time, preferably their physician, and have ready access to them. This is often challenging in a busy practice as the treatments can span for several weeks and mixed nonsurgical and surgical responsibilities must be met. What is possible, however, is to individualize the treatment plans, as outlined earlier, and provide a named nurse and IVF coordinator (team) to look after a group of patients under the overall supervision of the physician, who makes the key decisions. This will improve continuity and the communication of care.

A Genuinely Multidisciplinary Team (MDT) Approach

Although there usually is a "multidisciplinary team (MDT) meeting" that takes place from time to time, a genuine MDT approach is needed for each case. This means two-way interaction between key professionals at the diagnostic and treatment stages. For example, for women over 40 a psychological assessment and a nutritional assessment should take place along with preconceptional obstetric assessment and the core infertility investigations during the diagnostic/exploratory stages, before the problem is fully mapped and the treatment strategy is built. In addition to age and poor ovarian reserve, many patients may have other medical and psychological issues.

Business Growth

How to grow the service without compromising patient support and patient experience? A good model is the "fern": there should be different teams of doctors/nurse/administrators, each looking after limited segments of the patient population within the organization, all connected though a stem of shared resources, such as the embryology laboratory or the operating theatre. Trying to grow a business without this structure in place usually leads to reduced patient and staff satisfaction.

Treatment Packages and Structured Pathways

Many clinics offer treatment packages, for example two or more IVF cycles, which are useful as they provide some clarity about the overall cost and some discounts. These, however, are mostly quantitatively packages. They focus only on *number* of IVF cycles rather than elements that would create value and improve the experience [21].

Using the model of patient experience architecture, the aim should be to develop structured pathways, leading patients from point A to point B as outlined in Table 9.1. In designing various pathways within the fertility service, the element of the patient experience at each step needs to be the central focus and the most strategic consideration. Therefore, a good framework to use is the patient experience architecture to deliver optimal experiences to the different patient groups (segments): Table 9.2.

The pathways need to break down organizational silos (nurses, doctors, etc.) and address the diversity of patients and their needs, to produce unique and compelling experiences. Overall, realizing the organizational values with consistency at every touchpoint of patient contact should be a strategic priority.

Interactive Communication with Other Players in the Ecosystem

The structured pathways need to include active communication with other key players in the patient's ecosystem (Figure 9.1). Some examples include preconceptional advice, Early Pregnancy Unit, nutrition, psychology, support groups, organizations such as Fertility Network UK, financial advice and support, employment law, life coaching, and campaigning.

Digitalization of the Structured Pathways

Providing the above framework in a consistent and cost-effective manner may seem like a daunting task. Integration of digital technology offers its greatest value here. Many organizations are already advanced in digital transformation and several platforms and apps have been introduced on various services. To build more value in each pathway within the fertility service, reduce the cost and improve consistency, digital platforms such as specifically developed fertility clinic apps do exist. Some of them have integrated artificial intelligence and can automate clinic workflows while guiding patients through fertility treatment. The content of treatment pathways needs to be codesigned with patients and other stakeholders. Connections with other important partners within the ecosystem need to be activated and nurtured. Typically, a platform has two parts:

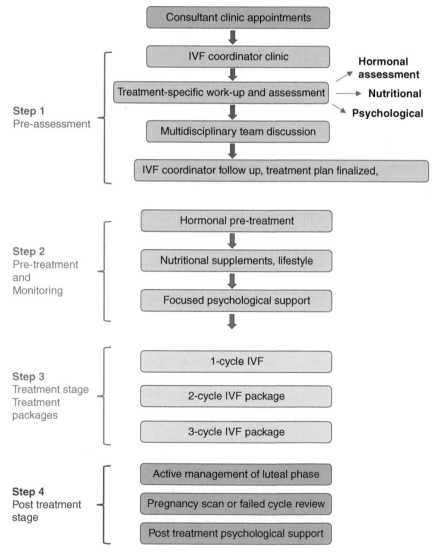

Figure 9.1 Example of an IVF pathway for women over 40

- A patient mobile application (mobile app) leading to a patient portal.
- A web-based clinic dashboard for the clinic staff.

Such platforms provide real-time onboarding materials, information documents and videos, pretreatment medical questionnaires, electronic consents, automated and personalized treatment guidance, medical appointment reminders, embryology results, access to medical records and letters, secure messaging between clinic and patient, mobile payments for clinic and cryostorage, and post-treatment outcomes capture.

The clinic staff can build customized patient pathways and journeys such as the ones previously outlined. The system has configurable logic for each clinic to automatically deliver notifications, messages, and content to guide them through each step of treatment, for example, consents, payments, and preparation reminders before various procedures. It reduces the need for follow-up and handholding of the patients along the way.

Digital platforms also provide real-time patient sentiment analysis using artificial intelligence, so the clinic can map the parts of the pathway where the patients are happy or unhappy. This is achieved through analysis of patterns in the content of messages [22]. Data on patient experience from using the service need to be collected, through client engagement platforms, at each point of contact, ideally at each interaction [23]. These should be analyzed and fed-back, in a constructive way, to operational meetings, staff appraisals, and job-planning.

Significant chunks of work in the Fertility Unit and the patient's journey can be automated and digitalized, freeing up time and resources, for example, electronic booking of appointments and payment of bills through digital platforms, electronic consents, and electronic prescribing and pharmacy service complete with home-delivery of drugs. Using artificial intelligence, the treatment pathways can be automated utilizing videos, prompts, and reminders about next steps. Virtual clinics, meetings, and training can become permanent features.

The nature of work the fertility clinic staff perform will change, as they will spend more quality time supervising and developing largely automated processes, instead of performing traditional tasks such as chasing down blood results, transcribing phone messages, or printing patient records. This work will not be an "extra supporting activity"; it will be *the core* of the clinical care in the near future. In essence, however, the main responsibility of the operators and management will remain the same: serve the patient's needs and deliver a fertility service with compassion, quality, speed, and flexibility, at competitive and affordable prices. From the business perspective, this approach is an optimal way to support the brand of the organization and add real value to the care that is provided.

The mere introduction of various clinic apps in clinics will not help unless they are used to support the development of experience architecture, with the central aim of optimizing patient support at every step through the journey. Additionally, the introduction of various client engagement platforms, usually in the context of marketing plans, not only does not improve much patient experience but also carries the risk of exposing all the deficiencies and weaknesses of the service.

Final Thoughts

"Patient support" is a wide concept that can be founded only on individualized clinical management strategies, appropriate clinical service organization, and staff support. The key requirements and practical steps to achieve this were discussed. It seems that digital transformation, if applied correctly, can offer a valued boost, by improving consistency, continuity and cost-effectiveness. "Patient experience" needs to be seen as a core strategic priority, as important as the service itself, to deliver the profession's core values at each interaction [24,25]. This requires leadership and the proper mentality and attitude of the entire staff in prioritizing the patient above all else by putting "patients first."

In the "client-segment" of women over 40 and women with poor prognosis, patient satisfaction is a far greater challenge, as it often needs to be achieved to provide "peace of mind" despite challenging odds.

"We are small worms, Zorba, very small worms on the tiniest leaf of a gigantic tree. This tiny leaf is our earth; the other leaves are the stars you see moving at night. We drag ourselves along on our tiny leaf, eagerly ferreting around in it. We smell it: it has an odor. We taste it: it can be eaten. We strike it: it resounds, shouting like a living thing. Some of us human beings, the most fearless, reach the edge of the leaf. We bend over this edge with open eyes and ears, observing chaos below. We shudder. We divine the terrible drop beneath us, occasionally hear a sound made by the gigantic tree's other leaves, sense the sap rising from the roots, swelling our hearts. In this way, leaning over the abyss, we realize with all our body and soul that we are being overcome by terror. What begins at that moment is—" I stopped. I had wanted to say, "What begins at that moment is poetry," but Zorba would not have understood, so I kept silent. "What begins?" asked Zorba eagerly. "Why did you stop?" "At that moment, Zorba, begins the great danger," I replied. "Some become dazed and delirious; others, growing afraid, take great pains to discover an answer that will brace their heart. These say, 'God.' Still others, calmly, bravely, look down at the drop from the leaf's edge and say, 'I like it.' "

Nikos Kazantzakis (1946), Zorba the Greek

Recommended Further Reading and Other Resources

- ESHRE: Routine psychosocial care in infertility and medically assisted reproduction – A guide for fertility staff. ESHRE psychology and counselling guideline development group. March 2015
- HFEA: Code of practice, ninth edition, December 2019
- HFEA: Pilot national fertility patient survey, 2018
- BICA: Guidelines for good practice in fertility counselling, fourth edition, 2019
- Fertility Network UK: https://fertilitynetwork uk.org/

References

1. ASRM. (2021). *COVID-19 updates and resources.* American Society for Reproductive Medicine. www .asrm.org/news-and-publications/covid-19/

2. Malave, A. (2020, April 3). *ASRM: tips on communicating with your patients during the COVID-19 pandemic.* American Society for Reproductive Medicine. www.asrm.org/news-and-publications/news-and-research/announcements/tips-on-communicating-with-your-patients–during-the-covid-19-pandemic/

3. ARCS/BFS. (2020). *ADDENDUM: COVID 19 VACCINATION ARCS-BFS Joint Working Group.* British Fertility Society. www.britishfertility society.org.uk/wp-content/uploads/2021/01/ARCS-BFS-COVID-19-vaccination-addendum-v2-13.1.20-rev2-FINAL.pdf

4. HFEA. (2020). *Directions given under the Human Fertilisation and Embryology Act 1990 (as amended) Covid-19 Treatment Commencement Strategy Ref: 0014 Version:2.* Human Fertilisation and Embryology Authority. https://portal.hfea.gov.uk/media/1543/2020-04-28-general-direction-0014-version.pdf

5. HFEA. (2021, January 5). *Coronavirus (COVID-19) guidance for professionals.* Human Fertilisation and Embryology Authority. www.hfea.gov.uk/treat ments/covid-19-and-fertility-treatment/corona virus-covid-19-guidance-for-professionals/

6. RCOG. (2021, January). *Coronavirus (COVID-19), pregnancy and women's health.* Royal College of Obstetricians & Gynaecologists. www.rcog.org.uk/en/guidelines-research-services/coronavirus-covid-19-pregnancy-and-womens-health/

7. Department of Health. (2021, January). *Joint Committee on Vaccination and Immunisation: advice on priority groups for COVID-19 vaccination, 30 December 2020.* GOV.UK. www.gov.uk/govern ment/publications/priority-groups-for-coronavirus-covid-19-vaccination-advice-from-the-jcvi-30-december-2020/joint-committee-on-vaccination-and-immunisation-advice-on-priority-groups-for-covid-19-vaccination-30-december-2020

8. Romanski, P. A., Bortoletto, P., Rosenwaks, Z., & Schattman, G. L. (2020). Delay in IVF treatment up to 180 days does not affect pregnancy outcomes in women with diminished ovarian reserve. *Human Reproduction, 35*(7), 1630–1636. https://doi.org/10.1093/humrep/deaa137

9. Bhattacharya, S., Maheshwari, A., Ratna, M. B., van Eekelen, R., Mol, B. W., & McLernon, D. J. (2020). Prioritizing IVF treatment in the post-COVID 19 era: a predictive modelling study based on UK national data. *Human Reproduction, 36*(3), 666–675. https://doi.org/10.1093/humrep/deaa339

10. WSP. (2020). *Hospitals after COVID-19: how do we design for an uncertain future?* WSP. www.wsp.com/en-GL/insights/hospitals-after-covid-19-how-do-we-design-for-an-uncertain-future

11. HFEA. (2019, December). *Read the Code of Practice.* Human Fertilisation and Embryology Authority. https://portal.hfea.gov.uk/knowledge-base/read-the-code-of-practice/

12. BICA. (2019). *Guidelines for Good Practice in Fertility Counselling 4th Edition 2019*. British Infertility Counselling Association. www.bica.net/item/1/BICA/Guidelines-for-Good-Practice-in-Fertility-Counselling-4th-Edition-2019.html

13. ESHRE. (2015, March). Routine psychosocial care in infertility and medically assisted reproduction – a guide for fertility staff. European Society of Human Reproduction and Embryology. www.eshre.eu/Guidelines-and-Legal/Guidelines/Psychosocial-care-guideline.aspx

14. Gameiro, S., Boivin, J., Dancet, E., Emery, M., Thorn, P., Van den Broeck, U., Venetis, C., Verhaak, C. M., Wischmann, T., & Vermeulen, N. (2016). Qualitative research in the ESHRE Guideline "Routine psychosocial care in infertility and medically assisted reproduction – a guide for staff." *Human Reproduction*, *31*(8), 1928–1929. https://doi.org/10.1093/humrep/dew155

15. HFEA. (2018). Pilot national fertility patient survey. Human Fertilisation and Embryology Authority. www.hfea.gov.uk/media/2702/pilot-national-fertility-patient-survey-2018.pdf.

16. Elrod, J. K., & Fortenberry, J. L. (2017). The hub-and-spoke organization design: an avenue for serving patients well. *BMC Health Services Research*, *17*(S1). https://doi.org/10.1186/s12913-017-2341-x

17. Hawkes, N. (2013). Hospitals without walls. *BMJ*, *347* (Sep 12), f5479–f5479. https://doi.org/10.1136/bmj.f5479

18. Shamshudin, M., & Nikolaou, D. (2015). *A national survey of organizational standards of fertility services*. Oral presentation, ESGE, Budapest, 2015. Annual meeting of the European Society of Gynaecological Endocrinology.

19. Poddar, S., Sanyal, N., & Mukherjee, U. (2014a). Psychological profile of women with infertility: a comparative study. *Industrial Psychiatry Journal*, *23*(2), 117. https://doi.org/10.4103/0972-6748.151682

20. Pistrui, J., & Dimov, D. (2018, October 26). *The role of a manager has to change in 5 key ways*. Harvard Business Review. https://hbr.org/2018/10/the-role-of-a-manager-has-to-change-in-5-key-ways

21. Hollebeek, L. D., & Macky, K. (2019). Digital content marketing's role in fostering consumer engagement, trust, and value: framework, fundamental propositions, and implications. *Journal of Interactive Marketing*, *45*, 27–41. https://doi.org/10.1016/j.intmar.2018.07.003

22. Campbell, C., Sands, S., Ferraro, C., Tsao, H.-Y. (Jody), & Mavrommatis, A. (2019a). From data to action: how marketers can leverage AI. *Business Horizons*, *63*(2), 227–243. https://doi.org/10.1016/j.bushor.2019.12.002

23. Bartolacci, G. (2019, September 12). *What is a customer engagement platform?* New Breed. www.newbreedmarketing.com/blog/what-is-a-customer-engagement-platform

24. Clark, N. (2016, June 15). *B2B communications is evolving – PR and marketing need to keep up*. Marketing Week. www.marketingweek.com/b2b-communications-is-evolving-pr-and-marketing-need-to-keep-up/

25. Yohn, D. L. (2015, February 3). *7 steps to deliver better customer experiences*. Harvard Business Review. https://hbr.org/2015/02/7-steps-to-deliver-better-customer-experiences?ab=at_articlepage_relatedarticles_horizontal_slot3

Chapter

10

Optimal Management of the First Trimester in Women over 40

Beth Cartwright and Aditi Naik

Introduction

Women over the age of 40 years are at a higher risk of early pregnancy complications such as miscarriage or ectopic pregnancy. They are also more likely to have pre-existing medical conditions, which further increase their risk of early pregnancy pathology, for example, previous pelvic inflammatory disease leading to a tubal ectopic, or uncontrolled diabetes increasing the risk of a miscarriage.

Women in this age group are also more likely to have conceived through fertility treatment, and may present with complications of this, such as multiple pregnancy or ovarian hyperstimulation syndrome. A woman's history of assisted reproductive technology and pre-existing subfertility is significant not only in accurately dating the pregnancy but also with regards to the psychological impact in case of a poor outcome.

The Role of the Early Pregnancy Unit

Early pregnancy units (EPUs) have become well established in most hospitals as a dedicated department providing specialist early pregnancy care. Women are referred by their GP or the A&E department with pain or bleeding in the first trimester and a transvaginal ultrasound scan is usually performed to assess the location and viability of the pregnancy. Women can also self-refer if they have a history of early pregnancy pathology for example a previous ectopic or molar pregnancy, or previous recurrent miscarriage. This model of care is recommended by the National Institute for Health and Care Excellence (NICE) [1] but local protocols may vary and some units have a full walk-in service.

NICE recommends that women with pain or bleeding in early pregnancy are seen in an early pregnancy assessment unit, and that this should be staffed by healthcare professionals specifically trained in the diagnosis and management of early pregnancy pathology [2].

General Points

Women should be advised to book their antenatal care early either by online self-referral, or through their GP. Women who have previously had poor outcomes may be eligible for a reassurance scan depending on the local EPU protocols.

Health and Lifestyle Advice

All women should be advised to maintain a healthy lifestyle in pregnancy by continuing a good diet and maintaining a healthy weight.

Folic acid 400 mcg should be taken from three months pre-conception until the end of the first trimester to reduce the risk of neural tube defects [3]. Women with certain medical conditions require a higher dose of 5 mg. These include epilepsy, diabetes, haematological conditions with a high cell turnover, women who are obese (body mass index, BMI, $\geq$30), as well as women who have previously had a child with a neural tube defect.

Vitamin D supplementation at a dose of 10 mcg should be encouraged routinely for pregnant and breastfeeding women. This is of particular importance in women of ethnic minority backgrounds, those with a raised BMI ($\geq$30) or limited mobility as they are at a higher risk of deficiency [4].

Some women may be eligible for free 'Health Start' vitamin supplements, which contain both folic acid and vitamin D, but these are also easily available over the counter at pharmacies.

Aspirin and Pre-Eclampsia Prophylaxis

Women who are above 40 years old are considered to be at a higher risk of developing pre-eclampsia and low dose aspirin should be offered to reduce the risk in women who meet the criteria as per the NICE guidance (Table 10.1) [5].

119

Table 10.1 Risk factors for pre-eclampsia [5]

High-risk factors Women with ONE of the following should be offered aspirin	Moderate risk factors Women with TWO of the following should be offered aspirin
Hypertensive disease during a previous pregnancy	First pregnancy
Chronic kidney disease	Age ≥40 years
Autoimmune disease such as systemic lupus erythematosus or antiphospholipid syndrome	Pregnancy interval >10 years
Type 1 or Type 2 diabetes	Body mass index (BMI) ≥35 kg/m^2 at first visit
Chronic hypertension	Family history of pre-eclampsia
	Multiple pregnancy

Women who have one high-risk factor, or two moderate-risk factors should be commenced on 75–150 mg once daily from 12 weeks of gestation to be continued until delivery.

A Cochrane review reported a reduction in risk of pre-eclampsia by 17% with the use of anti-platelet agents [6], although a more recent systematic review showed an absolute risk reduction of 2–5% depending on baseline risk [7].

Studies have shown no increase in maternal or neonatal bleeding risk, or congenital abnormalities with maternal low dose aspirin use [8]. Contraindications for use include allergy, NSAID-induced bronchospasm, or gastro-intestinal bleeding or ulcers.

Venous Thrombo-Embolism (VTE) Risk

Venous thrombo-embolism is the second highest cause of maternal mortality in the UK and age is a crucial risk factor.

The VTE risk score should therefore be assessed at booking and at every admission. Attendance at the EPU is an opportunity to commence low molecular weight heparin (LWMH) if required in order to reduce the risk.

Women who score 4 or more on the Royal College of Obstetricians and Gynaecologists (RCOG) risk stratification tool (Figure 10.1) require LMWH from the first trimester. Women over the age of 35 will score 1 for age, and women who have conceived via assisted reproductive technology (ART) will score an additional 1 [9].

Women who are on long-term anticoagulation, that is warfarin or direct acting oral anticoagulants (DOACs), should consider switching to an intermediate or treatment dose LMWH as soon as possible. Urgent discussion with a haematologist is required for these women if a plan is not already in place. A referral to the obstetric medicine clinic should be completed without delay.

Assessing Co-Morbidities

Women above the age of 40 are more likely to have co-morbidities than the younger patient. Ideally, women with significant medical problems will have had pre-conception counselling with an obstetrician or their GP but this is not always the case and the EPU may be the first opportunity for a healthcare professional to review their pregnancy in the context of their medical condition.

A thorough drug history should be taken to ensure that any drugs which are considered teratogenic or unsafe in pregnancy are identified, and it may be appropriate to change to an alternative known to be safe in pregnancy. For example, for the hypertensive patient with no end organ complications, ACE inhibitors should be stopped and labetalol can be used instead. Liaison with the GP or hospital specialist may be required because some medication will need to be continued or an alternative sought.

The patient may require an assessment by a different speciality, for example a neurology review in the case of poorly controlled epilepsy. An appropriate referral to the speciality as well as the dedicated obstetric medicine clinic should be made early. It may be worth considering if any further investigations may be required, for example an echocardiogram in women with known valvular disease, and again these should be requested in a timely fashion to better inform the care and management plans made at their first obstetric appointment.

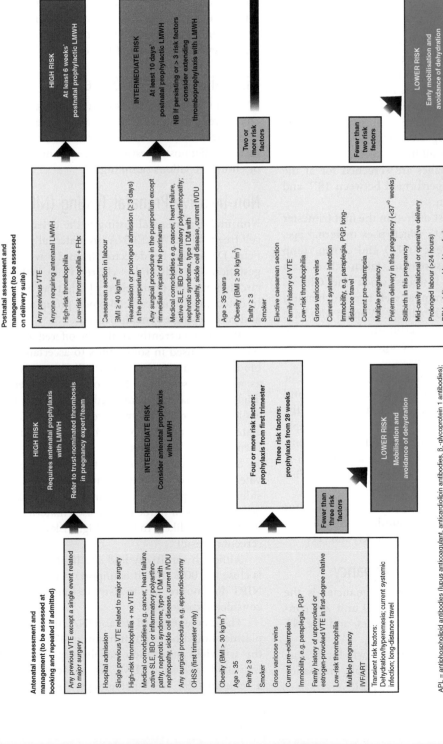

APL = antiphospholipid antibodies (lupus anticoagulant, anticardiolipin antibodies, β2-glycoprotein 1 antibodies); ART = assisted reproductive technology; BMI based on booking weight; DM = diabetes mellitus; FHx = family history; gross varicose veins = symptomatic, above knee or associated with phlebitis/oedema/skin changes; high-risk thrombophilia = antithrombin deficiency, protein C or S deficiency, compound or homozygous for low-risk thrombophilias; IBD = inflammatory bowel disease; immobility = ≥ 3 days; IVDU = intravenous drug user; IVF = in vitro fertilisation; LMWH = low-molecular-weight heparin; long-distance travel = > 4 hours; low-risk thrombophilia = heterozygous for factor V Leiden or prothrombin G20210A mutations; OHSS = ovarian hyperstimulation syndrome; PGP = pelvic girdle pain with reduced mobility; PPH = postpartum haemorrhage; thrombophilia = inherited or acquired; VTE = venous thromboembolism.

Figure 10.1 Royal College of Obstetricians and Gynaecologists venous thrombo-embolism risk stratification tool. *Source:* Reproduced from [9], with the permission of the Royal College of Obstetricians and Gynaecologists.

First Trimester Screening

Screening for aneuploidy forms part of the NHS Fetal Anomaly Screening Programme (FASP), which was established in 2001 [10]. Screening is offered routinely to all women in the UK. It is of particular importance in women above the age of 40 as the risk of aneuploidy increases with age. Conditions screened for are Trisomies 21 (Down's Syndrome), 13 (Patau's Syndrome) and 18 (Edward's Syndrome). The risk of a pregnancy affected by Trisomy 21 rises from 1:1500 at the age of 20 to 1:100 at the age of 40, and is almost 1:20 at 45 years of age [10]. The risks of Trisomies 13 and 18, although not as high, also rise exponentially with maternal age.

Women have the choice of no screening at all, and this must be respected, or screening for T21 only, T18/13 only or all three.

Structural anomalies are screened for at the fetal anomaly scan performed between 18^{+0} and 20^{+6} weeks' gestation.

The screening test offered in the first trimester is the 'combined test', which uses maternal age, the nuchal translucency (NT) and crown rump length (CRL) measurement taken at a scan between 11 and 14 weeks when the CRL is between 45 and 84 mm, as well two biochemical tests – free βhCG and PAPP-A. Women who have conceived via in vitro fertilisation (IVF) using donor eggs should use the age of the donor at the time of egg collection.

If an NT measurement cannot be obtained, or if a woman books her pregnancy too late and misses the window for the combined test, the recommended screening test is the 'quadruple test', which uses maternal age and four biochemical markers – AFP, hCG, uE3 and inhibin-A between 14^{+2} and 20^{+0} weeks' gestation. This screens for T21 only.

The detection rate is approximately 90% for Trisomy 21 and 95% for Trisomies 13 and 18, with a false positive rate of approximately 5% [11].

Screening in Multiple Pregnancy

The test of choice for twin pregnancies is the combined test. Each feto-placental unit will contribute to the biochemical markers, and the NT should be measured for each twin.

The risk will be calculated per twin for dichorionic pregnancies, and for the whole pregnancy for monochorionic pregnancies [12].

In the case of a viable first twin with a second empty sac, combined screening can still be used, as there is minimal contribution to the biochemical markers. In the case of a viable first twin, with a non-viable second twin, contribution to the biochemical markers from the non-viable twin may render the results inaccurate [10]. The patient should be made aware of this, and a referral to fetal medicine should be considered for further discussion on screening options.

Screening for higher order multiple pregnancies is beyond the scope of this chapter.

High Risk Combined Screening

Women who receive a risk of 1:150 or greater are considered 'high risk' [10] and are referred to the Fetal Medicine department for consideration of invasive diagnostic testing, either amniocentesis or chorionic villous sampling.

Non-Invasive Prenatal Testing (NIPT)

Non-invasive prenatal testing is the detection of cell free fetal DNA (cffDNA) in maternal plasma. Fetal DNA can be detected from 10 weeks of gestation onwards and is cleared from maternal circulation hours post-delivery [13]. It can be used to detect aneuploidies, fetal blood group and sex and certain single gene disorders.

It is not currently routinely offered on the NHS but is used in some units to ascertain fetal blood group in women who are RhD negative, or as a second screening test for women deemed 'high risk' based on combined screening. It may avoid the need for an invasive test and its associated risk of pregnancy loss if these women are then found to be low risk.

Some women opt to have this test in the private sector. Women may specifically wish to consider this if a previous pregnancy was affected by an aneuploidy or if due to increased maternal age, they are more likely to have a high risk combined screening result.

Although sensitivity and specificity for NIPT is close to 100% [14], it is important to note that NIPT does not replace invasive testing, and is not considered diagnostic.

The percentage of fetal DNA in maternal plasma should be at a minimum of 4%; less than this will yield an invalid or a false negative result. Increased maternal BMI is associated with a reduced fetal DNA percentage. As cffDNA is produced by the placenta, another source of potential error is placental mosaicism leading to a false positive result [14].

Non-invasive prenatal testing can be performed in twin pregnancies, where the pregnancy is known to be monozygotic (monochorionic pregnancies). Dichorionic pregnancies can be either dizygotic or monozygotic and this cannot be determined on ultrasound. The majority of dichorionic pregnancies are dizygotic. This poses challenges when it comes to NIPT as the levels of fetal DNA from each twin in maternal circulation may be discordant and lead to erroneous results [11]. The couple must be made aware of this as well as the lack of data on the accuracy of testing in dichorionic pregnancies.

Multiple Pregnancy

Increased maternal age is an independent risk factor for multiple pregnancy.

The rate of monozygotic twins has remained stable worldwide at approximately 3–5 per 1000 births. The rate of dizygotic twins varies geographically and is dependent on maternal age, ethnicity and other factors [15].

The rate of multiple pregnancies has increased over time due to the increased use and success of ART and correlates to the number of embryos transferred, with a rate of 18% with the transfer of two embryos increasing to 24% after four embryos are transferred [16].

In the US, the twin birth rate increased by 76% over 30 years from 1980 to 2009 [17]. The twin birth rate in the UK is approximately 15.8 per 1000 live births.

Multiple pregnancy significantly increases the risk of both maternal and perinatal morbidity and mortality, with higher order multiples at a higher risk than twin pregnancies.

The increased risk of preterm birth and low birthweight leads to an increased risk of cerebral palsy: 8 times higher in twins and 47 times higher in triplets compared with singletons, as well as stillbirth: 4.5 times higher in twins and 6.5 times higher in triplets compared with singletons [15].

Prevention strategies used in ART include limiting the number of embryos that can be transferred per cycle, and cancelling an ovulation induction cycle if there is evidence of hyperstimulation.

General Advice

Women pregnant with a multiple pregnancy should be advised to maintain a healthy balanced diet and lifestyle. Advice regarding nutritional supplements is similar to that for a singleton pregnancy.

Multiple pregnancy is an extra point in the VTE risk score, and women who score 4 or more should be commenced on LMWH in the first trimester [9].

Multiple pregnancy is also considered to be a moderate risk factor for pre-eclampsia, and aspirin 75–150 mg once daily should be recommended from 12 weeks for women who are over 40 with a multiple pregnancy [5].

Women should be counselled regarding the increased risk of medical conditions in pregnancy such as anaemia, pre-eclampsia, gestational diabetes, obstetric cholestasis, as well as obstetric complications such as preterm birth, stillbirth, operative delivery and postpartum haemorrhage.

Determining Chorionicity and Amnionicity

The chorionicity and amnionicity of a multiple pregnancy is determined by ultrasound, and the earliest time this can be done is around 6–8 weeks, although the most accurate time is during the 11–14 week scan [15].

Prior to 10 weeks the chorionicity is determined by the number of gestation sacs. Each gestation sac will develop its own placenta and chorion [18] and therefore two separate gestational sacs will represent a dichorionic pregnancy. The number of amniotic sacs within a gestational sac will determine the amnionicity.

At the 11–14 week or dating scan, NICE recommends the following to determine chorionicity and amnionicity: the number of placental masses; the presence of amniotic membranes and membrane thickness; the lambda or T-sign [12].

The lambda sign is a remnant of chorion in between the two amniotic sacs in a dichorionic placentation. The absence of a lambda sign along with paper thin inter-twin membrane, that is the 'T' sign, is specific for monochorionicity [15].

In the second trimester, discordant sex is a sign of dizygosity and therefore dichorionicity.

Determining the chorionicity and amnionicity is essential in a multiple pregnancy as it will inform the risk and therefore the management of the ongoing pregnancy, with dichorionic placentation being at significantly lower risk of complications than a monochorionic pregnancy. An assessment of this in the EPU will allow for earlier counselling of the patient, and timely referrals to appropriate departments such as fetal medicine.

Multifetal Pregnancy Reduction

This is the reduction of a higher order multiple pregnancy, that is triplets or quadruplets, to a twin pregnancy in order to mitigate the risk of a higher order multiple pregnancy as discussed previously [15].

This is an incredibly difficult decision to make for the couple and must be discussed sensitively and with empathy. It may not be acceptable to them depending on their belief system and social background, or particularly if they conceived via IVF after a history of subfertility.

It is important to note that this is different from selective fetal reduction where one fetus is terminated due to a chromosomal or structural anomaly [15]. In multifetal pregnancy reduction, the pregnancy that is terminated is usually the one easy to access for the procedure. The procedure is performed by injecting potassium chloride into the fetus' thorax under ultrasound guidance, either transabdominally or transvaginally. The procedure is not without risk, with the procedure-related loss rate ranging from 4.5% for triplets to 15% for sextuplets [15].

Studies have shown that a reduction from triplets to twins reduces the risk of complications, and outcomes are similar to those conceived spontaneously [16]

Miscarriage

Risk of Miscarriage

The majority of first trimester losses are caused by chromosomal abnormalities, most commonly Trisomies 16, 21 and 22 [19]. The risk of miscarriage increases with age due to the declining quality of the remaining oocytes, and therefore increased risk of aneuploidy.

The risk of a first trimester miscarriage is over 50% in women in their early 40s, rising to over 90% in women over the age of 45 (Table 10.2). Women should therefore be counselled appropriately, and expectations managed sensitively. The

Table 10.2 Age related risk of miscarriage [20]

Age, years	Risk of miscarriage, %
12–19	13
20–24	11
25–29	12
30–34	15
35–39	25
40–44	51
≥45	93

increased risk of miscarriage may influence the planned follow-up for a patient, for example, a further scan may be warranted for reassurance.

Diagnosis of Miscarriage

NICE has published guidance on the ultrasound diagnosis of a miscarriage [1]. A miscarriage can be diagnosed on the first ultrasound scan if the mean gestational sac diameter is >25 mm with no internal structures, or if CRL is >7 mm with no fetal heartbeat. If the dimensions are smaller than these, a repeat scan is required in 7–14 days. The ultrasound scan must be performed transvaginally, and the diagnosis must be confirmed by two trained clinicians. These guidelines are for pregnancies that are conceived spontaneously to allow for variations in cycle lengths and uncertainty regarding menstruation dates.

There is more certainty, however, when it comes to pregnancies conceived via IVF. The exact gestational age can be easily calculated once the date of embryo transfer and the age of the blastocyst is known. If the size of the pregnancy is not in keeping with the gestational age, the diagnosis of a miscarriage can be more confidently made on the first scan even if the criteria above are not met. However, if there is any uncertainty it is always best to repeat the scan a week later.

Management of Miscarriage

Women can be offered expectant, medical or surgical options for the management of miscarriage. Some units may have exclusion criteria for expectant and medical management based on the size of the pregnancy to reduce the risk of heavy bleeding requiring acute admission and emergency surgery. Ultimately, the choice is the woman's, and she should feel supported in her decision. Her choice may be influenced by previous experiences, the support network available to her and her psychological state.

Expectant management or 'waiting and watching' is successful in up to 60% of women by 14 days after the diagnosis [21]. This is higher in women who have already started bleeding and have an 'incomplete miscarriage.' The disadvantage of expectant management is heavy unpredictable bleeding at home and women should be warned about this. Women should be advised to perform a pregnancy test after three weeks, and to contact the EPU if they have ongoing bleeding beyond three weeks.

Medical management is the use of a single dose of misoprostol 800 mcg. This is usually inserted vaginally but can also be taken orally if that is the woman's preference. Success rates are between 80% and 90% [21] and most women will pass the pregnancy within the first 48 hours. A repeat dose can be considered if the first dose is unsuccessful. Analgesia should be provided and women should be informed of potential gastrointestinal side effects. Misoprostol is contraindicated in women with cardiovascular disease and should be used with caution in women with conditions that predispose to diarrhoea. Risks, as above, include heavy, unpredictable bleeding at home, infection and incomplete miscarriage. Again, women should be advised to perform a pregnancy test after three weeks, and to contact the EPU if they have ongoing bleeding beyond three weeks.

There is no evidence for the use of misoprostol in incomplete miscarriages; expectant or surgical management should be offered in these cases.

Surgical management can be performed under a general anaesthetic or local anaesthetic (known as manual vacuum aspiration). Risks are similar for both, and include bleeding, infection, retained products of conception, uterine adhesions, uterine perforation and cervical trauma. Cervical preparation with misoprostol may be useful in women with a delayed miscarriage who have not had any bleeding. Appropriate patient selection is vital for surgical procedures performed under local anaesthetic and the patient must be thoroughly counselled prior to the procedure.

Intrauterine adhesions are detected in up to 19% of women following a miscarriage but of these only 14% are severe [22]. The frequency and severity of adhesions is increased following multiple surgical procedures and recurrent miscarriage. Reproductive outcomes are similar following all forms of management of miscarriage. Therefore, women should be reassured that their choice of management of miscarriage will not affect the likelihood of scar tissue affecting future pregnancies. This may be a particular concern for women over 40 who are more likely to want to conceive again quickly.

Histology should be checked following surgical management in order to ensure gestational trophoblastic disease has been excluded. With expectant and medical management, where no histology is available, the EPU should contact the patient to ensure that a pregnancy test three weeks after the miscarriage is negative.

Recurrent Miscarriage

Recurrent miscarriage or recurrent pregnancy loss is defined by the RCOG as the loss of three or more consecutive pregnancies before the pregnancy has reached viability (24 weeks of gestation in the UK), and affects approximately 1% of couples [20].

The European Society of Human Reproduction and Embryology (ESHRE) guidance advises a diagnosis can be made after two consecutive miscarriages [23]. This may be a more pragmatic approach in women who are above 40 years of age, allowing for earlier diagnosis of treatable conditions such as antiphospholipid syndrome, thyroid dysfunction or certain anatomical abnormalities.

The RCOG recommends that women with recurrent miscarriage should be looked after by a healthcare professional with the necessary skills and expertise and that where available this might be within a recurrent miscarriage clinic.

Investigations that should be carried out include testing for antiphospholipid syndrome, thyroid function including thyroid peroxidase antibodies and a 3D ultrasound to assess for anatomical abnormalities [23]. Testing for inherited thrombophilias is contentious as there is, at best, a weak link to miscarriage, and LMWH has not been proven to be an effective treatment. Cytogenetic testing on products of conception is offered on the NHS after the third miscarriage in order to detect couples who are carrying a balanced translocation leading to recurrent miscarriage. If this is found in the pregnancy tissue then parental karyotyping is recommended to ascertain if a balanced translocation in the couple has led to the chromosomal abnormality in the fetus. A partner will carry a balanced structural chromosomal anomaly in approximately 2–5% of couples with recurrent miscarriages [20]. The risk of miscarriage depends on the size and genetic material of these segments. Referral to a geneticist is warranted in these situations to discuss further options.

Couples may want to opt for private cytogenetic testing prior to experiencing a third miscarriage, and although a positive result of a trisomy (the most common cause for miscarriage and more likely with increasing age) is unlikely to change management or impact future pregnancies, many couples find closure if they are able to understand the cause of the miscarriage.

There is no evidence for the routine use of progesterone in recurrent miscarriage despite its widespread use. The PROMISE trial was a multicentre double-blind randomised control trial, where women with a history of unexplained recurrent miscarriage were randomised to progesterone or placebo supplements to use through the first trimester. There was no significant difference in the live birth rate between the two groups (65.8% in the progesterone group and 63.3% in the placebo group; RR 1.04 (CI 0.94–1.15). The overall live birth rate was over 60% [24]. Women may find this reassuring – that even after three pregnancy losses the chance of having a live birth is higher than the chance of another miscarriage.

The PRISM trial, also a multicentre double-blind randomised control trial, investigated the use of progesterone in the context of a threatened miscarriage, that is bleeding in early pregnancy. Women were randomised to receive either progesterone or placebo supplements, which were commenced from initial presentation until 16 weeks of gestation. There was no benefit overall in terms of live births after 34 weeks of gestation with progesterone (75% in the progesterone group and 72% in the placebo group; RR 1.03; CI 1.00–1.07). Subgroup analysis showed a very small increase in live birth rate in women who had had three or more previous miscarriages [25]. However, this was a post-hoc analysis and further research is needed to confirm a benefit of progesterone in this particular group of patients.

There is no evidence for the use of levothyroxine in euthyroid women with thyroid peroxidase antibody (TPO) antibodies [26]. In this group thyroid function tests (TFTs) should be checked at approximately 7–9 weeks of gestation and treatment commenced if hypothyroid.

Some units have a dedicated recurrent miscarriage clinic that can investigate and manage these women in conjunction with the local EPU. The role of the EPU is key in providing advice and support, and reassurance scans in future pregnancies. Evidence has shown that support from a dedicated EPU can improve prognosis in the future pregnancy [20]. However, maternal age and number of previous miscarriages are both independent risk factors for further miscarriages, with the risk of a further pregnancy loss approximately 40% after three consecutive miscarriages.

Recurrent Implantation Failure

Recurrent implantation failure (RIF) is a term used specifically in women undergoing ART. There is no official definition, but most consider it a failure of three or more IVF embryo transfer cycles with good-quality embryos. Proposed mechanisms for implantation failure include immunological, infective, genetic and anatomical. Risk factors include smoking, BMI and crucially, maternal age. The risk of RIF increases with age due to the increased risk of aneuploidy and declining quality of embryos. Treatment of RIF is multifactorial and dependent on the cause.

Ectopic Pregnancy

An ectopic pregnancy is a pregnancy that has implanted outside the endometrial cavity. Of ectopic pregnancies, 95% are tubal, the majority of which are ampullary. Increased maternal age and ART are recognised as independent risk factors.

The overall incidence of a tubal ectopic is 1.1% [27]. Risk factors include increased maternal age, previous ectopic pregnancy, previous tubal surgery including sterilisation, smoking, previous pelvic inflammatory disease (PID) and ART. It is important to note that up to 50% of women with ectopic pregnancies do not have any risk factors.

The cause of an increased risk of ectopic pregnancies with maternal age is unclear; hypotheses include abnormal tubal function or scarring from previous PID. One study reported that women ≥39 years were nine times more likely to have an ectopic pregnancy compared with women aged

27–32 [28]. Older women are also more likely to have conceived through IVF which is an independent risk factor for ectopic pregnancy. Ectopic pregnancies have been reported in up to 5.4% of IVF pregnancies [29]. Known tubal factor infertility is a significant risk factor for ectopic pregnancies after IVF, along with previous pelvic surgery and previous PID.

A heterotopic pregnancy is one in which there are two simultaneous pregnancies with different implantation sites: one intrauterine and one extra-uterine. The background risk of a heterotopic pregnancy is 1 in 30,000 but the likelihood of a heterotopic pregnancy increases significantly with IVF to 1:100 and up to 1:45 if four embryos are transferred [30].

In the advanced maternal age population, women are more likely to have undergone ART in order to conceive and therefore it is essential to be aware of the possibility of a heterotopic pregnancy. An intrauterine pregnancy does not necessarily rule out another pregnancy which is an ectopic. The adnexae need to be thoroughly assessed if the woman remains persistently symptomatic.

Ectopic pregnancies can be managed expectantly, medically or surgically. There are national criteria set out by the RCOG and NICE based on symptoms, size of pregnancy, haemodynamic stability and βhCG levels. The role of the clinician in the EPU is to support the woman in her decision-making, allowing her to make an informed choice about the management option she has opted for. Her decision may be influenced by previous experience, future fertility aspirations or planned fertility treatments.

Expectant Management

Between 50% and 88% of ectopic pregnancies will resolve spontaneously [31], assuming appropriate patient selection, and this avoids the need for more invasive surgical or medical management. NICE recommends expectant management in women who are haemodynamically stable and pain-free with βhCG levels <1000 IU/l, and ectopic pregnancies measuring <35 mm with no fetal heartbeat [1]. Expectant management may be considered in women with βhCG levels up to 1500 IU/l.

Ectopic pregnancies managed expectantly can take weeks to resolve, and although this method of management confers the least morbidity to the patient, the patient may feel that she does want to wait for the pregnancy to resolve as she wishes to try to conceive again without delay, or in the case of women undergoing ART, commence another IVF cycle. Depending on the clinical situation it may also be appropriate to offer or recommend surgical management in women planning further IVF treatment to reduce the risk of a recurrent ectopic in the same tube. If the woman does not plan further spontaneous conception then there is little value in conserving the tube. On the other hand, other women over 40 may prefer to conserve the tube if they are not eligible for NHS-funded IVF treatment and are not in a position to self-fund.

Medical Management

Medical management with methotrexate is appropriate in women who meet the criteria as above, but with βhCG levels up to 5000 IU/l [1]. As methotrexate is a teratogenic drug, it is imperative that an intrauterine pregnancy has been ruled out and a definitive diagnosis of an ectopic pregnancy has been made prior to administration.

Ectopic pregnancies managed medically with methotrexate can take weeks to resolve. Due to its teratogenicity, women must not conceive for three months after administration. This again poses similar issues with regards to timing another pregnancy. If a woman over 40 wants to pursue another fresh IVF cycle then methotrexate will rarely be the management of choice due to the delay it imposes and the subsequent effect this may have on the quantity of eggs collected.

Methotrexate is a cytotoxic drug and can have significant side effects and potential end organ implications. It should be used with caution in women with known haematological, hepatic and renal disorders. The British National Formulary states that the risk of toxicity with regards to bone marrow suppression is increased with advanced age.

Surgical Management

Surgical management remains the definitive treatment for women who are haemodynamically unstable, do not meet the inclusion criteria for expectant or medical management, or have failed these methods. This is usually by laparoscopic salpingectomy.

A salpingotomy is considered when there is a history of fertility-reducing factors or damage to the contralateral tube due to, for example, PID or previous ectopic pregnancy as higher rates of subsequent intrauterine pregnancies have been found in these women compared with salpingectomy.

Women undergoing ART may prefer to have a salpingectomy over a salpingotomy to reduce the risk of a recurrence of ectopic pregnancy in the affected tube, as well as the risk of residual trophoblast which can lead to prolonged follow-up and potentially further treatment.

The ESEP study compared salpingotomy with salpingectomy for treatment of a tubal ectopic pregnancy with regards to impact on future fertility in women with a healthy contralateral tube. The cumulative ongoing pregnancy rate was 61% after a salpingotomy, and 56% after a salpingectomy, which was not clinically significant, confirming that a salpingectomy, in the presence of a healthy contralateral tube, does not impact on future fertility compared with a salpingotomy. Women are also at an increased risk of persistent trophoblast (7% versus <1%) and recurrent ectopic (8% versus 5%) following a salpingotomy compared with a salpingectomy [32].

Management of the Heterotopic Pregnancy

This will be decided on a case-to-case basis and is dependent on the site of the ectopic pregnancy, the viability of the intrauterine pregnancy, haemodynamic stability and the woman's wishes.

In the haemodynamically unstable woman, surgical management is essential. It is crucial that the uterus is not cannulated and manipulation avoided during surgery.

Methotrexate cannot be used, even locally, if there is an ongoing viable intrauterine pregnancy.

Pregnancy of Unknown Location

Definition

A pregnancy of unknown location (PUL) is the presence of a positive pregnancy test but no visible pregnancy on a transvaginal ultrasound scan [33]. The rate of PULs can vary between EPUs, ranging from 8% to 31% [34], and can depend on the experience of the sonographer and the quality of the machine used. The term PUL is not a final

diagnosis and further monitoring in the form of blood tests or scans will be required before a diagnosis can be made. Women should be referred to a dedicated EPU for appropriate monitoring and follow-up until a final diagnosis is reached.

The final outcomes of a PUL can be as follows:
1) intrauterine pregnancy, either viable or nonviable;
2) ectopic pregnancy;
3) persistent PUL;
4) failing PUL.

The majority of women will have either a failing PUL or an intrauterine pregnancy. Ectopic pregnancy will be diagnosed eventually in 8–16% of women [35].

Management

A thorough history is vital including symptoms of bleeding and pain, as well as risk factors for ectopic pregnancy and previous pregnancy history, as this will form part of the risk stratification tool.

Units will vary in their management of PULs and will have a local guideline or model they use. This may depend on local patient factors, scanning expertise and availability of the EPU services.

Biochemical investigations form a key component of the management of PULs.

βhCG

At the time of initial diagnosis βhCG should be tested. This may need to be repeated 48 hours later; the ratio will then inform further follow-up. A rise of over 66% predicts an intrauterine pregnancy with a positive predictive value of 96.5% [34]. A fall of over 15% is likely to be failing PUL. Anything in between this should be considered high risk of an ectopic pregnancy.

Progesterone

Progesterone is released by the corpus luteum, and the initial level indicates the viability of the pregnancy. A level of <20 nmol/l indicates a failing pregnancy with a positive predictive value of ≥95% [34]. A level >60 nmol/l strongly indicates a viable intrauterine pregnancy. Progesterone should not be used alone, but in conjunction with the βhCG ratio to form part of the clinical picture.

It is important to bear in mind that ongoing or live ectopic pregnancies can produce a biochemical picture which mimics that of an early IUP, and so a repeat scan should be considered once the βhCG is at a level at which an IUP would be expected to be visualised (approximately 1000 IU/l).

Patients should be counselled regarding the possibility of an ectopic pregnancy and risk of rupture. Appropriate safety net advice should be provided to instruct them to attend A&E in case of acute pain or collapse, and women should be advised against travel. The above outcomes should be explained to the patient, and it may be that one outcome is more likely than the others based on the clinical history and examination, so the woman's expectations should be appropriately managed.

The period of time between an initial diagnosis of PUL to when a final diagnosis is made can be a time of anxiety for women, as the unknown can sometimes lead to greater apprehension and fear than a diagnosis of a miscarriage or ectopic, and patients should be counselled sensitively.

The Psychological Impact of Early Pregnancy Pathology in Women over 40

A poor outcome in early pregnancy can be devastating at any age, regardless of previous obstetric and fertility history. Women above the age of 40 are more likely to have a history of subfertility and have conceived a much-wanted pregnancy via ART. Even if the pregnancy was conceived spontaneously, most women will be aware that fertility is reduced at this age and that the risk of miscarriage is increased, both reducing the likelihood of a further successful pregnancy. A poor outcome in these women can have a significant psychological impact on the couple and they should be treated with empathy and sensitivity.

Women and their partners may find it helpful to engage in support groups hosted by charities such as The Miscarriage Association or The Ectopic Pregnancy Trust. Some units may have direct access to counsellors, while those that do not can advise women and their partners to seek support via primary care.

It is also important to remember that not all pregnancies are planned and for some women this may be an unexpected pregnancy. It is always prudent to ask whether the pregnancy was planned, to sensitively explore the woman's feeling towards it and to provide contraception if required after early pregnancy loss. If the pregnancy is ongoing and the woman is considering abortion, provide her with information on the next steps to take to obtain this.

References

1. *Ectopic pregnancy and miscarriage: diagnosis and initial management (NG126).* NICE. 2019.

2. *Ectopic pregnancy and miscarriage; Quality standard (QS69).* NICE. 2014.

3. *Antenatal care for uncomplicated pregnancies (CG62).* NICE. 2008.

4. *Vitamin D: supplement use in specific population groups (PH56).* NICE. 2014.

5. *Hypertension in pregnancy: diagnosis and management (NG133).* NICE. 2019.

6. Duley L, Henderson-Smart DJ, Meher S, King JF. Antiplatelet agents for preventing pre-eclampsia and its complications. *Cochrane Database Syst Rev.* 2007, (**2**):CD004659.

7. Henderson JT, Whitlock EP, O'Connor E, et al. *Low-dose aspirin for prevention of morbidity and mortality from preeclampsia: a systematic evidence review for the U.S. Preventive Services Task Force.* Ann Intern Med. 2014, Vol. **160** (10):695–703.

8. American College of Obstetricians and Gynecologists. *Low-dose aspirin use during pregnancy. ACOG Committee Opinion No. 743. Obstet Gynecol.* 2018, Vol. **132**:e44–52.

9. *Reducing the Risk of Venous Thromboembolism during Pregnancy and the Puerperium. Green-top Guideline No. 37a.* Royal College of Obstetricians and Gynaecologists. 2015.

10. *Down's syndrome, Edwards' syndrome and Patau's syndrome. NHS Fetal Anomaly Screening Programme Handbook.* Public Health England. 2018.

11. Ashoor Al Mahri G, Nicolaides KH. Evolution in screening for Down syndrome. *Obstet Gynecol* 2019, Vol. **21**:51–57.

12. *Twin and triplet pregnancy (NG137).* NICE. 2019.

13. Gekas J, Langlois S, Ravitsky V, et al. Identification of trisomy 18, trisomy 13, and Down syndrome from maternal plasma. *Appl Clin Genet* 2014, Vol. **7**:127–131.

14. *Non-invasive Prenatal Testing for Chromosomal Abnormality using Maternal Plasma DNA.* Scientific Impact Paper No. 15. Royal College of Obstetricians and Gynaecologists. 2014.

15. Multiple Pregnancy. *StratOG*. [Online] [Cited: 06 July 2020.] https://elearning.rcog.org.uk/ multiple-pregnancy/epidemiology-multiple-pregnancy. Royal College of Obstetricians and Gynaecologists.

16. Dodd JM, Dowswell T, Crowther CA. Reduction of the number of fetuses for women with a multiple pregnancy. *Cochrane Database Syst Rev*. 2015, (**11**):CD003932.

17. The American College of Obstetricians and Gynecologists. *Multifetal Pregnancy Reduction*. 2017, Committee Opinion No. **719**.

18. Panagiotis A, Papamichail M, Theodora M, et al. *Early Pregnancy Ultrasound Assessment of Multiple Pregnancy*. 2018. DOI http://doi.org/10.5772/inte chopen.81498.

19. Levy B, Sigurjonsson S, Pettersen B, et al. *Genomic imbalance in products of conception: single-nucleotide polymorphism chromosomal microarray analysis*. Obstet Gynecol. 2014, Vol. **124**(2 Pt 1):202–209.

20. *The Investigation and Treatment of Couples with Recurrent First-trimester and Second-trimester Miscarriage. Green-top Guideline No. 17*. Royal College of Obstetricians and Gynaecologists. 2011.

21. Prine LW, MacNaughton H. *Office management of early pregnancy loss*. Am Fam Physician. 2011, Vol. **84**(1):75–82.

22. Hooker AB, Lemmers M, Thurkow AL, et al. *Systematic review and meta-analysis of intrauterine adhesions after miscarriage: prevalence, risk factors and long-term reproductive outcome*. Hum Reprod Update. 2014, Vol. **20**(2):262–278.

23. *Recurrent Pregnancy Loss*. Guideline. European Society of Human Reproduction and Embryology (ESHRE). 2017.

24. Coomarasamy A, Williams H, Truchanowicz E, et al. *PROMISE: first-trimester progesterone therapy in women with a history of unexplained recurrent miscarriages – a randomised, double-blind, placebo-controlled, international multicentre trial and economic evaluation*. Health Technol Assess. 2016, Vol. **20**(41):1–92.

25. Coomarasamy A, Devall AJ, Cheed V, et al. *A randomized trial of progesterone in women with bleeding in early pregnancy*. N Engl J Med. 2019, Vol. **380**:1815–1824.

26. Dhillon-Smith R, Middleton LJ, Sunner KK, et al. *Levothyroxine in women with thyroid peroxidase antibodies before conception*. N Engl J Med. 2019, Vol. **380**:1316–1325.

27. No authors listed. *Diagnosis and management of ectopic pregnancy: Green-top Guideline No. 21*. BJOG. 2016, Vol. **123**:e15–e55.

28. Moini A, Hosseini R, Jahangiri N, et al. *Risk factors for ectopic pregnancy: A case-control study*. J Res Med Sci. 2014, Vol. **19**(9):844–849.

29. Muller V, Makhmadalieva M, Kogan I, et al. Ectopic pregnancy following in vitro fertilization: meta-analysis and single-center experience during 6 years. *Gynecol Endocrinol*. 2016, Vol. **32**:69–74.

30. Talbot K, Simpson R, Price N, Jackson SR. *Heterotopic pregnancy*. J Obstet Gynaecol. 2011, Vol. **31**(1):7–12.

31. Ectopic Pregnancy. *DynaMed*. [Online] [Cited: 07 07 2020.] https://www.dynamed.com/condition/ ectopic-pregnancy#EXPECTANT_ MANAGEMENT_CONSIDERATIONS.

32. Mol F, van Mello NM, Strandell A, et al. *Salpingotomy versus salpingectomy in women with tubal pregnancy (ESEP study): an open-label, multicentre, randomised controlled trial*. Lancet. 2014, Vol. **383**(9927), 1483–1489.

33. Boyraz G, Bozdağ G. *Pregnancy of unknown location*. J Turk Ger Gynecol Assoc. 2013, Vol. **14** (2):104–108.

34. Sagili H, Mohamed K. *Pregnancy of unknown location: an evidence-based approach to management*. Obstet Gynaecol. 2008, Vol. **10**: 224–230.

35. Bobdiwala S, Al-Memar M, Farren J, Bourne T. Factors to consider in pregnancy of unknown location. *Women's Health (Lond)*. 2017, Vol. **13**: 27–33.

Optimal Management of Pregnancy beyond 12 Weeks, Labour and the Puerperium for Women over 40

Shane Duffy and Pritha Dasmahapatra

Introduction

Advanced maternal age (AMA) is defined as pregnancy at 35 years or older [1] and is associated with medical, social, and economic implications for both mother and her baby [2,3]. However, studies have generally observed that most women over the age of 45 have good pregnancy outcomes and are able to cope with the physical and psychological stresses of pregnancy and parenting [4]. In 2013, 20% of births in England and Wales were to women aged 35 years or over and 4% to women over 40 years compared with 6% and 1%, respectively, in 1980 [5]. The mean age of first-time mothers in other developed countries has increased as well: Canada (mean age 29.6 years), Sweden (mean age 28.3 years), and the Netherlands (28.7 years)

Advanced artificial reproductive techniques and introduction of oocyte donation have also enabled women at advanced ages to become pregnant. In 2016 in Canada, women over 45 years accounted for 0.9 of 1000 births [6]. A study conducted in the USA also showed doubling of birth rate in the age group 40–44 years from 1990 to 2012 [7]. Advanced maternal age is particularly observed in high-income countries [8] and is thought to be due to lifestyle choices in delaying pregnancy, subfertility, and desire for bigger families [9]. In this chapter we will review the effects a woman's age may have on a pregnancy, and suggest clinical management that can help optimize the pregnancy for women and children.

Early Pregnancy Issues

Chromosomal Abnormalities

Karyotype analysis from spontaneous abortions, pregnancy terminations, genetic amniocenteses, and liveborn and stillborn infants shows a steady increase in the risk of aneuploidy as a woman ages (Table 11.1).

Congenital Malformations

The risk of having a child with a congenital anomaly may increase with increasing maternal age. It was thought that an increase in congenital anomalies with advancing maternal age had been attributed to the recognized increase of aneuploidy with advancing maternal age and the association of aneuploid fetuses with structural anomalies. However, several analyses have suggested that the risk of nonchromosomal anomalies also increases as women age.

The US National Birth Defects Prevention study reviewed the association between birth defects and maternal age. When compared with the reference group of women of 25–29 years of age, offspring of women ≥40 years of age were at increased risk of several types of cardiac defects (aOR 2.2–2.9), as well as for oesophageal atresia (aOR 2.9, 95% CI 1.7–4.9), hypospadias (aOR 2.0, 95% CI 1.4–3.0), and craniosynostosis (aOR 1.6, 95% CI 1.1–2.4) [11].

In the FASTER trial, the rates of major congenital anomalies for offspring of women <35, 35–39, and ≥40 years of age were 1.7%, 2.8%, and 2.9%, respectively [12].

It should be noted that results worldwide have not been consistent with all of these findings.

Later Pregnancy Issues

Advanced maternal age has been shown to be associated with risks to mother and the fetus, with studies suggesting more adverse effects with rise in maternal age. Epidemiological studies have demonstrated higher rates of obstetric complications such as small for gestational age (SGA) babies, pre-eclampsia, pre-term birth,

Table 11.1 Crude maternal age-specific rates for trisomy 21, Down syndrome, and all chromosome abnormalities

Maternal age, years	Data from livebirths		Data from second trimester amniocentesis	
	Trisomy 21	All chromosome abnormalities	Trisomy 21	All chromosome abnormalities
33	1/625	1/345	1/416	1/208
34	1/500	1/277	1/333	1/151
35	1/385	1/204	1/250	1/132
36	1/303	1/167	1/192	1/105
37	1/227	1/130	1/149	1/83
38	1/175	1/103	1/115	1/65
39	1/137	1/81	1/89	1/53
40	1/106	1/63	1/69	1/40
41	1/81	1/50	1/53	1/31
42	1/64	1/39	1/41	1/25
43	1/50	1/30	1/31	1/19
44	1/38	1/24	1/25	1/15
45	1/30	1/19	1/19	1/12

Source: Data from [10].

and stillbirth with AMA [12–16]. Advanced maternal age can be associated with pre-existing medical conditions such as diabetes and hypertension, the increased risks are thought to be independent of any co-morbidity [17–19].

Hypertensive Disorders

Maternal physiology causes blood pressure to drop in the first trimester, reaching a nadir at mid-pregnancy and reaching pre-conception level at term [20–23]. Advanced maternal age was found to be associated with four-fold increase in incidence of hypertension in pregnancy [24–26]. While pre-existing chronic hypertension, often found in AMA, is an independent risk factor for pre-eclampsia [27–32], resistance of endothelial lining to vasodilators with advancing age could also contribute to the risk of pre-eclampsia in AMA. The incidence of pre-eclampsia in the general obstetric population is 3–4%; this increases to 5–10% in women over age 40 and is as high as 35% in women over age 50 [33,34].

In our practice we recommend the use of low-dose aspirin for women over 40 throughout pregnancy following a Cochrane meta-analysis in 2019 [35], which demonstrated a reduced risk of developing pre-eclampsia and its consequences:

- Reduction in proteinuric pre-eclampsia – 16 fewer cases per 1000 women treated, risk ratio (RR) 0.82, 95% CI 0.77–0.88.
- Reduction in fetal or neonatal death – 5 fewer deaths per 1000 women treated, RR 0.85, 95% CI 0.76–0.95.
- Reduction in overall pre-term birth <37 weeks – 16 fewer cases per 1000 women treated, RR 0.91, 95% CI 0.87–0.95.
- Reduction in SGA infants – 7 fewer cases per 1000 women treated, RR 0.84, 95% CI 0.76–0.92.
- Reduction in composite serious adverse maternal and neonatal outcomes – 20 fewer cases per 1000 women treated, RR 0.90, 95% CI 0.85–0.96.

Gestational Diabetes

The association of AMA and gestational diabetes is unclear. Some studies have suggested an increased risk [36,37], while a study conducted in Northern Ethiopia found no change in risk profile [25]. There have been suggestions of assisted reproductive technologies (ART) contributing to gestational diabetes mellitus (GDM) [38]. At present, in the UK, an evidence-based guideline of the National Institute for Clinical Excellence (NICE guideline on diabetes in pregnancy) does not recommend routine glucose tolerance testing (GTT) for AMA [39]. However, women at advanced age can have pre-existing diabetes which can have additional adverse maternal and fetal implications.

Cardiac Complications

Pregnancy is a cardiovascular compromised state and can have potentially serious effects on older women with pre-existing cardiac conditions. Cardiac complications are the leading cause of death in the UK [40], with mortality having a linear relationship with age [41].

Venous Thromboembolism

The risk of venous thromboembolism (VTE) with AMA is unclear. A large population-based cohort study from the UK showed non-pregnant women 35–44 years were at 50% higher risk of VTE compared with those of age 25–34 years [42]. However, data from case control studies showed only a modest increase in women over 35 years [43–45]. Even though age probably does not play a part in increasing VTE risk in the antenatal period, postnatally the risk can increase by 70% in those over 35 years compared with 25–34 year olds. The Royal College of Obstetricians and Gynaecologists (RCOG) has classed maternal age more than 35 years as a risk for VTE in the antenatal and postnatal periods [46].

Placental Disorders

Mothers at advanced age are at increased risk of antepartum haemorrhage [26,37].

Risk of placental abruption has been shown to be increased with AMA in multiple studies [12–16]. Pre-existing chronic hypertension further increases the incidence of abruption [27–31].

Rates of placenta previa are also higher in AMA. This could partially be confounded by increased gravidity, which is a risk for placenta previa [36]. Numerous epidemiological studies have shown higher risk of placenta previa with ART [47].

Small for Gestational Age

There is a risk of SGA with AMA with poorer APGAR scores and adverse effect on perinatal health [48–54]. A prospective population-based Swedish cohort study restricted to healthy nulliparous women (n = 173,715) delivering singletons

compared birth outcome in women age 35–40 with those age 20–24 years [55]. Demographic characteristics, smoking, history of infertility, and other medical conditions were taken into account when calculating risk. After adjusting for these factors, older age was associated with a significantly higher risk of low birth weight (LBW) and pre-term delivery (PTD): very LBW (OR = 1.9); moderate LBW (OR = 1.7); very pre-term birth (OR = 1.7); moderately pre-term birth (OR = 1.2); and SGA infant (OR = 1.7).

Pre-Term Delivery

Various studies have shown increased rates of PTD in AMA [26,37,56]. A multi-country assessment by WHO also supports this finding [2]. This may in part be due to iatrogenic prematurity in view of increased maternal and fetal complications indicating earlier delivery. A population-based study from Sweden evaluated outcome in women at more advanced ages and confirmed the increased risk of PTD in older women, after adjustment for confounders such as multiple gestation, smoking, parity, and maternal medical disease. This series included over 32,000 women ≥40 years of age. The rates of PTD <32 weeks for women 20–29, 40–44, and ≥45 years of age were 1.01%, 1.80%, and 2.24%, respectively [57].

Stillbirth

Systematic reviews and meta-analyses have proven that AMA is associated with increased risk of stillbirth [58,59]. The risk is more pronounced with advancing gestational age irrespective of the parity [59–63]. The role of co-morbidities in the rise of rate of stillbirth is unclear, and further investigations are needed. Compromised placental function with 'ageing' and vascular changes could be a factor [64,65], but little is known about the patho-physiology. Even though SGA has been demonstrated in AMA, a retrospective cohort study showed no increase in SGA in stillbirths at >35 years compared with <35 years [66]. This suggests that placental insufficiency may not be the primary cause. Diminished oocyte quality can be a contributing cause [67]; however, the theory is contradicted by the finding that oocyte donation with a younger oocyte is an independent risk factor [68]. Advanced paternal age, often associated with AMA has also been suggested to increase the risk of stillbirth. The excess perinatal

133

mortality experienced by older women is largely unexplained, even after controlling for risk factors such as hypertension, diabetes, antepartum bleeding, smoking, and multiple gestation [69]. An analysis of over 5 million singleton gestations in the United States found the risk of stillbirth at 37–41 weeks for primiparous women increased significantly with maternal age. The risk of stillbirth for women under age 35, age 35–39 years old, and >40 years old was 3.73, 6.41, and 8.65 per 1000 ongoing pregnancies, respectively. The increased risk of stillbirth with increasing age persisted after accounting for medical disease and race/ethnicity. The risk increased sharply at 40 weeks of gestation, which suggests that older women are 'post-term' sooner than younger women [70].

Caesarean Section

Systematic review and meta-analysis suggest that AMA is associated with increased Caesarean delivery [59]. The rates were significantly higher at >50 years compared with 45–49 years, irrespective of parity and co-morbidity. Rates of Caesarean delivery have been shown to increase from as early as 30 years of age [71]. Caesarean delivery is often considered to be safer for the fetus when compared with vaginal delivery and could be the chosen mode of delivery in the background of subfertility and poor obstetric history. Also, maternal and fetal complications associated with AMA may necessitate expedited delivery by Caesarean section. Myometrial activity diminishes at an advanced age with studies showing increased rates of emergency Caesarean section for labour dystocia in both spontaneous and induced labour [52,72–76]. In addition to Caesarean section, prolonged labour and instrumental delivery are higher in the nulliparous [75,76].

Post-Partum Haemorrhage

Incidence of post-partum haemorrhage is thought to be higher in AMA [77], possibly from higher rates of placental and hypertensive disorders. Multifetal pregnancy from ART should be considered when assessing the risk. Possibility of retained placenta needing operative intervention is also increased with ART in AMA. Uterine pathology such as fibroids and adenomyosis, found more in older women, increases chances of post-partum haemorrhage.

Malpresentation

Malpresentation is also said to be higher in AMA and can be a result of multiparity, multifetal pregnancy and submucous uterine fibroid.

Maternal Death

Several studies have linked AMA with an increased risk of maternal mortality. A large international multi-centre study found women older than 35 years had a higher maternal mortality ratio (MMR) than women in any younger age group (>700 maternal deaths/100,000 livebirths), and the MMR in adolescents (260 maternal deaths/100,000 livebirths) was higher than in women ages 20–24 years, who had the lowest MMR (190 maternal deaths/100,000 livebirths) [78]. Age-specific MMRs vary significantly among countries and regions: in Southeast Asia, adolescents had the lowest MMR of any age group. In the AMA age group, myocardial infarction and heart failure are the primary contributing factors to maternal deaths. Women must be informed about the risks of young and old maternal age during the pre-conception visits [40,41].

Practical Management of AMA

Advanced maternal age is a risk indicator of pregnancy and needs appropriate antenatal, intrapartum, and postnatal care. The exact age at which the adverse effects are increased is unclear. Some studies suggest women more than 40 years are at increased risk [79], while others set the mark at 35 years [55,80]. However, in the UK, antenatal care is not usually any different at less than 40 years unless there are other confounding factors.

Antenatal Care

Women at advanced age booking for pregnancy should have a thorough risk assessment to ascertain risk of hypertensive diseases of pregnancy and those at higher risk should be started on 150 mcg aspirin from 12 weeks till until 36 weeks [81]. The NICE guideline on hypertensive diseases in pregnancy [81] does not recommend additional monitoring of blood pressure and urinalysis, unless evidence of hypertension in pregnancy emerges.

In our practice the booking visit is performed by a midwife and an appointment is made for the woman to see an obstetrician. We offer shared care with the midwifery and medical staff.

Increased surveillance for GDM is not recommended in the UK based on age alone [39]. However, it should be noted that AMA is associated with an increased background incidence of diabetes and it is our practice to offer a mini glucose tolerance test.

Risk of VTE should be assessed at booking and at each encounter. Thromboprophylaxis is not started based on age alone; however, maternal age of more than 35 years is a minor risk factor and is to be included in the calculation. See Figure 11.1 for the antenatal risk assessment that we use in our practice for antenatal patients.

Chromosomal anomaly is one of the prime concerns of AMA and surveillance should be started in first trimester with nuchal scan/quad testing/ fetal DNA tests. A routine anomaly scan is recommended between 18+0 and 21+6 weeks [82,83].

In addition, serial growth scans with doppler studies are to be performed starting from 26–28 weeks of gestation in women more than 40 years. For mothers between 35 and 39 years this is considered a minor risk for SGA and if present with two other minor risks or one major risk, in our practice we perform an umbilical artery doppler measured at 20–24 weeks. If normal, we offer one additional scans at 28 and 34 weeks. However, if umbilical artery doppler at 20–24 weeks has pulsatility index >95% and/or notching, we perform serial growth scans with doppler studies at 24, 28, 32, and 36 weeks of gestation [84].

Care in Labour

There is enough evidence to suggest that the risk of stillbirth increases with AMA. For women more than 40 years the risk at 39–40 weeks of gestation is 2 in 1000 compared to 1 in 1000 at less than 35 years [85]. For women more than 40 years the risk of stillbirth at 39 weeks is similar to the risk at 41 weeks for women in their mid-20s. Based on these findings, induction of labour is recommended between 39 and 40 weeks when maternal age is more than 40 years [66,85,86]. There is insufficient evidence to comment on the possible effect on perinatal mortality and rates of operative delivery from this intervention, and

this should be mentioned when counselling for induction of labour. We have provided an educational video for our patients that can also be accessed online. Some older women may request Caesarean delivery, particularly if this is their first pregnancy. Discussion of risks and benefits of both should then be arranged [86].

Management of labour does not need to be modified in view of maternal age; however, due to the possible compromise in uteroplacental blood flow and myometrial function, continuous electronic fetal monitoring is recommended for women more than 40 years. Decision for operative delivery should be taken for obstetric reasons and not based on age alone.

Postnatal Care

If additional risk for VTE is present, thromboprophylaxis should be arranged.

Conclusion

Most women with AMA have successful pregnancy outcomes; however, women and health care professionals must be aware that AMA has higher risk associated with pregnancy. We have described above the preventative and extra monitoring needed for AMA pregnancies. As risk factors can develop, we recommend reviewing the care plan (Figure 11.2) at each antenatal visit.

References

1. Dekker R. Evidence on: Pregnancy at Age 35 and Older. https://evidencebasedbirth.com/advanced-maternal-age/?msclkid=4ab20ad8b01611ecb492f79cf6a22536

2. Laopaiboon M, Lumbiganon P, Intarut N, et al. Advanced maternal age and pregnancy outcomes: a multi country assessment. BJOG 2014; **121** Suppl 1:49–56

3. Olusanya B O, Solanke OA. Perinatal correlates of delayed childbearing in a developing country. Arch Gynecol Obstet 2012;**285**(4):951–7

4. Dildy GA, Jackson GM, Fowers GK, et al. Very advanced maternal age: pregnancy after age 45. Am J Obstet Gynecol. 1996;**175**(3 Pt 1):668

5. ONS. Birth Summary Tables, England and Wales, 2013. Office for National Statistics. 2014

6. Martin JA, Hamilton BE, Osterman M. National Center for Health Statistics Data Brief, no. 318. *Natl Cent Heal Stat* 2018;**318**(318):415–6

Risk	Antenatal VTE Risk Factors			Antenatal Score (WMUH-OMC: Obstetric Medicine Clinic)
Pre-existing Risk Factor(s)	Any previous recurrent VTE			**4 and OMC**
	Any previous VTE e.g. unprovoked VTE, VTE related to oestrogen-containing contraception/pregnancy (excluding a single previous VTE related to major surgery, provoking factors and no other risk factors)			**4 and OMC**
	Any previous VTE provoked by major surgery			**3 and OMC**
	Medical comorbidities e.g. cancer, heart failure, active systemic lupus erythematosus, inflammatory polyarthropathy or active inflammatory bowel disease, nephrotic syndrome, type 1 diabetes mellitus with nephropathy, sickle cell disease, current intravenous drug user, urinary tract infection, heart disease			**3**
	Thrombophilia	Heritable:	Antithrombin deficiency	**See Table 2** Seek further advice from Haematology (C&W)/ OMC (WMUH) as appropriate
			Protein C deficiency	
			Protein S deficiency	
			Factor V Leiden	
			Prothrombin gene mutation	
		Acquired:	Antiphospholipid antibodies	
			Persistent lupus anticoagulant and/or persistent moderate/high titre anticardiolipin antibodies and/or β2-glycoprotein 1	
	Family history of VTE (first-degree relative with unprovoked VTE or oestrogen-provoked VTE)			1
	Age ≥35 years old			1
	Obesity at booking (**BMI ≥40 kg/m²**)			2
	Obesity at booking (**BMI 30–39 kg/m²**)			1
	Parity ≥3 (a woman becomes para 3 after her third delivery)			1
	Smoker			1
	Gross varicose veins (symptomatic or above knee or with associated phlebitis, oedema/skin changes)			1
	Paraplegia			**Refer to Consultant Obstetrician**
Obstetric Risk Factor(s)	Pre-eclampsia in current pregnancy			1
	Multiple pregnancy			1
	Assisted reproductive technology (ART)/In vitro fertilisation (IVF)-antenatal only			1
Transient Risk Factor(s)	Ovarian hyperstimulation syndrome (OHSS) Thromboprophylaxis in 1st trimester			**4**
	Any surgical procedure in pregnancy or puerperium except immediate repair of the perineum e.g. appendicectomy, postpartum sterilisation			3
	Hyperemesis			**3**
	Current systemic infection (requiring intravenous antibiotics or hospital			1
	Immobility e.g. pelvic girdle pain with reduced mobility, long-distance travel			1
	All long-distance travel (all forms ≥4 hours (not exclusively by air) within the last 2–4 weeks)			1
	Dehydration			1
No Risk	No known risk			**0**

Antenatal VTE Score	Antenatal Thromboprophylaxis Management
≥4	○ Enoxaparin thromboprophylaxis (use booking weight) **from the first trimester** if no contraindications present ○ Offer anti-embolism stockings, unless contraindicated, if an inpatient
3	○ Enoxaparin thromboprophylaxis (use booking weight) **from 28 weeks** if no contraindications present ○ Offer anti-embolism stockings, unless contraindicated, if an inpatient
≥2	○ Antenatal enoxaparin thromboprophylaxis is not indicated ○ Offer anti-embolism stockings, unless contraindicated, if an inpatient ○ Encourage mobilisation ○ Avoid dehydration
Antenatal admission to hospital	○ Review risk(s) and consider enoxaparin thromboprophylaxis (use booking weight) **during hospital admission** if no contraindications present ○ Offer anti-embolism stockings, unless contraindicated, if an inpatient

Figure 11.1 Antenatal venous thromboembolism risk factors, score, and management

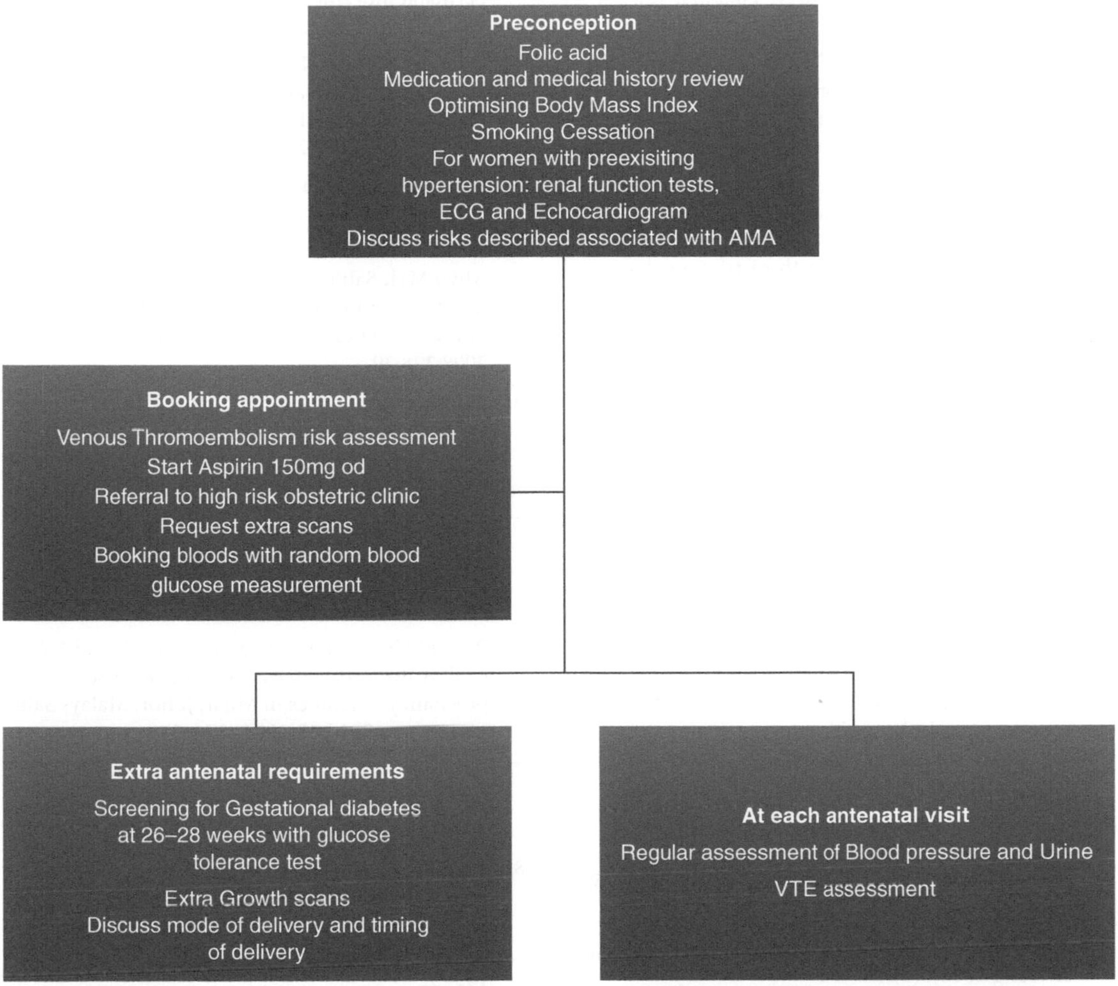

Figure 11.2 Quick reference flow diagram for care of pregnant women at advanced maternal age (AMA)

7. Matthew Ts, Hamilton Be, First births to older women continue to rise. *NCHS Data Brief* 2014; (**152**):1–8

8. Royal College of Obstetricians and Gynaecologists. Reproductive Ageing (Scientific Impact Paper No. 24.2011. https://www .rcog.org.uk/guidance/browse-all-guidance/scien tific-impact-papers/reproductive-ageing-scientific-impact-paper-no-24/

9. Guedes M, Canavarro MC. Characteristics of primiparous women of advanced age and their partners: a homogenous or heterogenous group? Birth 2014;**41**:46–55

10. Schreinemachers DM, Cross PK, Hook EB. Rates of trisomies 21, 18, 13 and other chromosome abnormalities in about 20,000 prenatal studies compared with estimated rates in live births. Hum Genet 1982;**61**:318

11. Gill SK, Broussard C, Devine O, et al. Association between maternal age and birth defects of unknown etiology: United States, 1997–2007. Birth Defects Res A Clin Mol Teratol 2012;**94**(12):1010

12. Cleary-Goldman J, Malone FD, Vidaver J, et al. Impact of maternal age on obstetric outcome. Obstet Gynecol 2005;**105**: 983–90

13. Kenny LC, Lavender T, McNamee R, et al. Advanced maternal age and adverse pregnancy outcome: evidence from a large contemporary cohort. *PloS* One 2013;**8**: e56583

14. Khalil A, Syngelaki A, Maiz N, et al. Maternal age and adverse pregnancy outcome: a cohort study. Ultrasound *Obstet Gynecol* 2013;**42**:634–43

15. Salihu HM, Wilson RE, Alio AP, Kirby RS. Advanced maternal age and risk of antepartum and intrapartum stillbirth. *J Obstet Gynaecol Res* 2008;**34**: 843–50

16. Giri A, Srivastav VR, Suwal A, Tuladhar AS. Advanced maternal age and obstetric outcome. Nepal *Med Coll J* 2012;**15**: 87–90

17. Bahtiyar M, Funai E, Norwitz E, et al. Advanced maternal age (AMA) is an independent predictor of intrauterine fetal death at term. Am J Obstet Gynecol 2006;**195**:S209

18. Odibo AO, Nelson D, Stamilio DM, et al. Advanced maternal age is an independent risk factor for intrauterine growth restriction. Am J Perinatol 2006;**23**:325–8

19. Lamminpaa R, Vehvilainen-Julkunen K, Gissler M, Heinonen S. Preeclampsia complicated by advanced maternal age: a registry-based study on primiparous women in Finland 1997–2008. BMC Pregnancy Childbirth 2012;**12**:47

20. Gabbe S. Obstetrics: Normal and problem pregnancies. Philadelphia: Elsevier/Saunders; 2012

21. Page EW, Christianson R. The impact of mean arterial pressure in the middle trimester upon the outcome of pregnancy. Am J Obstet Gynecol 1976;**125**:740–6

22. Halligan A, O'Brien E, O'Malley K, et al. Twenty-four-hour ambulatory blood pressure measurement in a primigravid population. J Hypertens 1993;**11**:869–73

23. Clapp JF 3rd, Seaward BL, Sleamaker RH, Hiser J. Maternal physiologic adaptations to early human pregnancy. Am J Obstet Gynecol 1988;**159**: 1456–60

24. Yılmaz E, Tosun ÖA, Tarhan N, et al. Perinatal outcomes in advanced age pregnancies. J Clin Exp Investig 2016;**7**(2):157–62

25. El-Gilany A-H, Hammad S. Obstetric outcomes of teenagers and older mothers: experience from Saudi Arabia. Int J Collab Res Intern Med Public Health. 2012;**4**(6):901–9

26. Mehari M-A, Maeruf H, Robles CC, et al. Advanced maternal age pregnancy and its adverse obstetrical and perinatal outcomes in Ayder comprehensive specialized hospital, Northern Ethiopia, 2017: a comparative cross-sectional study. BMC Pregnancy Childbirth 2020;**20**:60

27. Haddad B, Sibai BM. Chronic hypertension in pregnancy. Ann Med 1999;**31**:246–52

28. Rey E, Couturier A. The prognosis of pregnancy in women with chronic hypertension. Am J Obstet Gynecol 1994;**171**:410–6

29. McCowan LM, Buist RG, North RA, Gamble G. Perinatal morbidity in chronic hypertension. Br J Obstet Gynaecol 1996;**103**:123–9

30. Steer PJ, Little MP, Kold-Jensen T, et al. Maternal blood pressure in pregnancy, birth weight, and perinatal mortality in first births: prospective study. BMJ 2004;**329**:1312

31. Orbach H, Matok I, Gorodischer R, et al. Hypertension and antihypertensive drugs in pregnancy and perinatal outcomes. Am J Obstet Gynecol 2013;**208**:301 e1–6

32. Livingston JC, Sibai BM. Chronic hypertension in pregnancy. Obstet Gynecol Clin N Am 2001;**28**:447–64

33. Aliyu MH, Salihu HM, Wilson RE, et al. The risk of intrapartum stillbirth among smokers of advanced maternal age. Arch Gynecol Obstet 2008;**278**:39.

34. Paulson RJ, Boostanfar R, Saadat P, et al. Pregnancy in the sixth decade of life: obstetric outcomes in women of advanced reproductive age. JAMA 2002;**288**:2320.

35. Duley L, Meher S, Hunter KE, et al. Antiplatelet agents for preventing pre-eclampsia and its complications. Cochrane Database Syst Rev 2019;**10**:CD004659.

36. Rashed HEM, Maria Awaluddin S, Ahmad NA, et al. Advanced maternal age and adverse pregnancy outcomes in Muar, Johor. Malays Sains Malaysiana 2016;**45**(10):1537–42

37. Koo Y-J, Ryu H-M, Yang J-H, et al. Pregnancy outcomes according to increasing maternal age. Taiwan J Obstet Gynecol 2012;**51**:60–5

38. Ashrafi M, Gosili R, Hosseini R, et al. Risk of gestational diabetes mellitus in patients undergoing assisted reproductive techniques. Eur J Obstet Gynecol Reprod Biol 2014;**176**: 149–52

39. National Institute for Health and Care Excellence (NICE). Diabetes in pregnancy: management from preconception to the postnatal period. NICE guideline NG3. London: NICE; 2015

40. GBD 2016 Mortality Collaborators. Global, regional, and national under-5 mortality, adult mortality, age-specific mortality, and life expectancy, 1970–2016: a systematic analysis for the Global Burden of Disease Study 2016. Lancet 2017;**390**:1084–150

41. Gelson E, Gatzoulis M, Steer P, Johnson M. Heart disease – why is maternal mortality increasing? BJOG 2008;**116**:609–11

42. Sultan AA, West J, Tata LJ, et al. Risk of first venous thromboembolism in and around pregnancy: a population-based cohort study. Br J Haematol 2012;**156**:366–73

43. Lindqvist P, Dahlbäck B, Marŝál K. Thrombotic risk during pregnancy: a population study. Obstet Gynecol 1999;**94**:595–9

44. Liu S, Rouleau J, Joseph KS, et al. Epidemiology of pregnancy-associated venous thromboembolism: a population-based study in Canada. J Obstet Gynaecol Can 2009;**31**:611–20

45. Simpson EL, Lawrenson RA, Nightingale AL, Farmer RD. Venous thromboembolism in pregnancy and the puerperium: incidence and additional risk factors from a London perinatal database. BJOG 2001;**108**:56–60

46. Royal College of Obstetricians and Gynaecologists. Reducing the Risk of Venous Thromboembolism during Pregnancy and the Puerperium Green-top Guideline No. 37a April 2015

47. Franklin SS, Larson MG, Khan SA, et al. Does the relation of blood pressure to coronary heart disease risk change with aging? Circulation 2001;**103**:1245

48. Karami M, Jenabi E, Fereidooni B. The association of placenta previa and assisted reproductive techniques: a meta-analysis. J Matern Fetal Neonatal Med 2018;**31**(14):1940–7

49. Amarin V. Effect of maternal age on pregnancy outcome: a hospital based study. J Med Res 2013;**1**(4):28–31

50. Salem Yaniv S, Levy A, Wiznitzer A, et al. A significant linear association exists between advanced maternal age and adverse perinatal outcome. Arch Gynecol Obstet 2011;**283**:755–9

51. Wang Y, Tanbo T, Abyholm T, Henriksen T. The impact of advanced maternal age and parity on obstetric and perinatal outcomes in singleton gestations. Arch Gynecol Obstet 2011;**284**:31–7

52. Carolan M, Davey MA, Biro MA, Kealy M. Older maternal age and intervention in labor: a population-based study comparing older and younger first-time mothers in Victoria, Australia. Birth 2011;**38**:24–9

53. Hoffman MC, Jeffers S, Carter J, et al. Pregnancy at or beyond age 40 years is associated with an increased risk of fetal death and other adverse outcomes. Am J Obstet Gynecol 2007;**196**:11–3

54. Hoque ME. Advanced maternal age and outcomes of pregnancy: a retrospective study from South Africa. Biomed Res 2012;**23**(2):281–5

55. Cnattingius S, Forman MR, Berendes HW, Isotalo L. Delayed childbearing and risk of adverse perinatal outcome. A population-based study. JAMA 1992;**268**(7):886

56. Almeida NK, Almeida RM, Pedreira CE. Adverse perinatal outcomes for advanced maternal age: a cross-sectional study of Brazilian births. J Pediatr (Rio J) 2015;**91**(5):493–8

57. Jacobsson B, Ladfors L, Milsom I. Advanced maternal age and adverse perinatal outcome. Obstet Gynecol 2004;**104**:727

58. Huang L, Sauve R, Birkett N, et al. Maternal age and risk of stillbirth: a systematic review. CMAJ 2008;**178**:165–72

59. Lean SC, Derricott H, Jones RL, Heazell AEP. Advanced maternal age and adverse pregnancy outcomes: A systematic review and meta-analysis. PLoS ONE 2017;**12**(10):e0186287

60. Hilder L, Costeloe K, Thilaganathan B. Prolonged pregnancy: evaluating gestation-specific risks of fetal and infant mortality. Br J Obstet Gynaecol 1998;**105**:169–73

61. Haavaldsen C, Sarfraz AA, Samuelsen SO, Eskild A. The impact of maternal age on fetal death: does length of gestation matter? Am J Obstet Gynecol 2010;**203**:554:1–8

62. Nybo Andersen AM, Wohlfahrt J, Christens P, et al. Maternal age and fetal loss: population based register Linkage study. BMJ 2000;**320**:1708–12.

63. Flenady V, Koopmans L, Middleton P, et al. Major risk factors for stillbirth in high-income countries: a systematic review and meta-analysis. Lancet 2011;**377**:1331–40

64. Lean SC, Heazell AEP, Dilworth MR, et al. Placental dysfunction underlies increased risk of fetal growth restriction and stillbirth in advanced maternal age women. Sci Rep 2017;**7**(1):9677

65. Miller DA. Is advanced maternal age an independent risk factor for uteroplacental insufficiency? Am J Obstet Gynecol 2005;**192**:1974–80

66. Wyatt PR, Owolabi T, Meier C, Huang T. Age-specific risk of fetal loss observed in a second trimester serum screening population. Am J Obstet Gynecol 2005;**192**:240–6

67. Hunt PA, Hassold TJ. Human female meiosis: what makes a good egg go bad? Trends Genet 2008;**24**:86–93

68. Younis JS, Laufer N. Oocyte donation is an independent risk factor for pregnancy complications: the implications for women of advanced age. J Womens Health (Larchmt) 2015;**24**(2):127–30

69. Alio AP, Salihu HM, McIntosh C, et al. The effect of paternal age on fetal birth outcomes. Am J Mens Health 2012;**6**:427–35

70. Reddy UM, Ko CW, Willinger M. Maternal age and the risk of stillbirth throughout pregnancy in the United States. Am J Obstet Gynecol 2006;**195**(3):764

71. Bell JS, Campbell DM, Graham WJ, et al. Do obstetric complications explain high caesarean

rates among women over 30? A retrospective analysis. BMJ 2001;**322**:894–5

72. Wang Y, Tanbo T, Abyholm T, Henriksen T. The impact of advanced maternal age and parity on obstetric and perinatal outcomes in singleton gestations. Arch Gynecol Obstet 2011;**284**:31–7

73. Gilbert WM, Nesbitt TS, Danielsen B. Childbearing beyond age 40: Pregnancy outcome in 24,032 cases. Obstet Gynecol 1999;**93**:9–14

74. Patel RR, Peters TJ, Murphy DJ, ALSPAC Study Team. Prenatal risk factors for Caesarean section. Analyses of the ALSPAC cohort of 12 944 women in England. Int J Epidemiol 2005;**34**:353–67

75. Ecker JL, Chen KT, Cohen AP, et al. Increased risk of cesarean delivery with advancing maternal age: Indications and associated factors in nulliparous women. Am J Obstet Gynecol 2001;**185**:883–7

76. Smith GC, Cordeaux Y, White IR, et al. The effect of delaying childbirth on primary cesarean section rates. PLoS Med 2008;**5**:e144

77. Yogev Y, Melamed N, Bardin R, et al. Pregnancy outcome at extremely advanced maternal age. Am J Obstet Gynecol 2010;**203**:558:1–7

78. Nove A, Matthews Z, Neal S, Camacho AV. Maternal mortality in adolescents compared with women of other ages: evidence from 144 countries. Lancet Glob Health 2014;**2**(3):e155

79. Nybo Andersen AM, Wohlfahrt J, Christens P, et al. Maternal age and fetal loss: population based register linkage study. BMJ 2000;**320**:1708–12

80. Delbaere I, Verstraelen H, Goetgeluk S, et al. Pregnancy outcome in primiparae of advanced maternal age. Eur J Obstet Gynecol Reprod Biol 2007;**135**:41–6

81. National Institute for Health and Care Excellence (NICE). Hypertension in pregnancy: diagnosis and management. NICE guideline NG133. London: NICE; 2019

82. National Institute for Health and Care Excellence (NICE). Antenatal care for uncomplicated pregnancies (CG62). London 2016

83. Public Health England. Fetal Anomaly Screening Programme. 2015. https://www.gov.uk/govern ment/publications/fetal-anomaly-screening-programme-handbook? msclkid=480d63b4b02911ecbd2db90bf6d6a1b6

84. The Investigation and Management of the Small–for–Gestational–Age Fetus Green–top Guideline No. 31 2nd Edition | February 2013 | Minor revisions – January 2014. https://rcog.org.uk/med ia/t3lmjhnl/gtg_31.pdf

85. Reddy UM, Ko CW, Willinger M. Maternal age and the risk of stillbirth throughout pregnancy in the United States. Am J Obstet Gynecol 2006;**195**:764–70

86. Royal College of Obstetricians and Gynaecologists. Induction of Labour at Term in Older Mothers (Scientific Impact Paper No. 34). 2013. https://www.rcog.org.uk/guidance/browse-all-guidance/scientific-impact-papers/induction-of-labour-at-term-in-older-mothers-scientific-impact-paper-no-34/

Chapter

12

What Do We Know about the Children of Women over 40 and What Can Older Mothers Do to Optimize Their Children's Development?

Winifred Mak and Vickie Schafer

Health and Development of Children with Mothers over 40

Introduction

The number of women over 40 who are becoming mothers for the first time is growing. This growth has been spurred by various factors such as public acceptance of assisted reproductive technology (ART) and donor gametes, the increasing availability of donor oocytes and improved affordability of frozen donor oocytes. As providers, we will be taking care of women over 40 preconceptionally and they are likely to ask especially if they use ART: "Is my baby going to have any issues?" We will need the basic knowledge on how to counsel these women on potential adverse health and developmental outcomes that could affect their future child. The first part of this chapter will focus on an overview of the literature on the health of children of older mothers conceiving spontaneously, using ART with autologous oocytes and donor oocytes. These age and ART associated outcomes are largely beyond the control of women and their partners. However, the second part of this chapter will be dedicated to the literature surrounding the influences of parental aging on family interactions and several practical "tips" on older parenting from a licensed psychologist who has worked extensively with couples with infertility and third-party counseling. This part can aid older parents with optimizing their family interactions with their child and may influence their child's development. These outcomes can be controlled by women. The majority of the literature surrounding these topics are level III evidence such as retrospective cohort or case-control studies and are heterogeneous.

Comprehensive reviews regarding each topic if available will be cited for readers needing more detailed information.

Perinatal and Neonatal Outcomes

There has been a wealth of literature published including a chapter in this book on the increased risk of obstetrical complications of women of advanced maternal age (>35 years old) and, more recently, new categories of very advanced maternal aged women (>45 years old) and extremely advanced maternal age (>50 years old) (Figure 12.1). Several hypotheses have been suggested that could predispose older mothers to worsening obstetrical outcomes such as purely aging itself, having preexisting comorbidities such as hypertension, diabetes and using ART.

After managing a high-risk obstetrical course as an older woman, what are the outcomes of their babies? One of the earliest studies to answer this question is a large population-based cohort (n=487,000) study using prospectively collected data from the Swedish Medical Birth Register

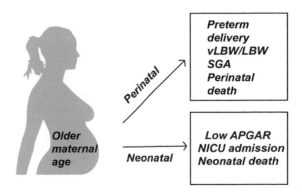

Figure 12.1 Perinatal and neonatal outcomes of older maternal age

between 1983 through 1987 [1]. The registry did not accurately document mode of conception; therefore, this confounder could not be adjusted for. However, the likelihood that ART was used extensively in the 1980s as a method of conception is likely low. These investigators found that women aged 40 and over were significantly at higher risk of having a baby that was very low birth weight (adjusted OR (aOR) 1.8, CI 1.04–3.0), low birth weight (aOR 2.0, CI 1.5–2.5), very preterm (aOR 1.9, CI 1.2–2.9), preterm (aOR 1.5, CI 1.2–1.8) and small-for-gestational age (aOR 1.4, CI 1.01–2.0) than women aged 20–24 years old, even after adjusting for maternal complications and other potential confounders (such as maternal education, infertility and hypertensive disease). Importantly, this study shows that increasing maternal age alone is a risk factor for adverse perinatal outcomes.

A decade later, another study was published that provided more granularity on the risk for women over 40 by investigating subgroups of women who were 40–44 and over 45 years old at delivery [2]. Again, this study used the Swedish Medical Birth Registry and they used an extended time period of 15 years (1987–2001) of data. Similarly, the authors noted that mode of conception could not be reliably documented so ART births could not be separated out. The control group were women between 20 and 29 years old (n=876,361) and the study groups were women between 40 and 44 years (n=31,662) and over 45 years old (n=1205). Consistent with the prior study, the authors found that as women aged, they were more likely to be at risk of adverse perinatal morbidities (preterm birth, etc.) and that women over 45 had the highest risk for all adverse outcomes. Also, perinatal mortality and death was significantly more likely in infants born to women in both older age groups. For example, the risk of perinatal mortality of infants born to women 40–44 years had aOR 1.7 (CI 1.5–1.9) and infants born to women over 45 years had aOR 2.4 (CI 1.5–4.0). Reassuringly, the absolute risk of perinatal mortality was extremely low in all three age groups, 0.5% (20–29), 1.0% (40–44) and 1.4% (≥45). Interestingly, the risk of neonatal death was significantly increased in women in the 40–44 age group (aOR 1.29 CI 1.08–1.64) and there was a trend towards increased risk in women over 45 (aOR 1.42 CI 0.62–3.23), which was not statistically significant. Adjustments for confounders

included nulliparity, significant malformations, smoking, maternal disease and multiple pregnancy, and therefore the authors concluded that the adverse perinatal outcomes were found to be associated with age alone and not due to concurrent illnesses or pregnancy complications.

A subsequent study using a Finnish Birth Registry studied two time points (1991 and 2008) and again found an increase in perinatal morbidity and mortality in babies with advanced maternal age with highest risk in the over 40 age group compared with women aged 20–34 [3]. Additionally, these authors reported a significantly increased risk of low (<7) 1 and 5 min APGAR and increased risk of baby going to the neonatal intensive care unit (NICU)/observation with increasing age. For example in the 2008 cohort, the infants of women ≥40 had increased risk of 63% for low 1 min APGAR, two-fold increase for low 5 min APGAR and 64% increase in risk of being admitted into the NICU. In this study, they were able to document the proportion using in vitro fertilization (IVF) in the over 40 age group; in 1991 only 3% used IVF, which rose to 15% in 2008. Therefore, the majority of this cohort were from spontaneous conceptions. The large population cohort studies cited above most likely represent the relationship between perinatal outcomes of children and advanced maternal age with minimal confounding by ART use. One could argue that these prior studies are not representative of the present day given there have been major advances in obstetrical and neonatal care.

More recent studies [4–7] have shown consistent trends in adverse perinatal/neonatal outcomes. Wu et al. [6] carried out a population-based retrospective cohort study in Ontario, in which they studied three age groups: the control group of women aged 20–34 (n=298,844), 35–42 (n=83,913) and ≥43 (n=3266) (time period 2012–2015). The primary outcomes studied were pregnancy and neonatal outcomes. In this study, the authors showed consistent findings of increased risk of adverse perinatal and neonatal outcomes such as low APGAR and increased risk of neonatal death in the over 43 age group. In this study, they were also able to document method of conception and they performed a subanalysis comparing spontaneous and ART conceived births in the different age groups.

As more women are contemplating motherhood at not only over 40 but 50 and over, is there additional risk for these women? A recent publication carried a population-based retrospective cohort investigating the perinatal outcomes of women stratified by the following age groups: <39 (reference population n=234,824), 40–44 (n=7321), 45–49 (n=558) and ≥50 (n=68) (time period 1991–2014) [7]. Interestingly, the reported use of IVF in all age groups was low, at 2.7% for the 40–44 age group, 9.9% for those aged 45–49 and only 13.2% for the over 50 age group, with the majority of the over 50 women reported to be grand-multiparous women, who therefore may be more fertile. This group found that increasing maternal age is associated with adverse perinatal outcomes; however, their main finding is that women over the age of 50 are not at additional risk compared with women of age 40–49 years. For example, the risk of preterm delivery compared with the <39 group was aOR 1.4 (CI 1.37–1.62) for age 40–44, aOR 1.5 (CI 1.19–2.12) for age 45–49 and aOR 1.4 (CI 0.63–3.37) for age ≥50. Limitations in interpreting these findings include the small number of women over 50 considered, who were assumed more fertile; therefore, these women may be overall genetically "younger" too. There was likely underreporting of use of donor oocytes, which could confound these findings. Ideally, comparing women over 50 who have conceived spontaneously with women over 50 using donor oocytes would help to clarify this. However, such a study is unlikely to be feasible due to the small number of women conceiving naturally at ages over 50. Later we will discuss studies of women using donor oocytes and whether this provides a protective effect.

Lastly, one systematic review investigated the association of adverse maternal, perinatal and neonatal outcomes with maternal aging; however, the authors specifically chose to include studies addressing only very advanced maternal aged women defined as ≥45 years [8]. This systematic review confirmed the findings discussed above such as an increased risk of preterm delivery for women over 45 years (aOR 1.96 CI 1.16–2.39) and greater risk of their neonates having abnormal 5 min APGAR score (aOR 2.49 CI 1.37–4.54). However, the authors reported significant heterogeneity in the studies and inconsistent reporting of method of conception, therefore the results should be interpreted with caution.

In summary, neonates born to women over 40 are at increased risk of perinatal morbidities such as preterm delivery, low birth weight, neonatal complications such as low APGAR scores and admission to the NICU, and there is an increased risk of perinatal and neonatal mortality. However, the absolute risk is very low, which should be reassuring news to older women. Older women should be aware that their baby may be more likely to be admitted to the NICU.

Perinatal and Neonatal Outcomes of Children Born to Women over 40 after Using ART with Their Own Oocytes

Since the first paper by Schieve et al. in 2002 [9] showing increased risk of low birth weight and very low birth weight of singleton infants conceived by IVF compared to spontaneously conceived infants, numerous studies have established that children conceived using ART procedures have increased risk of both adverse perinatal and neonatal outcomes. Therefore, as more women are seeking ART especially in the over 40 age group, does ART have an additive adverse effect for women over 40? There have been several studies over the years that address this important question [6,10,11].

A large retrospective population-based cohort study was published that included data from three Nordic countries: Denmark, Finland and Norway from these countries' national ART and Medical Birth Registries collected from 1982 to 2007 [11]. The ART cohort included only fresh autologous IVF cycles with singleton births. For each ART child, four spontaneously conceived children were used as matched controls. The spontaneous conception (SC) cohort comprised 260,166 singleton births and there were 39,919 singleton births in the ART cohort. When comparing the ART cohort with the SC cohort in all age groups, as expected, the ART children had an increased occurrence of perinatal complications such as preterm birth, low birth weight, very low birth weight, SGA and perinatal mortality. The authors performed the same analysis for different age cut-offs (Table 12.1) comparing the ART conceived with SC conceived infants.

Interestingly, overall, the ART babies were at increased risk of perinatal complications; however, with increasing age, the risk between the ART and SC population was less pronounced such that at age 40, there was no difference in risk between ART and SC conceived infants with

Table 12.1 Comparison of select perinatal outcomes for infants conceived after assisted reproductive technologies versus spontaneous conceptions (reference group) at different maternal ages.

Outcome	Adjusted OR (95% Confidence Interval) P value				
	Age 25 y	Age 30 y	Age 35 y	Age 40 y	Age 45 y
Preterm birth <37wk	**2.19** **(1.94–2.47)** **P<.0001**	**1.58** **(1.45–1.71)** **P<.0001**	**1.45** **(1.33–1.59)** **P<.0001**	**1.23** **(1.05–1.43)** **P<.0086**	0.84 (0.44–1.61) P<.60
Low birth weight <2500 g	**2.35** **(2.05–2.68)** **P<.0001**	**1.76** **(1.60–1.94)** **P<.0001**	**1.44** **(1.30–1.59)** **P<.0001**	1.08 (0.91–1.28) P<.41	0.63 (0.30–1.34) P<.23
Perinatal mortality ≥ 28wk	**1.68** **(1.02–2.77)** **P<.040**	**1.53** **(1.12–2.10)** **P<.0083**	1.00 (0.74–1.37) P<.98	1.00 (0.64–1.56) P<.99	1.00 (0.38–2.65) P<1.00

Adjusted odds ratios and 95% confidence intervals included. P values shown are for assisted reproductive technologies versus spontaneous conceptions. Adjustment made for parity, year of birth, sex of offspring and country. Bolded text indicates statistically significant data.

Adapted from Wennberg et al. 2016 [11].

Table 12.2 Association of maternal age and preterm delivery in assisted reproductive technologies (ART) and spontaneous conception.

Method of conception	Adjusted OR (95% Confidence Interval) P Value			
	< 30 y	30 to <35 y	35 to <40 y	≥ 40 y
ART	**0.70** **(0.60–0.81)** **P<.0001** **n = 948**	1.06 (0.94–1.20) P<.32 n = 1,494	1.07 (0.92–1.25) P<.37 n = 983	0.73 (0.40–1.33) P<.31 n = 90
Spontaneous	0.97 (0.94–1.00) P<.090 n = 9,461	**1.15** **(1.08–1.23)** **P<.0001** **n = 3,699**	**1.27** **(1.13–1.44)** **P<.0001** **n = 1,309**	1.07 (0.74–1.52) P<.73 n = 198

Adjusted odds ratios and 95% confidence intervals and number of study subjects included. P values shown calculated by piecewise logistic regression model. Bolded text indicates statistically significant data.

Adapted from Wennberg et al. 2016 [11].

respect to low birth weight and perinatal mortality and preterm delivery by age 45 and over. The authors performed another analysis to investigate the effect of increasing maternal age on the ART and SC cohorts separately (Table 12.2). Their main findings were that the adverse neonatal outcomes did not increase in women over 35 in the ART cohort, whereas in the SC group, preterm delivery, very preterm delivery, low birth weight and SGA increased with maternal age. For example, for preterm delivery, in the ART cohort, there was a decrease in risk if the mother was under 30 years old and no increased risk after that. Whereas in the SC group, the risk for preterm delivery increased between ages 30 and 40, and there was

no significant increase in risk after age 40. In conclusion, in both SC and ART conceptions it appears that the risk of adverse perinatal outcomes does not increase significantly after the age of 40.

The strength of this study is that it is the largest to date and excluded donor oocyte pregnancies. There were a few limitations reported by the authors including the small number of women who were very advanced maternal age (>45) and although more than 1,000 women over 40 were included in the ART group, the number of adverse events was low, which reduced the statistical power for this group. Another limitation was the inability to adjust for socioeconomic status and this could have confounded the data. In the Nordic countries IVF is not provided free to women over 40, so the women over 40 in the ART group could have been from higher socioeconomic status compared with those in the SC group and may have had better overall health.

Others have investigated specifically the population of women of very advanced maternal age and use of ART. In a small retrospective cohort study from one single center that compared 185 women over 45 who used ART (± donor oocytes) with 193 women over 45 who conceived naturally, the authors found the only significant difference was in increased cesarean delivery rate in the women who had ART. They did not find any significant differences in fetal outcomes such as mean birth weight, mean gestational age, APGAR or NICU admission [10]. They also compared the outcomes between pregnancies with autologous oocytes and donor oocytes and did not find any significant differences. A limitation is that their sample size was small, low birth weight and preterm delivery were not assessed, and the ART group had a mixture of autologous and donor oocytes used, which could have confounded their findings. In another study discussed above by Wu and colleagues [6], they performed a subgroup analysis comparing ART versus spontaneously conceived pregnancies across different age groups, 20–34, 35–42 and ≥43. Consistent with the above Nordic study, all adverse perinatal outcomes were more likely in younger women undergoing ART than those conceiving naturally, whereas this association was not observed in women over 43. Of note, this study did adjust for socioeconomic status such as neighborhood income level and educational level, which were not adjusted for in the Nordic study; therefore, the hypothesis that women undergoing ART could be of higher socioeconomic status and therefore healthier is somewhat adjusted for in this study. Specifically, the authors found that apart from preterm delivery, there were no significant differences in risk for other perinatal outcomes, SGA and NICU admission between women over 43 undergoing ART versus natural conception.

In summary, the age-related increased risk of adverse perinatal outcomes is not present in women undergoing ART. Advancing maternal age impacts the risk of poor perinatal outcomes in women who conceived naturally to a greater extent than those who conceived by ART. Less is known about very advanced maternal age (>45) with use of ART compared with spontaneous conceptions due to the small numbers available for such analysis. Positively, it seems that on the basis of the available data, women over 40 can be reassured that using ART does not significantly increase their child's risk of having adverse perinatal outcomes over conceiving naturally. Furthermore, the data also indicate that, generally, there is no significant increase in adverse perinatal outcomes in pregnancies over 40, regardless of the mode of conception.

Perinatal and Neonatal Outcomes of Children Born to Women over 40 Who Used Donor Oocytes

The use of donor oocytes for women in perimenopause and menopause started in the early 1990s. A case report by Check et al. reported successful uncomplicated livebirths in two postmenopausal women who delivered at age 52 using donor oocytes [12]. Since then, use of donor oocytes as an acceptable form of family building has grown. The CDC (Centers for Disease Control and Prevention) reported in 2016 that 24,300 ART cycles used donor oocytes and the percentage of ART cycles using donor oocytes increased after age 40. Therefore, understanding whether there are differences in perinatal outcomes in women using donor oocytes or their own oocytes is increasingly becoming an important question. A well-documented obstetrical complication of donor oocyte pregnancies versus autologous oocyte IVF/intracytoplasmic sperm injection (ICSI) pregnancies is the increased risk of pregnancy-induced hypertension and preeclampsia, which has been hypothesized due to immunological differences between donor embryos and recipients [13]. Two meta-analyses have been performed to investigate the perinatal and neonatal outcomes of donor oocyte pregnancies versus both ART/spontaneous conception with autologous oocytes [14,15]. Adams and colleagues [14] searched for articles up until 2012 and included 23 studies in their analysis, and Storgaard et al. [15] included 35 articles published up till 2016. Both meta-analyses found similar conclusions, that infants born after donor oocyte cycles had increased risk of preterm delivery and low birth weight when compared with both IVF/ICSI and spontaneously conceived infants, these findings adjusted for maternal age. The increased risk of adverse neonatal outcomes remained when only singleton births were investigated. Additionally, Adams et al. found increased risk of very low birth weight. Neither meta-analysis found an increase in risk in small-for-gestational age in the donor oocyte conceived infants, but Adams et al. [14] mentioned that one study showed an increased number of infants conceived by donor oocytes admitted to the NICU and longer NICU admissions; more studies are needed to explore this. A more recent study [16] using the SART-CORS database, investigated the neonatal outcomes of infants from autologous oocyte frozen embryo cycles versus donor oocyte frozen embryo cycles in women aged 40–43 and found consistent results to the prior meta-analysis. Interestingly, when the authors analyzed only single blastocyst transfer cycles, the increased perinatal risks associated with donor oocyte cycles were ameliorated. Therefore, these authors recommended that single blastocyst transfer would be preferable for donor oocyte cycles to minimize the associated adverse outcomes.

Using donor oocytes to conceive at any age has increased adverse perinatal and neonatal outcomes compared with using IVF/ICSI with autologous oocytes or spontaneous conception. However, there is evidence that single embryo transfer can minimize these associated risks with donor oocyte cycles.

Childhood Outcomes

This next section will focus on what is known about parental aging and childhood illnesses. Many different studies of varying quality on various disorders associated with parental age have been published. In this part of the chapter, the literature on the more commonly studied and most impactful diseases on the child and family will be reviewed. For a comprehensive detailed review, the reader should refer to the review by Bergh and colleagues [17], which covers the entire spectrum of maternal and paternal age and association with various childhood diseases ranging from birth defects to schizophrenia.

Childhood Cancers

Cancer is one of the commonest causes of death in children aged 0–14 years old. Several investigators have addressed the relationship between advanced parental age and risk of childhood cancers. Theoretically, the accumulation of chromosomal aberrations such as de novo mutations could occur in aged gametes leading to an increased likelihood of cancer in children conceived from these gametes. Other factors that are hypothesized to have an effect are transgenerational epigenetic mutations in gametes and increased use of ART.

Two large studies have been published, one involving a California-based population case-control study of all pediatric cancers (n=24,734 cancer cases) [18] and the other Danish case-control study (n=5,856 cancer cases) [19]. The California study included pediatric cancer cases (0–19 years) occurring between 1978 and 2009 and found significant increase in pediatric cancer risk with increase in maternal age. The referent maternal age group was 20–24 years and the adjusted OR of the ≥40 age group was 1.53 (CI 1.26–1.84). The Danish group used the national Danish Cancer Registry to identify children with cancer aged 0–16 years between 1968 and 2015. This study had the referent age group at 25–29 and found that with every 5-year increase in maternal age, there was a significant increase in risk of all childhood cancers, aOR 1.05 (CI 1.01–1.18) after adjustment with paternal age. Interestingly, an increase in paternal age showed minimal to no association with the risk of childhood cancers. Therefore, in agreement with the review by Bergh et al., we conclude that the association between advanced maternal age and increased risk of childhood cancer is significant but a small contributor. Lastly, the likelihood of ART treatment additionally exacerbating the risk of childhood cancer is low, as using ART alone for conception has not been found to significantly increase childhood cancer risk [20].

With respect to specific childhood cancers, such as the two most common childhood cancers, acute lymphoblastic leukemia (ALL) and central nervous system (CNS) tumors, there are numerous studies that show significant though weak association with advancing maternal age and others that show no association (reviewed in [17]). Therefore, the association with ALL and CNS tumors is present, although weak. For example, the above California-based study [18] showed that each 5-year increase in maternal age was associated with an increase in risk of ALL, aOR

1.06 (CI 1.02–1.10) and that ≥40 age group had an aOR 1.40 (CI 1.13–1.74).

With advancing maternal age, there is an associated increased risk of childhood cancers; however, this risk is overall low, and the risk also varies depending on the type of childhood cancer.

Childhood Morbidity and Hospitalizations

The prior sections focused on specific diseases; however, are children of older mothers more likely to have increased overall morbidity or be admitted to the hospital more frequently than children of younger mothers? One large cohort study from Denmark using National Registry databases, studied 352,027 first-born singletons and 18 disease categories [21]. The data were stratified by age groups 15–24, 25–29, 30–34 and ≥35, with 25–29 being the referent group. Children of mothers over 35 had significant increase of risk in 8 of the 18 disease categories studied: mental disorders, cerebral disease, eye diseases, heart diseases, circulatory diseases, rheumatic diseases, neonatal diseases and congenital malformations. The incidence relative ratios varied from 1.06 to 1.29. Advanced maternal age was protective for respiratory diseases. Interestingly, increased childhood morbidity was also found for the youngest age group; therefore, there is a U-shaped age distribution for childhood morbidity. A recent cohort study included 202,709 deliveries in a region in Israel and investigated the long-term morbidity (up to 18 years) including hospitalization in six categories: cardiovascular, respiratory, endocrine, hematological, neurological and gastrointestinal [22]. The maternal age categories compared were 20–34, 35–39 and 40–50, and the authors found that the cumulative incidence did not differ significantly between the age groups. The seemingly conflicting data between these two studies is likely due to the latter study considering hospitalizations only, so there could be reporting bias towards the most serious morbidities.

There are sparse data on this topic; however, there is evidence that an increased risk of childhood morbidity not requiring hospitalization is associated with advanced maternal age.

Neurodevelopmental Diseases

Numerous studies have focused on the physical health outcomes of children born to older mothers; however, less is known about the neurodevelopment aspects. A review by Tearne provides a comprehensive review of the latter; however, it also highlights the paucity of data that exists [23].

General Behavior and Cognition

There have been a few studies investigating the behavioral development of children who have older mothers (summarized in [21]). The consensus from these studies showed a trend toward fewer behavioral problems (externalizing – disruptive, internalizing – withdrawal, conduct disorders) in children with older mothers; however, when maternal family background is accounted for, the detrimental effects of younger age are improved, which suggests that maternal family background is a more important factor than age itself. Similarly, several studies have looked at the relationship between cognitive ability and maternal age. Overall, the studies have found that children with older mothers have increased IQ and cognitive scores; however, there is a complex interplay with socioeconomic factors which could also account for these differences [21].

Being an older mother appears to positively affect their children's behavior and cognitive abilities, although age alone cannot explain all these observations.

Autism Spectrum Disorder

Autism spectrum disorder (ASD) encompasses a range of chronic neurodevelopmental disorders characterized by difficulties with social interactions, ability to communicate and by a restrictive, stereotyped, repetitive repertoire of interests and activities [24]. In the past two decades, the incidence of ASD has increased and is mirrored by the increase in parental age, therefore there have been many studies to investigate the relationship between the risk of ASD and parental age. This has been reviewed by Bergh et al. [17] and there has been a meta-analysis by Wu and colleagues [25]. The meta-analysis included 27 studies (6 cohort studies and 21 case-control studies) and had 66,948 autism events in total. As different studies had different age cut-offs, the authors of the meta-analysis used the midpoint of parental age as the reference age and calculated the risk of the lowest and highest parental age. For the highest maternal age category there was increased risk of ASD with aOR 1.41 (CI 1.29–1.55) and similarly increased paternal age was a risk factor aOR

1.55 (CI 1.39–1.73). The authors also investigated the dose-response of increasing parental age and found that a 10-year increase in maternal age was associated with 18% increased risk of ASD and paternal age was associated with 21% increased risk. One limitation of several of the studies in the meta-analysis is that there was no adjustment for partner's age, therefore there may be potential unadjusted confounders of both older mother and father contributing to increased risk of ASD.

There is a well-documented increased risk of ASD associated with both increasing maternal and paternal age although the age cut-off for this increase is unknown. Mothers and fathers 40 and over will have the highest associated risk.

Attention Deficit/Hyperactivity Disorder

Attention deficit/hyperactivity disorder (ADHD) is one of the commonest psychiatric disorders in childhood and is characterized by inattention, hyperactivity and impulsivity. There have been numerous studies examining the association of ADHD and parental age and the majority show that young parental age increases the risk of ADHD, while older parents have a reduced risk. There is no meta-analysis of the studies regarding ADHD; however, a recent large nested case-control study by Chudal et al. [26] provides a succinct summary of the studies in its introduction. This study investigated 10,409 cases versus 39,125 controls and showed that maternal age ≥40 had a significant protective effect against ADHD (aOR 0.79, CI 0.64–0.97).

There is significant decreased risk of ADHD associated with advanced maternal age (Table 12.3).

Strategies to Optimize the Development of Children Born to Women over 40

Introduction

Physicians (including Reproductive Endocrinology and Infertility specialists (REIs), Ob/Gyns, pediatricians) are increasingly presented with individuals who are intending to, or have, become parents over 40 years of age. Most are familiar with the literature regarding increased risks of "advanced maternal age," but may need information and guidance regarding recommendations for parenting after conceiving beyond 40. Even when individuals do not ask, it will be helpful to provide them information about what to expect once the baby has arrived.

Parenting at Age 40 and Over

Compared with parenting in the teens to mid-20s, parenting over 40 carries many advantages. Research indicates that humans do not complete development of their frontal lobes until the mid-to-late 20s [27]. The frontal lobes of the human cortex are responsible for managing oneself and one's resources to achieve a goal, and include flexible thinking, working memory and self-control. Although there are challenges associated with parenting over 40, these parents can fully utilize their strengths in executive functioning to plan for and address these challenges. Indeed, the planful nature that is often required to become a parent over 40 allows individuals to prepare for the challenges of parenting, and to optimize their child's development.

Recent research [28] has defined advantages and disadvantages from the parents' viewpoints of

Table 12.3 Summary of the relationship of advanced maternal age (≥35 years) and childhood health outcomes.

Childhood disorder	Effect of advanced maternal age
All childhood cancers	Increased risk
Leukemias	Increased risk
Central nervous system tumors	Conflicting results
General behavior disorders	Decreased risk externalizing behaviors Increased risk internalizing behaviors
Autistic spectrum disorder (ASD)	Increased risk
Attention deficit/hyperactivity disorders (ADHD)	Decreased risk

having a child after 40. Interviews with 117 parents who conceived through IVF at age 40 or older indicated several advantages of the experience including feeling more emotionally ready for parenthood, mature and financially secure. They reported strong relationships in support of coparenting. The respondents indicated that parenting in later life made them feel young for longer and motivated them to stay physically fit. Later life parents reported having more flexibility in balancing work and family due to their better-established careers, which allowed them to reorient their lives more easily as they adopted a parenting role. Despite these advantages, the later life parents in this study also described many challenges, including lack of physical energy (feeling depleted), awareness of having fewer years to spend with their children and concern that their own illness or physical well-being could impact their child. Of those interviewed for this study, 90% indicated that the optimal timing for becoming a parent was prior to the age of 40.

Those who opt to become parents after 40 should be encouraged to consult with a psychologist or other mental health professional with expertise in assisted reproduction, parenting and child development. A referral to a mental health professional can help to develop parenting skills, address concerns and challenges of later life parenting, and ensure when couples are coparenting that expectations are clearly defined. Medical providers may not have time for lengthy discourse regarding parenting, but they can share the following resources and encourage consultation with an appropriate mental health professional.

Parenting a Child Conceived by Donor Oocytes and Sperm

Those who are using donor gametes (sperm, egg or embryo) to have a child have additional considerations. Guidelines from the American Society for Reproductive Medicine (ASRM) indicate that those using donor gametes should have a consultation with a qualified mental health professional to discuss the impact of using donor gametes [29]. In this consultation, the recipient(s) will consider issues such as whether to use a known or de-identified (previously referred to as anonymous) donor. In the age of direct to consumer genetic testing, anonymity no longer exists [30]. Recipients can be encouraged to explore options such as an open identity, wherein the child has access to the identity of the donor when the child reaches the age of majority. The mental health professional will also provide the language (e.g., the donor is never referred to as the biological "mother" or "father," but simply as the donor) and examples for the recipients on how to share their child's story with them. As many professionals with experience working with donor conceived children advise, it is best to "tell early and often." Parents can learn how to share their child's story in a way that celebrates how wanted the child was and the parts that were necessary to bring the child into the family. Additional issues such as how to share the idea of donor-related others (others conceived from gametes from the same donor) with their child are also discussed in the donor recipient consultation. Some parents worry that they will feel less connection with their child because of their donor origins, or they worry that the child will feel "different." These complex issues can be explored and validated in the consultation session, and with additional counseling support if needed.

Later Life Parenting Tips to Optimize the Development of the Child

Consider and Plan for the Full Lifespan of the Child

Many who are yearning to become parents have a hard time imagining that fertility treatments will result in a baby in their arms, making it difficult to consider what it will be like to parent a child throughout the child's lifespan. However, capitalizing on their strengths, later life parents can plan and prepare for each stage of development, to optimize their child's outcomes and their parenting experience.

Preparing for an Infant

Parents should be encouraged to make plans to address the sleep deprivation that necessarily accompanies infants' needs for feedings throughout the night. If coparenting, the couple can work together on a plan to ensure each parent is able to get an extended period of uninterrupted sleep. New parents often need encouragement to seek and accept help. The new parent should have a plan in place to support adequate sleep for each partner, utilizing friends, family and paid help as needed. Parents should be made aware that prolonged sleep deprivation can increase postpartum mood and anxiety disorders, for which women over 40 are already at greater risk (compounded further if they have a history of infertility, pregnancy loss and/or failed fertility treatments)[31,32]. New parents should be made aware of resources such as night nurses and postpartum doulas. Additional planning and education surrounding nourishment of the baby (including options related to breastmilk and formula) and infant care (diaper changing, swaddling, bathing, etc.) should be provided. For those who are coparenting, education about the impact of having a child on the marriage should be encouraged. There are resources such as Gottman and Gottman's *And Baby Makes Three* and a workshop called *Bringing Baby Home* that are available to help couples as they anticipate the change in their family when they have a baby. Couples should be encouraged to clearly define expectations surrounding maternity/paternity leave, returning to work and childcare decisions.

Preparing to Parent a Toddler

In the transition from infancy to toddlerhood, parents should be encouraged to have a clear understanding of the parenting style they wish to adopt. Extensive research has supported that a positive authoritative parenting style results in the best outcomes for children [33]. Parents that are positive and authoritative balance warmth, behavioral control and responsiveness. As infants become toddlers, their behavior will naturally be more challenging and will require parents to determine how they want to guide their child's behaviors. It is true that children do not come with instruction manuals, and it is also true that there are innumerable conflicting books about how to best parent a child. In general, the goal is to develop a nurturing, warm and responsive parent-child relationship with appropriate boundaries to ensure behavioral control. This in turn helps the child develop a secure attachment [34]. Parents may need to reflect on their own upbringing and obtain guidance from a mental health professional with knowledge about parenting and child development.

Preparing to Parent a School-Aged Child

Parents are encouraged to reflect on the age they will be as their child enters elementary school. Later life parents can be encouraged to find other families with whom they connect, to share the joy and challenges of parenting. Parents should continue to ensure that their activity level supports their children's energy level, and that there is a community of others who also engage with the child.

Preparing to Parent a Tween and Teen

This stage is difficult for parents to imagine prior to the birth of their child, particularly when they have struggled to conceive or have had pregnancy loss. Later life parents should be encouraged to imagine their own stage of life as their child enters the preteen and teen years. At this stage, they may have already been faced with the failing health of their own parents, which can be particularly difficult as they have their own parenting demands.

Preparing to Parent beyond 18 Years of Age

Later life parents should consider and plan for the possibility that their child will be presented with illness or loss of their parents at a relatively young age. It will be important to develop a community of family and/or friends so that their child has support in the case of having to manage parental death at an early age. Research has found that the death of a parent before a child reaches the age of 35 shortens the lifespan of the child [35]. Helping to mitigate the stress that is sure to accompany such a loss will be important.

Finding a Community

Parenting can be isolating, particularly if later life parents' friends are not in the same stage of family building. The reality that later life parents are more likely to have fewer years with their children means that expanding the network of those your child knows and trusts will be vital. Later life parents can be encouraged to begin to create their community prior to their child's birth. Their village may include friends and a range of family members. Asking for others to be part of their village as they raise their child can help ensure that the child has many who love them and will be part of their lives in myriad ways. Research indicates that children of later life parents appreciate their parents' emotional and financial stability, recognize that they were wanted and view their parents as wise, devoted and patient [36]. However, they also experience worries of their parents' mortality, so ensuring that they are surrounded by many people who love and care for them eases some of the concern for parents and children alike.

Closing Remarks

The goal of this chapter is to inform women over 40 of potential adverse health outcomes that their child may be at risk of, which represent factors beyond their control (nature), balanced with informing them of strategies to nurture their child, over which they have absolute control.

Further reading

Gottman, J.M. and Gottman, J.S. *And Baby Makes Three: The Six-Step Plan for Preserving Marital Intimacy and Rekindling Romance After Baby Arrives*. CA: Three Rivers Press; 2008.

The Gottman Institute. Bringing Baby Home Educator Training. www.gottman.com/professionals/training/bringing-baby-home/

References

1. Cnattingius, S., et al., *Delayed childbearing and risk of adverse perinatal outcome. A population-based study.* JAMA, 1992. **268**(7): p. 886–90.

2. Jacobsson, B., L. Ladfors, and I. Milsom, *Advanced maternal age and adverse perinatal outcome.* Obstet Gynecol, 2004. **104**(4): p. 727–33.

3. Klemetti, R., et al., *At what age does the risk for adverse maternal and infant outcomes increase? Nationwide register-based study on first births in Finland in 2005–2014.* Acta Obstet Gynecol Scand, 2016. **95**(12): p. 1368–75.

4. Zapata-Masias, Y., et al., *Obstetric and perinatal outcomes in women ≥40 years of age: Associations with fetal growth disorders.* Early Hum Dev, 2016. **100**: p. 17–20.

5. Kahveci, B., et al., *The effect of advanced maternal age on perinatal outcomes in nulliparous singleton pregnancies.* BMC Pregnancy Childbirth, 2018. **18**(1): p. 343.

6. Wu, Y., et al., *Adverse maternal and neonatal outcomes among singleton pregnancies in women of very advanced maternal age: a retrospective cohort study.* BMC Pregnancy Childbirth, 2019. **19**(1): p. 3.

7. Maoz-Halevy, E., et al., *Perinatal outcomes of women aged 50 years and above.* Am J Perinatol, 2020. **37**(1): p. 79–85.

8. Leader, J., et al., *The effect of very advanced maternal age on maternal and neonatal outcomes: a systematic review.* J Obstet Gynaecol Can, 2018. **40**(9): p. 1208–18.

9. Schieve, L.A., et al., *Low and very low birth weight in infants conceived with use of assisted reproductive technology.* N Engl J Med, 2002. **346**(10): p. 731–7.

10. Jackson, S., et al., *Pregnancy outcomes in very advanced maternal age pregnancies: the impact of assisted reproductive technology.* Fertil Steril, 2015. **103**(1): p. 76–80.

11. Wennberg, A.L., et al., *Effect of maternal age on maternal and neonatal outcomes after assisted reproductive technology.* Fertil Steril, 2016. **106**(5): p. 1142–9.e14.

12. Check, J.H., et al., *Successful delivery after age 50: a report of two cases as a result of oocyte donation.* Obstet Gynecol, 1993. **81**(5 (Pt 2)): p. 835–6.

13. Masoudian, P., et al., *Oocyte donation pregnancies and the risk of preeclampsia or gestational hypertension: a systematic review and metaanalysis.* Am J Obstet Gynecol, 2016. **214**(3): p. 328–39.

14. Adams, D.H., et al., *A meta-analysis of neonatal health outcomes from oocyte donation.* J Dev Orig Health Dis, 2016. **7**(3): p. 257–72.

15. Storgaard, M., et al., *Obstetric and neonatal complications in pregnancies conceived after oocyte donation: a systematic review and meta-analysis.* BJOG, 2017. **124**(4): p. 561–72.

16. Yu, B., et al., *Comparison of perinatal outcomes following frozen embryo transfer cycles using autologous versus donor oocytes in women 40 to 43 years old: analysis of SART CORS data.* J Assist Reprod Genet, 2018. **35**(11): p. 2025–9.

17. Bergh, C., A. Pinborg, and U.B. Wennerholm, *Parental age and child outcomes.* Fertil Steril, 2019. **111**(6): p. 1036–46.

18. Wang, R., et al., *Parental age and risk of pediatric cancer in the offspring: a population-based record-linkage study in California.* Am J Epidemiol, 2017. **186**(7): p. 843–56.

19. Contreras, Z.A., et al., *Parental age and childhood cancer risk: A Danish population-based registry study.* Cancer Epidemiol, 2017. **49**: p. 202–15.

20. Levi-Setti, P.E. and P. Patrizio, *Assisted reproductive technologies (ART) and childhood cancer: is the risk real?* J Assist Reprod Genet, 2018. **35**(10): p. 1773–5.

21. Hviid, M.M., et al., *Maternal age and child morbidity: A Danish national cohort study.* PLoS One, 2017. **12**(4): p. e0174770.

22. Pariente, G., et al., *Advanced maternal age and the future health of the offspring.* Fetal Diagn Ther, 2019. **46**(2): p. 139–46.

23. Tearne, J.E., *Older maternal age and child behavioral and cognitive outcomes: a review of the literature.* Fertil Steril, 2015. **103**(6): p. 1381–91.

24. World Health Organization. Autism. 2022. https://www.who.int/news-room/fact-sheets/detail/autism-spectrum-disorders

25. Wu, S., et al., *Advanced parental age and autism risk in children: a systematic review and meta-analysis.* Acta Psychiatr Scand, 2017. **135**(1): p. 29–41.

26. Chudal, R., et al., *Parental age and the risk of attention-deficit/hyperactivity disorder: a nationwide, population-based cohort study.* J Am Acad Child Adolesc Psychiatry, 2015. **54**(6): p. 487–94.e1.

27. Sowell, E.R., et al., *In vivo evidence for post-adolescent brain maturation in frontal and striatal regions.* Nat Neurosci, 1999. **2**(10): p. 859–61.

28. Mac Dougall, K., Y. Beyene, and R.D. Nachtigall, *'Inconvenient biology:' advantages and disadvantages of first-time parenting after age 40 using in vitro fertilization.* Hum Reprod, 2012. **27**(4): p. 1058–65.

29. *Recommendations for gamete and embryo donation: a committee opinion.* Fertil Steril, 2013. **99**(1): p. 47–62.

30. Harper, J.C., D. Kennett, and D. Reisel, *The end of donor anonymity: how genetic testing is likely to drive anonymous gamete donation out of business.* Hum Reprod, 2016. **31**(6): p. 1135–40.

31. Boivin, J., et al., *Associations between maternal older age, family environment and parent and child wellbeing in families using assisted reproductive techniques to conceive.* Soc Sci Med, 2009. **68**(11): p. 1948–55.

32. Carlson, D.L., *Explaining the curvilinear relationship between age at first birth and depression among women.* Soc Sci Med, 2011. **72**(4): p. 494–503.

33. Kuppens, S. and E. Ceulemans, *Parenting styles: a closer look at a well-known concept.* J Child Fam Stud, 2019. **28**(1): p. 168–81.

34. Karavasilis, L., A.B. Doyle, and D. Markiewicz, *Associations between parenting style and attachment to mother in middle childhood and adolescence.* Int J Behav Dev, 2003. **27**(2): p. 153–64.

35. Myrskylä, M., et al., *The association between advanced maternal and paternal ages and increased adult mortality is explained by early parental loss.* Soc Sci Med, 2014. **119**: p. 215–23.

36. Yarrow, A.L., *Latecomers: children of parents over 35.* 1991, New York: Free Press; Oxford: Maxwell Macmillan International.

Chapter

13

Practical Egg Donation in Women over 40

James P. Toner and Lauren Rouleau

Donor eggs can overcome age-related decline in egg quality, premature ovarian insufficiency, and transmission of genetic disease in those carrying gene mutations [1,2]. Among recipients over 40, while success rates remain excellent with this approach, certain age-related risks of pregnancy increase [3]. This chapter reviews the practical management of these cycles, and the age-related risks.

Source of Donor Eggs

Most egg donors are not known to the recipients of their eggs (formerly termed "anonymous" but the term is no longer apt due to widespread personal genetic testing [4]), and the donors are in their 20s. Before oocyte vitrification was developed, most donations of eggs were "fresh," that is, the eggs were immediately inseminated to produce embryos, which in turn were transferred to the intended carrier without first freezing the embryos. This required synchronization of the recipient endometrium to the donor's egg retrieval, which was cumbersome but avoided the expense and risk of cryopreservation. Alternatively, some programs froze all embryos to avoid the need for synchronization; embryos were then thawed at the appropriate time in the recipient's cycle. Some limitations of working with fresh eggs included an uneven number of available eggs across recipients (some donors produced many eggs and some few), delayed treatment (while waiting for donor to be stimulated) and higher cost.

With the development of effective egg vitrification, a more effective form of cryopreservation [5], many recipients now choose to use frozen eggs. As the eggs are already banked, they are immediately available. Synchronization of donor and recipient are not required, the number of eggs is fixed, and cost is typically lower as the donor-related costs can be spread over several recipients. In the United States today, a cycle of egg donation with fresh eggs typically costs about $32,000, whereas a cycle using a batch of frozen embryos from an outside egg bank costs about $26,000. Some clinics have their own egg banks, and thereby are able to charge a lower amount, typically around $22,000 (personal experience of JPT).

Success Rates

The use of donor eggs largely eliminates the age-related decline of fertility [6]. In a retrospective analysis of donor egg cycles, small increases in miscarriage rates and small decreases in implantation, pregnancy, and liveborn delivery rates, were noted to occur in the late 40s (Figure 13.1) [7]. A 2013 report confirms the same trends in tabular form [8].

Pregnancy Risks

Age-related pregnancy risks rise whether the eggs involved are autologous or donor. These risks include many serious medical and obstetric conditions and are especially high in women at or above age 45. For instance, maternal death and cardiac arrest are 10 times more common in women over 44 versus women under 35 (Table 13.1) [9–12]. Accordingly, most programs require preconceptual clearance from an internist and obstetrician before proceeding with donor egg therapy [12]. Moreover, most programs also have age limits for recipients of donor eggs due to these increased risks [13]. The American Society for Reproductive Medicine (ASRM)'s Ethics Committee concludes that treatment of women above age 55 should generally be discouraged [14].

Fresh versus Frozen Donor Eggs

The advent of vitrification has allowed highly successful survival of both eggs and embryos [15]. Several reports, but not all, indicate that the implantation rates per embryo, as well as the "egg to baby" rate, are similar for fresh and frozen eggs

Table 13.1 Medical and obstetric events at delivery among women age 34–44 and ≥45 compared with women aged <35 y old [6]

Condition/event	Age 35–44 y	Age ≥45 y
Medical condition		
Maternal death	2.07 (1.78–2.40)	9.90 (5.60–15.98)
Transfusion	1.21 (1.20–1.23)	2.46 (2.27–2.68)
Myocardial infarction	4.05 (3.29–4.98)	21.38 (11.46–39.88)
Cardiac arrest	2.07 (1.82–2.42)	10.84 (6.48–18.14)
Pulmonary embolism	1.83 (1.69–1.98)	5.01 (3.47–7.23)
Deep vein thrombosis	2.02 (1.91–2.14)	4.38 (3.26–5.89)
Acute renal failure	1.86 (1.76–1.97)	6.38 (5.06–8.04)
Obstetric event		
Cesarean delivery	1.62 (1.61–1.62)	2.51 (2.44–2.57)
Gestational diabetes	2.42 (2.41–2.44)	3.5 (3.37–3.62)
Gestational hypertension	1.11 (1.10–1.12)	2.17 (2.09–2.25)
Preterm labor	1.16 (1.15–1.17)	1.91 (1.84–1.98)
Fetal growth restriction	0.92 (0.91–0.93)	1.53 (1.42–1.64)
Fetal demise	1.30 (1.27–1.33)	1.5 (2.22–2.89)
Premature rupture of membranes	1.10 (1.09–1.11)	1.38 (1.30–1.46)

Values are odds ratio (95% confidence interval). All *P* values <.001 compared with women aged <35 y.

Source: Modified from [12], with permission from Elsevier.

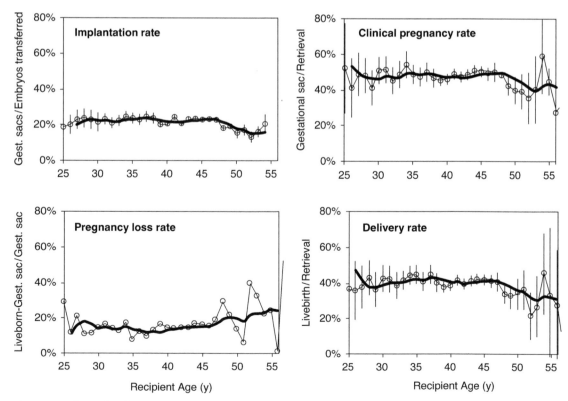

Figure 13.1 Rates of implantation, clinical pregnancy, miscarriage, and delivery among recipients of donor eggs. Each panel shows mean ± SEM as the line with markers and error bars, and a moving average as the line without markers to show the general trend
Source: Reprinted from [5], with permission from Elsevier.

[16–21]. Other studies report reduced blastulation rates with vitrified oocytes [17,22,23].

While overall delivery rates with fresh eggs exceed those using frozen eggs, some of this advantage is due to a larger number of eggs being available. Moreover, use of frozen donor eggs has several advantages [15,16]: it is quicker (eggs are already available so there is no delay in [18,19] stimulating the donor to obtain eggs), there is no need for synchronization of donor and recipient, it is often less expensive, and provides a fixed "dose" of eggs. Most Egg Banks in the United States provide six to eight eggs per batch, with some guaranteeing that at least one high-quality blastocyst develops. Modelling suggests the probability of having at least one live-born child with the use of donor eggs is above 50% with as few as five frozen donor eggs [17]. The use of frozen eggs also allows clinics without their own egg donors to offer this option to their patients.

An ASRM Committee Opinion exists with data showing improved pregnancy rates after blastocyst (day 5) transfer versus cleavage stage (day 3) transfer [24]. This practice has become widely accepted. Although there are less data focused specifically on donor oocytes, similar improvements are seen in implantation and pregnancy rates using blastocyst transfer over cleavage stage transfer [25,26]. The ASRM Practice Committee recommends that no more than one embryo be transferred at the cleavage and blastocyst stage for cycles involving donor eggs [27].

Preparation of Recipient's Endometrium and Support of Pregnancy

During a medicated recipient cycle, a corpus luteum does not form, thus, exogenous estradiol and progesterone are required to support the pregnancy until the placenta can produce enough on its own, typically around 8 weeks of gestation [28]. During a natural cycle, the corpus luteum provides sufficient estrogen and progesterone until the placental production takes over (the "luteoplacental shift"). Early experience in donor egg recipient cycles confirmed that this shift occurs at around 7 weeks of gestation [28]. In

routine in vitro fertilization (IVF), the multiple corpora lutea are sufficient, rendering additional progesterone supplementation unnecessary [29–32]. In natural cycle FETs, the data are conflicting. A small randomized controlled trial by Eftekhar et al. demonstrated that during a natural FET cycle there was no difference with or without use of progesterone for luteal phase support in clinical pregnancy rate [33]. This contrasts with a randomized controlled trials by Bjuresten et al., which showed an increase in live birth rate after luteal progesterone supplementation during a natural FET cycle [34]. Given the conflicting data, more investigation in this area is needed. One specific population in which luteal progesterone support has shown a positive effect is in women with recurrent pregnancy loss [35].

The recipient's endometrium can be made receptive via programmed cycles or natural cycles [36,37]. Programmed (or medicated) cycles employ estradiol and progesterone to prepare the endometrium. The dose and route of administration can vary, and studies have been unable to show that one approach is better than another. Estradiol can be given transdermally, vaginally, intramuscularly, or orally. Progesterone can be given intramuscularly or vaginally. Embryo transfer typically occurs on the sixth day of progesterone if blastocysts are being transferred, or on the fourth day if cleavage stage embryos are being transferred. The primary advantage of programmed FETs is predictability of office visits; the primary disadvantage is use of intramuscular progesterone (at least in the United States, where it is the most common route). Among recipients with ovulatory cycles, embryo transfer can be timed to ovulation, based on luteinizing hormone (LH) surge or human chorionic gonadotropin (hCG) trigger. In this case, transfer is scheduled for the seventh day after LH surge is detected in the morning or eighth day after hCG trigger given in the evening. There is no evidence that maternal age affects the success of these approaches.

Programmed versus Natural Cycle Endometrial Prep

Estrogen and progesterone are sufficient to prepare the endometrium for pregnancy. Due to the historical pattern of trying to get fresh embryos into the uterus without freezing, synchronization of the donor and recipient cycles was done by providing exogenous estradiol and progesterone [38,39]. Synchronization was often challenging but is moot when transfer of frozen embryos from either fresh or frozen eggs is being planned. Medicated or natural cycle FETs can be planned independent of the date of egg retrieval. While medicated FETs have historically been more common, recent studies suggest that natural cycles can also be used, timing the thaw of oocytes to the day of ovulation. Recently, studies have suggested increased neonatal and maternal risks following programmed versus natural cycles. Hypertensive disorders were especially increased [40–46]. As the human corpus luteum also secretes relaxin, oxytocin, and other vasoactive compounds [47], it is possible that these other substances influence the course of pregnancy [44,45,48].

Other Considerations
Donor and Recipient Screening

Egg donors undergo a comprehensive screening process to assure the donors are physically and mentally healthy, do not have serious genetic conditions, have no relevant infectious disease, have a sufficient supply of eggs, and are not being coerced to donate [49]. In the United States, the Food and Drug Administration specifies the required screening tests [50].

In assessing the ability of the recipient to engage in this therapy, it is essential to optimize the uterine environment for successful implantation. This would include addressing fibroids that are large or distort the cavity, communicating hydrosalpinges, and intracavity adhesions. In the United States currently, in the absence of pain or endometriomas, the presence of endometriosis is no longer assessed by routine laparoscopy, so some recipients with endometriosis go undetected. Even so, the effect of endometriosis on IVF is uncertain.

Postmenopausal Donor Oocyte Recipients

Many recipients of donor eggs are beyond normal reproductive age, and some are even menopausal. In guidance with the ASRM's Ethics Committee Opinion, offering oocyte donation to women over age 55 should be discouraged [51]. Additionally, a full health evaluation should be performed for women 45 and older. If a major health concern is apparent, a comprehensive discussion of risks and benefits must be undertaken. There are ample data showing a significantly increased rate of obstetric complications for women age 45 and older. Menopausal recipients will need hormone replacement prior to endometrial preparation. Those menopausal for an extended period may suffer from atrophy of the genital tract and uterus [52,53] and thus may benefit from estrogen replacement for several months before embryo transfer. Hormone replacement therapy can restore the endometrial appearance to a premenopausal state [54]. Overall, there are few data examining the safety or efficacy of this approach, but it is reasonable to consider, especially if a mock or prep cycle does not produce the desired hormonal levels or endometrial thickness.

Legal Considerations

Both donors and recipients sign contracts outlining the process and risks with this form of third-party reproduction. If the donor is not known to the recipients, these contracts are with the treating clinic. If the donor is known to the recipient, then the contract is between the donor and recipient. In all cases the language specifies that the eggs obtained, and the children resulting from those eggs, become the recipient's. The donor has no parental rights or responsibilities, and the recipient assumes these rights and responsibilities.

Legal and ethical implications of oocyte donation are complex. The ASRM has Ethics Committee guidelines surrounding this issue, and statutory laws also exist [55]. The laws include both uniform laws/model acts and enacted state laws. The National Organ Transplant Act, created in 1984, prohibits the sale of certain tissues and organs but excludes renewable tissues such as sperm and blood. Oocytes are not technically renewable, but this act does not address them directly. It is widely accepted that oocyte donation and compensating oocyte donors is not prohibited or illegal.

Reproductive law must be enacted by each state individually. The uniform parentage act (UPA) was created in 1973 and has been revised several times. Initially, the UPA legitimized individuals born from donor sperm, but at the time did not mention oocyte donation, as it was not yet an established practice. It now incorporates same-sex parents' right to be named on birth certificates and equal recognition of intended parents regardless of gender, sexual orientation, or marital status. Most recently, it was revised to include the right of donor-conceived persons to access de-identified medical data about their donor. As of the date of this publication, the UPA has been enacted in four states and introduced in three others. There are several other acts, which have not yet been enacted in any states including the Model Act Governing Assisted Reproductive Technology, which states a gamete donor without intent to parent is not considered a parent and additionally requires all third-party reproductive participants to meet with a licensed mental health professional. Less than 15 states have laws surrounding oocyte donation [56,57].

Full discussion/description of the laws surrounding oocyte donation is out of the scope of this text, but it is evident that the legal landscape is changing and having difficulty keeping up with the pace of technological advancement. Considering this, we must be vigilant with how we counsel patients.

Epigenetic Changes

Epigenetics is defined as the study of gene expression changes rather than the alterations of the gene sequence itself. This includes any process that may alter gene expression including DNA methylation changes, histone modifications, alterations in imprinting, and variations in the level of microRNA expression. These effects are imparted by the woman carrying the pregnancy, not the woman supplying the eggs. Highlighting this effect can allow recipients to feel more connected to any donor egg pregnancy, knowing that they influence which genes are turned on and which off.

Epigenetics has become especially important in the field of reproductive medicine as there has been an increase in rare imprinting disorders tied to use of ART including Beckwith-Wiedemann syndrome, Angelman syndrome, and Silver-Russell syndrome [58]. As imprinting occurs during the early days of embryo development and coincides with the window of embryo culture in IVF, it is not surprising that such effects may occur. An extensive literature review by Barberet et al. suggests that there may be specific epigenetic changes that occur during oocyte vitrification, but

the data are limited, especially in reference to fetal programming and long-term outcomes [59]. One study by Cobo et al. examined over 1,000 children born using vitrified oocytes and suggests favorable obstetric and neonatal outcomes, but no long-term follow-up is yet available [60].

Preimplantation Genetic Testing

There are few data on preimplantation genetic testing for aneuploidy (PGT-A) with regard to oocyte donation. Given that aneuploidy increases with age and most oocyte donors are young, it follows that the rate of aneuploidy is lower in this population. Thus, it may not be beneficial to use PGT for these embryos unless there is an autosomal dominant or shared autosomal recessive condition involving the gametes that PGT-M could identify. A recent study by Doyle et al. examined data from 1,291 cycles from 223 donors which showed no difference in the live birth rate from vitrified oocyte donors whether PGT-A was used or not [61]. There is an additional study from 2017, which reports a lower rate of live birth with PGT-A [62]. More data are needed to make a final determination, but it is likely PGT-A is unnecessary in most cases when using donor oocytes. The decision to use PGT-A should be discussed in a shared decision-making model with the patient.

Recurrent Implantation Failure

Recurrent implantation failure describes the situation in which a sustained implantation has not occurred after the transfer of several high-quality embryos (three or more is a common cutoff). Theoretically, endometritis or abnormal endometrial development could shift or alter the window of receptivity, leading to failed implantation [63,64].

Although several aspects of the endometrium may in principle lead to implantation failure, it has been difficult to define their prevalence or importance. Evaluation of endometrial histology to identify a luteal phase defect has not proved reliable [65]. The Endometrial Receptivity Assay (ERA) examines an array of endometrial gene expression and correlates them to receptive, prereceptive, or postreceptive endometria. Unfortunately, the data are mixed on whether this assay improves implantation rates in the following FET cycle [66,67]. The Endometrial Function Test (EFT) examines both histology and molecular function. The molecular aspect examines levels of cyclin E and p27, a proliferative and anti-proliferative marker, respectively, to assess endometrial development. The result of the assay itself has not been shown to increase implantation rates, but an abnormal test does correlate with likely implantation failure, and may allow for specific adjustments to be made in stimulation protocols for individual women [68,69]. Another test is ReceptivaDx, which can suggest endometriosis as a cause for recurrent implantation failure by examining an inflammatory marker BCL-6, which is known to be increased in, though not specific for, endometriosis [70,71]. There are some promising data showing improved pregnancy rates once treatment of endometriosis is performed (typically via laparoscopy) in patients with severe disease who have failed prior attempts at IVF [72,73]. This assay can improve diagnostic accuracy of endometriosis leading to appropriate treatment and theoretically improved implantation rates.

These tests require endometrial biopsy and should not be performed during a transfer cycle. Initial testing for obvious causes such as endometrial polyps, endometritis, or hyperplasia should be addressed prior to these more expensive assays. The use of these tests is still controversial and can be costly, but if an individual has had recurrent implantation failure and the number of embryos remaining is few, it may be worth considering.

Protocols

The goal is to transfer embryos into the uterus at the appropriate time of a natural or medicated menstrual cycle. For blastocyst transfers, this will be on the sixth day of progesterone supplementation in a medicated cycle, the seventh day after an hCG injection that induces ovulation, or the sixth day after a urinary LH surge if detected in the morning. Serum progesterone levels are often checked in the midluteal phase, and supplementation provided if the level is <15 ng/mL (47.7 nmol/L).

Endometrial Preparation Using Exogenous Estradiol and Progesterone

Taking control of the menstrual cycle with leuprolide in the mid-luteal phase of the prior cycle is a common strategy that facilitates the timing of embryo transfer and prevents undesired interference from ovarian activity. Normally the leuprolide is continued daily until progesterone is begun.

Alternatively, oral contraceptives can also be used, but should be stopped a few days before beginning the estradiol replacement to permit shedding of the endometrial lining.

Estradiol is essential for endometrial development. It can be given orally, vaginally, or transdermally, all to good effect. The dose regimen can be fixed or escalating without an evident difference in pregnancy outcome. Adequate response is indicated on ultrasound by a trilaminar endometrium at least 7 mm thick. If this goal is not achieved at the first midcycle check, the estradiol dosing can be extended or increased. If pregnancy occurs, the estradiol is continued through 9 weeks of pregnancy to allow time for onset of sufficient placental production.

A common medication schedule and options (Figure 13.2) is:

- Leuprolide

  ○ 20 units subcutaneously daily from cycle day 21, drop dose to 10 units once estradiol begun, and stop altogether once progesterone is started.

- Estradiol

  ○ One 0.1 mg patch × 2 days, then two 0.1 patches × 2 days, then three 0.1 patches × 2 days, then four 0.1 mg patches every other day through 9 weeks of pregnancy

  ○ Four 0.1 mg patches every other day through 8–10 weeks of pregnancy

  ○ Oral estradiol 1 mg twice daily for 4 days, then 2 mg twice daily for 4 days, then 2 mg three times daily through 9 weeks of pregnancy

  ○ Vaginal estradiol 2 mg daily through weeks 8–10 of pregnancy.

- Progesterone

  ○ Progesterone in oil 50–100 mg daily intramuscularly through 8–10 weeks of pregnancy

  ○ Progesterone capsules 200 mg vaginally three times daily until 8–10 weeks of pregnancy

  ○ Endometrin 100 mg vaginally three times daily until 8–10 weeks of pregnancy

  ○ Crinone 90 mg vaginally twice daily until 8–10 weeks of pregnancy.

If frozen donor eggs are being used, once the desired endometrial response is evident, progesterone can be added. The eggs are thawed and

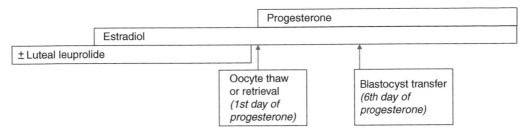

−7 −6 −5 −4 −3 −2 −1 0 1 2 3 4 5 6 7 8 9 10 11 12 13 14 1 2 3 4 5 6 7 8 9 10 11 12 13 14 15

Progesterone

Estradiol

± Luteal leuprolide

Oocyte thaw
or retrieval
*(1st day of
progesterone)*

Blastocyst transfer
*(6th day of
progesterone)*

Figure 13.2 Endometrial preparation using exogenous estradiol and progesterone

inseminated that same day to synchronize the eggs and endometrium. If eggs are fresh, then progesterone is added the same day the eggs are retrieved from the donor. If pregnancy occurs, progesterone continues until placental production is sufficient.

Embryo transfer is scheduled for the sixth day of progesterone if blastocysts are to be transferred, or the fourth day if day 3 (cleavage stage) embryos are to be transferred.

Endometrial Preparation Using a Natural Cycle

Endometrial preparation in a natural cycle is an option for women with ovulatory cycles, especially those who wish to avoid progesterone injections. This approach does not work for anovulatory women, or recipients using fresh donor eggs. In this approach, the thawing of the donor eggs is timed to the day of ovulation, as determined by the LH surge or hCG injection given 2 days before (Figure 13.3).

Ultrasound monitoring of folliculogenesis commences around cycle day 10. Once the follicle reaches 18 mm, an hCG trigger shot can be given, or twice daily urine checks for the LH surge can begin. It is common to also provide some progesterone support vaginally after embryo transfer.

Summary

- Donor eggs can be fresh or frozen.
- Endometrial preparation can be based on a natural or programmed cycle.
- The uterus functions well until the late 40s.
- Preconceptual counseling and evaluation above age 45 is prudent.
- Embryo transfer past age 50 is associated with significant risks.

Recommendations

- Preconceptual clearance for women over 44 (or over 40 for those with comorbidities).
- Source of eggs can be fresh or frozen. No significant differences in success are reported.
- Programmed or natural cycles both produce a receptive environment.
- Do not assert that donor's identity will remain anonymous.

References

1. Melnick, A.P. and Z. Rosenwaks, *Oocyte donation: insights gleaned and future challenges.* Fertil Steril, 2018. **110**(6): p. 988–93.

2. Christianson, M.S. and J. Bellver, *Innovations in assisted reproductive technologies: impact on contemporary donor egg practice and future advances.* Fertil Steril, 2018. **110**(6): p. 994–1002.

3. Yeh, J.S., et al., *Pregnancy rates in donor oocyte cycles compared to similar autologous in vitro fertilization cycles: an analysis of 26,457 fresh cycles from the Society for Assisted Reproductive Technology.* Fertil Steril, 2014. **102**(2): p. 399–404.

4. Braverman, A.M. and W.D. Schlaff, *End of anonymity: stepping into the dawn of communication and a new paradigm in gamete donor counseling.* Fertil Steril, 2019. **111**(6): p. 1102–4.

5. Cobo, A., *Oocyte vitrification: a watershed in ART.* Fertil Steril, 2012. **98**(3): p. 600–1.

6. Kawwass, J.F., et al., *Trends and outcomes for donor oocyte cycles in the United States, 2000–2010.* JAMA, 2013. **310**(22): p. 2426–34.

7. Toner, J.P., D.A. Grainger, and L.M. Frazier, *Clinical outcomes among recipients of*

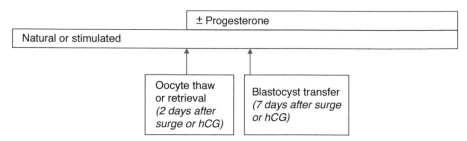

-7 -6 -5 -4 -3 -2 -1 0 1 2 3 4 5 6 7 8 9 10 11 12 13 14 1 2 3 4 5 6 7 8 9 10 11 12 13 14 15

Figure 13.3 Endometrial preparation using a natural cycle

donated eggs: an analysis of the U.S. national experience, 1996–1998. Fertil Steril, 2002. **78**(5): p. 1038–45.

8. Kawwass, J.F., et al., *Trends and outcomes for donor oocyte cycles in the United States, 2000–2010.* JAMA, 2013. **310**(22): p. 2426–34.

9. Wennberg, A.L., et al., *Effect of maternal age on maternal and neonatal outcomes after assisted reproductive technology.* Fertil Steril, 2016. **106**(5): p. 1142–9.e14.

10. Ginström Ernstad, E., et al., *Neonatal and maternal outcome after blastocyst transfer: a population-based registry study.* Am J Obstet Gynecol, 2016. **214**(3): p. 378.e1–e10.

11. Kamath, M.S., et al., *High-risk of preterm birth and low birth weight after oocyte donation IVF: analysis of 133,785 live births.* Reprod Biomed Online, 2017. **35**(3): p. 318–324.

12. Sauer, M.V., *Reproduction at an advanced maternal age and maternal health.* Fertil Steril, 2015. **103**(5): p. 1136–43.

13. Kort, D.H., et al., *Pregnancy after age 50: defining risks for mother and child.* Am J Perinatol, 2012. **29**(4): p. 245–50.

14. Ethics Committee of the American Society for Reproductive Medicine. *Oocyte or embryo donation to women of advanced reproductive age: an Ethics Committee opinion.* Fertil Steril, 2016. **106**(5): p. e3–e7.

15. Crawford, S., et al., *Cryopreserved oocyte versus fresh oocyte assisted reproductive technology cycles, United States, 2013.* Fertil Steril, 2017. **107**(1): p. 110–18.

16. Duarte, C.M., et al., *Clinical pregnancy in frozen embryo transfer with fresh versus vitrified metaphase II oocytes in an egg donation program: a retrospective study.* Fertil Steril, 2020. **114**(3): p. e167.

17. Goldman, K.N., et al., *Oocyte efficiency: does live birth rate differ when analyzing cryopreserved and fresh oocytes on a per-oocyte basis?* Fertil Steril, 2013. **100**(3): p. 712–17.

18. Patrizio, P., et al., *Ongoing implantations and baby per vitrified oocyte during third party reproduction.* Fertil Steril, 2011. **96**: p. S53.

19. Patrizio, P. and D. Sakkas, *From oocyte to baby: a clinical evaluation of the biological efficiency of in vitro fertilization.* Fertil Steril, 2009. **91**(4): p. 1061–6.

20. Shah J., et al., *Fresh versus frozen embryo transfer in frozen donor egg IVF and preimplantation screening cycles.* Fertil Steril, 2016. **106**: p. e136.

21. Trokoudes, K.M., C. Pavlides, and X. Zhang, *Comparison outcome of fresh and vitrified donor oocytes in an egg-sharing donation program.* Fertil Steril, 2011. **95**(6): p. 1996–2000.

22. Arian S., et al., *Comparison of vitrified versus fresh donor oocytes.* Fertil Steril, 2014. **101**(2): p. e31.

23. Hosseini Nasab S., et al., *Are outcomes from fresh donor oocytes still superior to frozen donor oocytes?* Fertil Steril, 2018. **110**(4): p. e340.

24. *Blastocyst culture and transfer in clinically assisted reproduction: a committee opinion.* Fertil Steril, 2018. **110**(7): p. 1246–1252.

25. Kontopoulos, G., et al., *Cleavage stage versus blastocyst stage embryo transfer in oocyte donation cycles.* Medicina (Kaunas, Lithuania), 2019. **55**(6): p. 293.

26. Schoolcraft, W.B. and D.K. Gardner, *Blastocyst culture and transfer increases the efficiency of oocyte donation.* Fertil Steril, 2000. **74**(3): p. 482–6.

27. Practice Committee of the American Society for Reproductive Medicine. *Guidance on the limits to the number of embryos to transfer: a committee opinion.* Fertil Steril, 2017. **107**(4): p. 901–903.

28. Scott, R., et al., *A human in vivo model for the luteoplacental shift.* Fertil Steril, 1991. **56**(3): p. 481–4.

29. Jiang, L., et al., *Effects of intramuscular and vaginal progesterone supplementation on frozen-thawed embryo transfer.* Sci Rep, 2019. **9**(1): p. 15264.

30. Nyboe Andersen, A., et al., *Progesterone supplementation during early gestations after IVF or ICSI has no effect on the delivery rates: a randomized controlled trial.* Hum Reprod, 2002. **17**(2): p. 357–61.

31. Pan, S.-P., et al., *Early stop of progesterone supplementation after confirmation of pregnancy in IVF/ICSI fresh embryo transfer cycles of poor responders does not affect pregnancy outcome.* PloS one, 2018. **13**(8): p. e0201824-e0201824.

32. Kyrou, D., et al., *Does cessation of progesterone supplementation during early pregnancy in patients treated with recFSH/GnRH antagonist affect ongoing pregnancy rates? A randomized controlled trial.* Hum Reprod, 2011. **26**(5): p. 1020–4.

33. Eftekhar, M., M. Rahsepar, and E. Rahmani, *Effect of progesterone supplementation on natural frozen-thawed embryo transfer cycles: a randomized controlled trial.* Int J Fertil Steril, 2013. **7**(1): p. 13–20.

34. Bjuresten, K., et al., *Luteal phase progesterone increases live birth rate after frozen embryo transfer.* Fertil Steril, 2011. **95**(2): p. 534–7.

35. Stephenson, M.D., et al., *Luteal start vaginal micronized progesterone improves pregnancy success in women with recurrent pregnancy loss.* Fertil Steril, 2017. **107**(3): p. 684–90.e2.

36. Paulson, R.J., *Hormonal induction of endometrial receptivity.* Fertil Steril, 2011. **96**(3): p. 530–5.

37. Paulson, R.J., *Introduction: Endometrial receptivity: evaluation, induction and inhibition.* Fertil Steril, 2019. **111**(4): p. 609–10.

38. Pabuçcu, E., et al., *Luteal phase support in fresh and frozen embryo transfer cycles.* J Gynecol Obstet Hum Reprod, 2020. **49**(10): p. 101838.

39. Casper, R.F., *Frozen embryo transfer: evidence-based markers for successful endometrial preparation.* Fertil Steril, 2020. **113**(2): p. 248–51.

40. Ginstrom Ernstad, E., et al., *Neonatal and maternal outcome after frozen embryo transfer: Increased risks in programmed cycles.* Am J Obstet Gynecol, 2019. **221**(2):p. 126 e1–126 e18.

41. Luke, B., et al., *In vitro fertilization and risk for hypertensive disorders of pregnancy: associations with treatment parameters.* Am J Obstet Gynecol, 2020. **222**(4):p. 350 e1–350 e13.

42. Peeraer, K., et al., *Frozen-thawed embryo transfer in a natural or mildly hormonally stimulated cycle in women with regular ovulatory cycles: a RCT.* Hum Reprod, 2015. **30**(11): p. 2552–62.

43. Saito, K., et al., *Endometrial preparation methods for frozen-thawed embryo transfer are associated with altered risks of hypertensive disorders of pregnancy, placenta accreta, and gestational diabetes mellitus.* Hum Reprod, 2019. **34**(8): p. 1567–75.

44. von Versen-Hoynck, F., et al., *Absent or excessive corpus luteum number is associated with altered maternal vascular health in early pregnancy.* Hypertension, 2019. **73**(3): p. 680–90.

45. von Versen-Hoynck, F., et al., *Increased preeclampsia risk and reduced aortic compliance with in vitro fertilization cycles in the absence of a corpus luteum.* Hypertension, 2019. **73**(3): p. 640–9.

46. Zong, L., et al., *Increased risk of maternal and neonatal complications in hormone replacement therapy cycles in frozen embryo transfer.* Reprod Biol Endocrinol, 2020. **18**(1): p. 36.

47. Khan-Dawood, F.S., et al., *Human corpus luteum secretion of relaxin, oxytocin, and progesterone.* J Clin Endocrinol Metab, 1989. **68**(3): p. 627–31.

48. Singh, B., et al., *Frozen-thawed embryo transfer: the potential importance of the corpus luteum in preventing obstetrical complications.* Fertil Steril, 2020. **113**(2): p. 252–7.

49. American Society for Reproductive Medicine, *Guidelines for oocyte donation.* Fertil Steril, 2004. **82 Suppl 1**: p. S13–5.

50. Administration, F.a.D. *Donor Eligibility Final Rule and Guidance Questions and Answers.* 2018; Available from: Donor Eligibility Final Rule and Guidance Questions and Answers.

51. *Oocyte or embryo donation to women of advanced reproductive age: an Ethics Committee opinion.* Fertil Steril, 2016. **106**(5): p. e3–e7.

52. Cano, F., et al., *Effect of aging on the female reproductive system: evidence for a role of uterine senescence in the decline in female fecundity.* Fertil Steril, 1995. **64**(3): p. 584–9.

53. Pellicer, A., C. Simon, and J. Remohi, *Effects of aging on the female reproductive system.* Hum Reprod, 1995. **10**(suppl 2): p. 77–83.

54. Adams, S.M., et al., *Endometrial response to IVF hormonal manipulation: Comparative analysis of menopausal, down regulated and natural cycles.* Reprod Biol and Endocrinol, 2004. **2**(1): p. 21.

55. *Recommendations for gamete and embryo donation: a committee opinion.* Fertil Steril, 2013. **99**(1): p. 47–62.e1.

56. Madeira, J.L. and S.L. Crockin, *Legal principles and seminal legal cases in oocyte donation.* Fertil Steril, 2018. **110**(7): p. 1209–15.

57. Rinehart, L.A., *Storage, transport, and disposition of gametes and embryos: legal issues and practical considerations.* Fertil Steril, 2021. **115**(2): p. 274–81.

58. Vermeiden, J.P. and R.E. Bernardus, *Are imprinting disorders more prevalent after human in vitro fertilization or intracytoplasmic sperm injection?* Fertil Steril, 2013. **99**(3): p. 642–51.

59. Barberet, J., et al., *What impact does oocyte vitrification have on epigenetics and gene expression?* Clin Epigenetics, 2020. **12**(1): p. 121.

60. Cobo, A., et al., *Obstetric and perinatal outcome of babies born from vitrified oocytes.* Fertil Steril, 2014. **102**(4): p. 1006–15.e4.

61. Doyle, N., et al., *Donor oocyte recipients do not benefit from preimplantation genetic testing for aneuploidy to improve pregnancy outcomes.* Hum Reprod, 2020. **35**(11): p. 2548–55.

62. Barad, D.H., et al., *Impact of preimplantation genetic screening on donor oocyte-recipient cycles in the United States.* Am J Obstet Gynecol, 2017. **217**(5): p. 576.e1–576.e8.

63. Bonhoff, A., E. Johannisson, and H.G. Bohnet, *Morphometric analysis of the endometrium of infertile patients in relation to peripheral hormone levels.* Fertil Steril, 1990. **54**(1): p. 84–9.

64. Lessey, B.A., et al., *Integrins as markers of uterine receptivity in women with primary unexplained infertility.* Fertil Steril, 1995. **63**(3): p. 535–42.

65. Scott, R.T., et al., *Evaluation of the impact of intraobserver variability on endometrial dating and the diagnosis of luteal phase defects.* Fertil Steril, 1993. **60**(4): p. 652–7.

66. Tan, J., et al., *The role of the endometrial receptivity array (ERA) in patients who have failed euploid embryo transfers.* J Assist Reprod Genet, 2018. **35**(4): p. 683–92.

67. Bassil, R., et al., *Does the endometrial receptivity array really provide personalized embryo transfer?* J Assist Reprod Genet, 2018. **35**(7): p. 1301–5.

68. Kliman, H.J. and D. Frankfurter, *Clinical approach to recurrent implantation failure: evidence-based evaluation of the endometrium.* Fertil Steril, 2019. **111**(4): p. 618–28.

69. Kliman, H.J., et al., *Optimization of endometrial preparation results in a normal endometrial function test (EFT) and good reproductive outcome in donor ovum recipients.* J Assist Reprod Genet, 2006. **23**(7–8): p. 299–303.

70. Evans-Hoeker, E., et al., *Endometrial BCL6 overexpression in eutopic endometrium of women with endometriosis.* Reprod Sci, 2016. **23**(9): p. 1234–41.

71. Almquist, L.D., et al., *Endometrial BCL6 testing for the prediction of in vitro fertilization outcomes: a cohort study.* Fertil Steril, 2017. **108**(6): p. 1063–9.

72. Soriano, D., et al., *Fertility outcome of laparoscopic treatment in patients with severe endometriosis and repeated in vitro fertilization failures.* Fertil Steril, 2016. **106**(5): p. 1264–9.

73. Littman, E., et al., *Role of laparoscopic treatment of endometriosis in patients with failed in vitro fertilization cycles.* Fertil Steril, 2005. **84**(6): p. 1574–8.

Chapter

14

Is It Likely That Reproductive Aging Could Be Delayed or Reversed Using Advanced Technologies in the Future?

Paula Amato and Dimitrios S. Nikolaou

The number of oocytes in the ovaries decreases through a process called atresia from a peak of 6–7 million at 20 weeks' gestation to 1–2 million at birth and approximately 400,000 at puberty [1]. The average age of menopause in the United States is 51 years [2]. The fecundity of women decreases gradually beginning in the early 30s and more rapidly after age 37 years. Furthermore, an estimated 10% of the general population will experience an accelerated decline of their ovarian reserve significantly earlier, before the age of 32 [3]. This represents a shift to the left of the curve of reproductive aging and has been described as "early ovarian aging." Risk factors include, among others, ovarian surgery, chemotherapy, radiotherapy and smoking. However, by far, the most important factors are believed to be genetic [3].

As seen in earlier chapters, women in the developed world have been having children at older ages. The age of first birth has been rising [4]. Women are delaying childbearing for various reasons including pursuit of education, participation in the workforce and other societal factors [5]. There is also a perception that assisted reproductive technologies (ART) can overcome age-related infertility.

In terms of fertility prognosis, by far, the most important factor is oocyte quality, which depends on age. The pregnancy success rate per embryo transfer has improved significantly in the past 20 years for women aged 35 or less. However, the success rates for women over 40 have remained extremely low, generally less than 10%, and there continue to be very few live births with autologous in vitro fertilization (IVF) beyond the age of 43 [6].

Improving the Quality of the Eggs

For women over 40, especially over 43, the chance of a healthy live birth with IVF using their own eggs remains extremely low regardless of ovarian stimulation protocol and gonadotropin dose. Previous chapters have examined the various approaches in detail. Currently, the emphasis is on pretreatment and optimization of health and diet. Traditional endocrinology, which had been slightly neglected with the advent of ART, has found a new application in this context, especially with the study of androgen profiles and supplementation with androgens for several weeks before the onset of ovarian stimulation [7]. This is explored in detail by Barad and Gleicher in Chapter 7, as well as the potential application of growth hormone supplementation. The chapter on nutrition highlights the role of supplements such as CoQ10 and others.

Potential future therapeutic approaches to treat infertility related to advanced maternal age are described in the following text.

Mitochondrial Replacement Therapy

Mitochondrial replacement therapy (MRT) has been used mainly for avoiding the transmission of mitochondrial diseases [8]. Details of the first live birth in a human were published in 2017, where nuclear transfer (NT) technology was used to overcome the transmission of Leigh syndrome to the offspring [9].

There has been increasing interest in the application of NT to overcome certain types of female infertility, the feasibility and safety of which is supported by some promising studies in animal models such as rhesus macaques. The macaque studies were conducted for 3 years after birth and no further follow-up has been reported.

The processes of fertilization and embryonic development require great amounts of energy. Mitochondria are, of course, the sites of energy production. Aging is associated with mitochondrial dysfunction. One approach, therefore, is to transfer young mitochondria to the aged oocyte.

Mitochondrial replacement therapy was initially achieved by cytoplasmic transfer from a donor, as first described by Cohen [10]. This was successful in improving the embryo quality and there were clinical pregnancies and live births. However, the Food and Drug Administration (FDA) has banned its application, since 2001, due to ethical and medical concerns. To avoid concerns related to including a heterologous donor, a new technique was developed involving autologous germline mitochondrial energy transfer (AUGMENT). This included isolation of mitochondria from the patient's ovarian stem cells, which were then injected into the patient's own oocytes during intracytoplasmic sperm injection [11]. This technique has not been shown to improve pregnancy and live birth rates in a small clinical trial.

There are four techniques available for MRT, pronuclear transfer (PNT), polar body transfer (PBT), maternal spindle transfer (MST) and germinal vesicle transfer (GVT) [8]. The three latter techniques are based on donor enucleated MII oocytes, whereas PNT requires a donor zygote following removal of the pronuclei and polar bodies. Maternal spindle transfer is the only technique currently being applied and investigated to address poor ovarian reserve. Human spindle transfer has yielded blastocyst development and derivation of karyotypically normal embryonic stem cell lines [12]. There have been several births reported worldwide from this technique (Figure 14.1).

Activation of Dormant Follicles (In Vitro Activation)

Some patients with a diagnosis of premature ovarian insufficiency contain residual dormant follicles in the ovaries. In murine and human ovaries, stimulation of the phosphatidyl inositol-3-kinase-AKT-forkhead box 03 pathway activated dormant primordial follicles in vitro [14]. Subsequent studies found that ovarian fragmentation suppressed the Hippo signaling pathway, leading to ovarian follicular growth [15]. The procedure involves laparoscopic removal of one or both ovaries and autotransplantation after treatment in vitro by combining P13K signal activation and Hippo signaling disruption.

Spontaneous recovery of menses, pregnancies and live births have been reported in premature ovarian insufficiency (POI) patients.

Autologous Activated Platelet-Rich Plasma Injection

It has been suggested that germline stem cells (GSCs) exist in adult ovaries and that such cells can be utilized to extend fertility, although the existence of such cells is controversial [16]. In recent years, clinical experience with a technique based on autologous activated platelet-rich plasma (PRP) treatment of the adult human ovary has been reported [17]. Previously, the technique had been applied successfully in various other systems [18]. Many physiological mechanisms and factors included in platelets could be contributing, including vascular endothelial growth factor (VEGF), platelet-derived growth factor AB (PDGF-AB) and TGF-β1. The rationale was to provide growth factors directly to the adult human ovary. Initial experiments in the ovaries of animals were encouraging. The first reports in humans involved perimenopausal women or women with premature ovarian insufficiency (POI). These patients were treated with intraovarian PRP injection. Restoration of the menstrual cycle was observed within 1–3 months post treatment. Subsequently, natural IVF cycles led to one to five oocytes being collected per retrieval-attempt. Reduced serum FSH and higher post-treatment levels of serum AMH have been observed which are clinically consistent with improved ovarian function. Frozen blastocysts and pregnancies have been reported [19]. The PRP is obtained from the same patient. The technique is not without its challenges as injecting the PRP into small ovaries can be difficult. There is also a theoretical concern that this may increase the risk of ovarian cancer.

In Vitro Gametogenesis (IVG)

There have been many studies on the possible use of stem cells in the treatment of factors involved in infertility [20]. The ability to produce human eggs entirely in vitro would be a significant advance. One approach that has shown promise is the derivation of gametes from human embryonic stem cells (ESC) in vitro [21]. This was based on our understanding of the way in which gametes develop in vivo from primordial germ cells

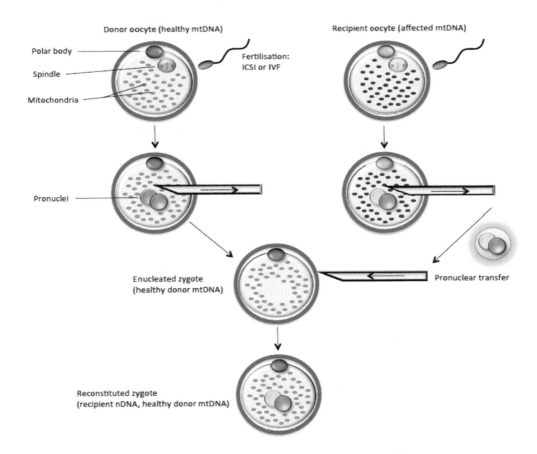

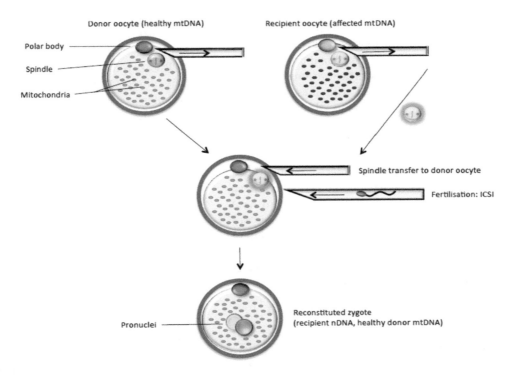

b. PRONUCLEAR TRANSFER (Post-fertilisation)

a. SPINDLE TRANSFER (Pre-fertilisation)

Figure 14.1 Spindle transfer. ICSI, intracytoplasmic sperm injection; mtDNA, mitochondrial DNA; nDNA, nuclear DNA.
Source: Reznichenko et al., 2015 [13]

(PGCs) within the embryo. Human embryonic stem cells (hES) can be derived from the inner cell mass of human blastocysts created via IVF. They can replicate themselves and are pluripotent. Detailed experiments of transcription factors active at around 6 days post coitum reveal that PGC specification is induced from the proximal epiblast by extrinsic factors secreted by the extra-embryonic ectoderm cells. These experiments suggest that "germcellness" is induced rather than being presegregated in the early embryo [22].

There have been attempts in mice to use the haploidization potential of the oocyte cytoplasm to direct somatic nuclei into a meiotic or pro-nuclear state.

Patient cells can be reprogrammed into iPSCs using optimized reprogramming protocols that involve small molecules, microRNAs and combinations of reprogramming factors. iPSCs can be differentiated into somatic cells that could be used either in transplantation therapies or alternatively to model human diseases [23] (Figure 14.2).

Takahashi and Yamanaka reported on the induction of pluripotent stem cells from mouse embryonic and adult fibroblast cultures by defined factors [24]. Their main hypothesis is that a small set of transcription factors, when expressed in a somatic cell, can reprogram it back into a pluripotent state.

Previously, in a study by Hayashi et al. [25], murine induced pluripotent stem cells (iPSCs) were differentiated into functional oocytes in the presence of specific growth factors resulting in live births. Mice transplanted with these cells were able to successfully reproduce through in vitro maturation (IVM) and fertilization.

Many issues need to be resolved, of course, before this technology can be applied clinically in humans; for example, there is still limited knowledge of the imprinting requirements during gametogenesis. Also, iPSCs are known to have mitochondrial DNA mutations even when isolated from healthy donors [26,27]. Derivation of human gametes in vitro is allowed under UK law, but the use of embryos created from such gametes to establish a pregnancy is not allowed

Aneuploidy Correction through Gene Editing

The 14-day rule, proposed in the UK in the Warnock Report (1984), and then enshrined in law in the Human Fertilisation and Embryology (HFE) Acts of 1990 and 2008, is a limit that prevents the in vitro culture of human embryos beyond 14 days after onset of embryo creation. The International Society for Stem Cell Research (ISSCR) has announced that it no longer endorses the prevailing international standard limiting human embryo research to 14 days after fertilization.

Genome editing is a way of making specific changes to the DNA of a cell or organism. It can be used for research, to treat disease or in biotechnology. It involves making cuts at specific DNA sequences with enzymes called "engineered nucleases" (Figure 14.3). Engineered nucleases are made up of two parts: a nuclease part that cuts the DNA and a DNA-targeting part that is designed to guide the nuclease to a specific sequence of DNA. After cutting the DNA in a specific place, the cell will naturally repair the cut. We can manipulate this repair process to make changes (or "edits") to the DNA in that location in the genome.

There are several different types of engineered nucleases used in genome editing. They mainly differ in how they recognize the DNA to cut:

- RNA-based: contain a short sequence of RNA that binds to the target DNA to be cut.
- Protein–based: contain a protein that recognizes and binds to the target DNA to be cut.

CRISPR-Cas9 is the most common system used for genome editing. CRISPR stands for "clustered regularly interspaced short palindromic repeats." CRISPR is the DNA-targeting part of the system which consists of an RNA molecule, or "guide," designed to bind to specific DNA bases through complementary base-pairing. Cas9 stands for CRISPR-associated protein 9 and is the nuclease part that cuts the DNA (Figure 14.4). The CRISPR-Cas9 system was originally discovered in bacteria that use this system to destroy invading viruses.

Recently, the application of human-induced pluripotent stem cells (hiPSCs) has been frequently associated with the use of gene editing, targeting the disease-causing gene to study the pathophysiology even more deeply, carry out drug screening and improve cell therapeutic potential (Figure 14.5) [27,28].

CRISPR/Cas9 has been used to conduct targeted trisomic chromosome elimination in murine culture

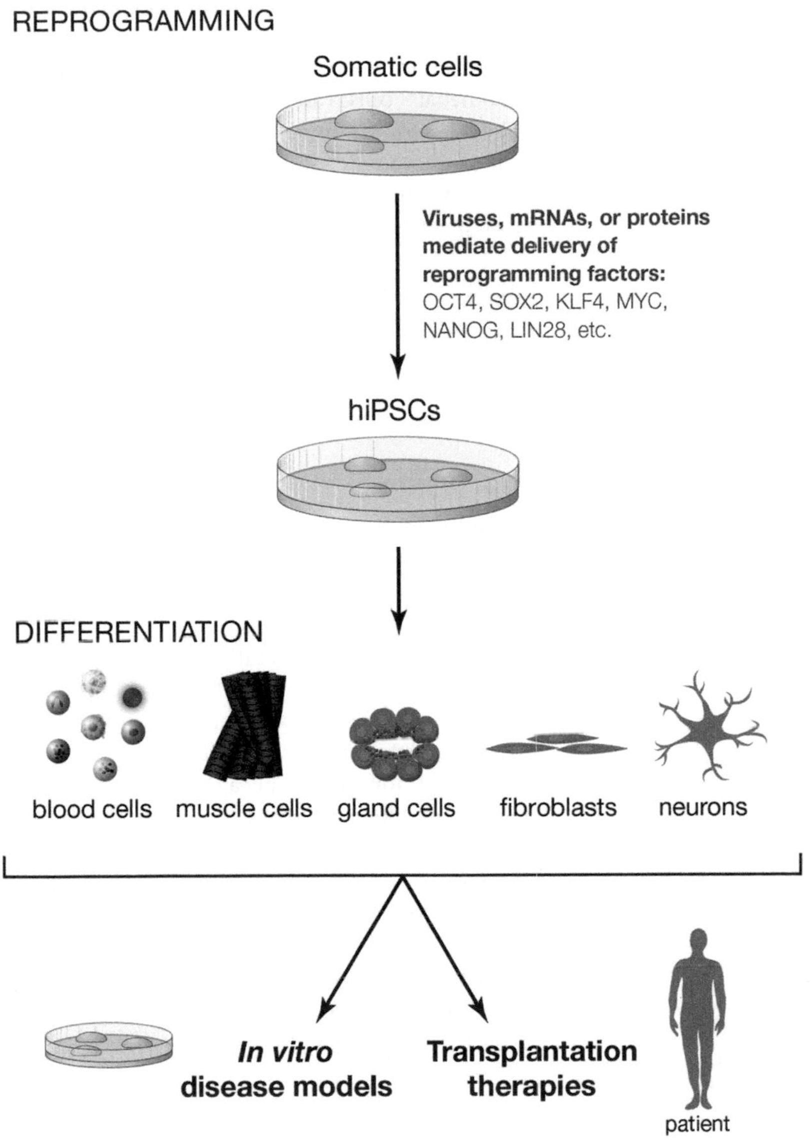

REPROGRAMMING

Somatic cells

**Viruses, mRNAs, or proteins
mediate delivery of
reprogramming factors:**
OCT4, SOX2, KLF4, MYC,
NANOG, LIN28, etc.

hiPSCs

DIFFERENTIATION

blood cells   muscle cells   gland cells   fibroblasts   neurons

In vitro
disease models

**Transplantation
therapies**

patient

Figure 14.2 Overview of the induced pluripotent stem cell (iPSC) technology.
Source: Reproduced from [27], with permission from Elsevier.

DNA-targeting part

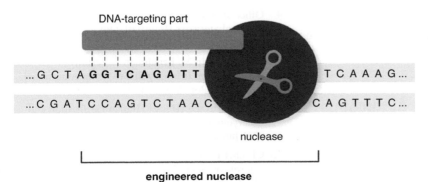

...G C T A **G G T C A G A T T**   T C A A A G...

...C G A T C C A G T C T A A C   C A G T T T C...

nuclease

engineered nuclease

Figure 14.3 Illustration
showing the basic structure and
function of engineered
nucleases used for genome
editing.
Source: Genome Research Ltd.

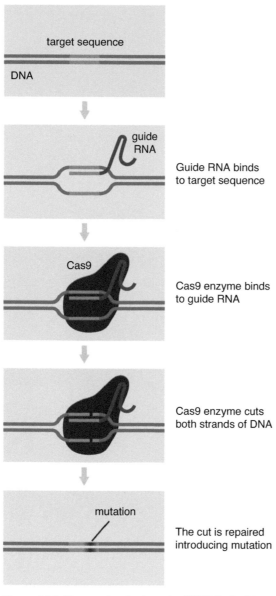

target sequence

DNA

Guide RNA binds
to target sequence

guide
RNA

Cas9

Cas9 enzyme binds
to guide RNA

Cas9 enzyme cuts
both strands of DNA

mutation

The cut is repaired
introducing mutation

Figure 14.4 Diagram showing how the CRISPR-Cas9 editing tool works.
Source: Genome Research Ltd.

cells, embryos and tissue in vivo, and iPSCs and cancer cells ex vivo.

The Artificial Ovary (Ovarian Tissue Cryopreservation and Autologous Transplantation)

This involves transplanting isolated ovarian follicles with or without biological scaffold [29]. Ovarian tissue or the whole ovary is removed

and cryopreserved. To achieve a pregnancy, the tissue is thawed, follicles are isolated and placed in a scaffold along with various growth factors, endothelial cells and ovarian stromal cells (Figure 14.6). Many obstacles are yet to be overcome. For example, designing a scaffold is a crucial step. The material used for producing scaffolds must meet various standards. And also development of techniques for higher follicular recovery rate and a better scaffold, better transplantation techniques and consideration of genetic safety. In animal studies the artificial ovary restored endocrine function, achieved in vitro follicular development and resulted in successful pregnancies.

Conclusion

There are numerous lines of research trying to overcome the problem of decreased ovarian reserve and some have shown promise. However, clinicians should exercise extreme caution in managing patient expectations regarding these novel technologies. Currently, the mainstay of treatment for premature ovarian insufficiency is oocyte donation. Clinical application of stem cell technology for maternal age-related infertility does seem likely at some point in the future; however, the timeline remains uncertain.

References

1. Faddy MJ, Gosden RG, Gougeon A, Richardson SJ, Nelson JF. Accelerated disappearance of ovarian follicles in mid-life: implications for forecasting menopause. Human Reproduction. 1992;**7**(10):1342–6.

2. Santoro N. The menopause transition: an update. Human Reproduction Update. 2002;**8**(2):155–60.

3. Nikolaou D. Early ovarian ageing: a hypothesis: Detection and clinical relevance. Human Reproduction. 2003;**18**(6):1137–9.

4. Office of National Statistics. Home – Office for National Statistics [Internet]. Ons.gov.uk. 2020. Available from: www.ons.gov.uk/

5. Ní Bhrolcháin M, Beaujouan É. Fertility postponement is largely due to rising educational enrolment. Population Studies. 2012;**66**(3):311–27.

6. Welcome to the HFEA | Human Fertilisation and Embryology Authority [Internet]. hfea.gov.uk. [cited 2021 Jun 29]. Available from: http://hfea.gov.uk

7. Gleicher N, Kushnir VA, Albertini DF, Barad DH. Improvements in IVF in women of advanced age. The Journal of Endocrinology. 2016;**230**(1):F1-6.

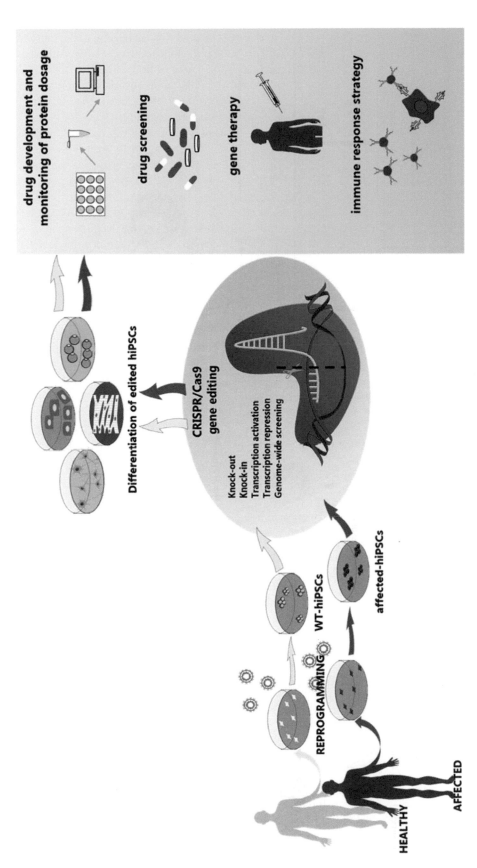

Figure 14.5 Workflow of the research involving hiPSCs and CRISPR/Cas9 gene editing for the investigation of new drugs and therapeutic alternatives. *Source:* Reproduced from [28].

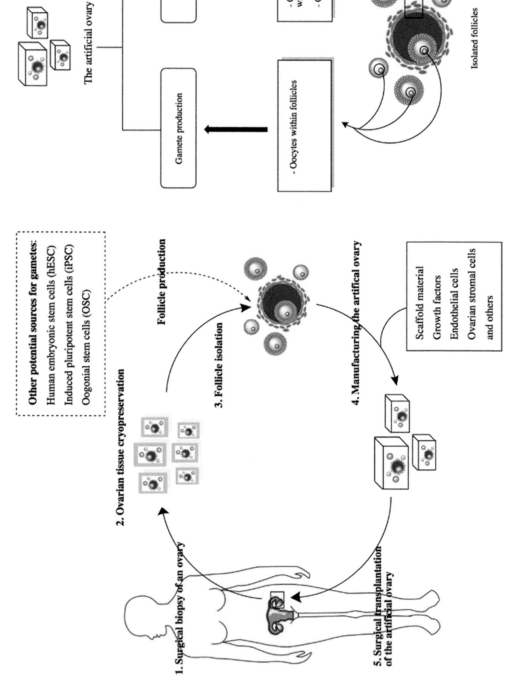

Figure 14.6 Manufacturing and transplanting of the artificial ovary.
Source: Reproduced from [29], with permission from John Wiley and Sons.

8. Reznichenko A, Huyser C, Pepper M. Mitochondrial transfer: Implications for assisted reproductive technologies. Applied & Translational Genomics. 2016;11:40–7.

9. Sfakianoudis K, Rapani A, Grigoriadis S, Retsina D, Maziotis E, Tsioulou P, et al. Novel approaches in addressing ovarian insufficiency in 2019: are we there yet? Cell Transplantation. 2020;29:096368972092615.

10. Cohen J. Ooplasmic transfer in mature human oocytes. Molecular Human Reproduction. 1998;4 (3):269–80.

11. Fakih MH. The AUGMENT^SM treatment: physician reported outcomes of the initial global patient experience. Journal of Fertilization: In Vitro – IVF-Worldwide, Reproductive Medicine, Genetics & Stem Cell Biology. 2015;03(03).

12. Tachibana M, Kuno T, Yaegashi N. Mitochondrial replacement therapy and assisted reproductive technology: A paradigm shift toward treatment of genetic diseases in gametes or in early embryos. Reproductive Medicine and Biology. 2018;17 (4):421–33.

13. Reznichenko A, Huyser C, Pepper MS. Mitochondrial transfer: Ethical, legal and social implications in assisted reproduction. South African Journal of Bioethics and Law. 2015;8 (2):32.

14. Ernst EH, Grøndahl ML, Grund S, Hardy K, Heuck A, Sunde L, et al. Dormancy and activation of human oocytes from primordial and primary follicles: molecular clues to oocyte regulation. Human Reproduction. 2017;32 (8):1684–700.

15. Hsueh AJW, Kawamura K. Hippo signaling disruption and ovarian follicle activation in infertile patients. Fertility and Sterility. 2020;114 (3):458–64.

16. Tilly JL, Telfer EE. Purification of germline stem cells from adult mammalian ovaries: a step closer towards control of the female biological clock? Molecular Human Reproduction. 2009;15 (7):393–8.

17. Sfakianoudis K, Simopoulou M, Grigoriadis S, Pantou A, Tsioulou P, Maziotis E, et al. Reactivating ovarian function through autologous platelet-rich plasma intraovarian infusion: pilot data on premature ovarian insufficiency, perimenopausal, menopausal, and poor responder women. Journal of Clinical Medicine. 2020;9(6).

18. Anitua E, Prado R, Padilla S, Orive G. Platelet-rich plasma therapy: another appealing technology for regenerative medicine? Regenerative Medicine. 2016;11(4):355–7.

19. Panda SR, Sachan S, Hota S. A systematic review evaluating the efficacy of intra-ovarian infusion of autologous platelet-rich plasma in patients with poor ovarian reserve or ovarian insufficiency. Cureus. 2020;12(12):e12037.

20. Fazeli Z, Abedindo A, Omrani MD, Ghaderian SMH. Mesenchymal stem cells (MSCs) therapy for recovery of fertility: a systematic review. Stem Cell Reviews and Reports. 2017;14 (1):1–12.

21. Thomson JA. Embryonic stem cell lines derived from human blastocysts. Science. 1998;282 (5391):1145–7.

22. Kimble J, Page DC. The mysteries of sexual identity: the germ cell's perspective. science. 2007;316(5823):400–1.

23. Nagy ZP, Chang C-C. Current advances in artificial gametes. Reproductive BioMedicine Online. 2005;11(3):332–9.

24. Takahashi K, Yamanaka S. Induction of pluripotent stem cells from mouse embryonic and adult fibroblast cultures by defined factors. Cell. 2006;126(4):663–76.

25. Hayashi K, Ogushi S, Kurimoto K, Shimamoto S, Ohta H, Saitou M. Offspring from oocytes derived from in vitro primordial germ cell-like cells in mice. Science. 2012 Oct 4;338(6109):971–5.

26. Prigione A, Lichtner B, Kuhl H, Struys EA, Wamelink M, Lehrach H, et al. Human iPSCs harbor homoplasmic and heteroplasmic mitochondrial DNA mutations while maintaining hESC-like metabolic reprogramming. Stem Cells. 2011;29(9):1338–1248.

27. Hockemeyer D, Jaenisch R. Induced pluripotent stem cells meet genome editing. Cell Stem Cell. 2016;18(5):573–86.

28. De Masi C, Spitalieri P, Murdocca M, Novelli G, Sangiuolo F. Application of CRISPR/Cas9 to human-induced pluripotent stem cells: from gene editing to drug discovery. Human Genomics. 2020 Jun 26;14(1).

29. Cho E, Kim YY, Noh K, Ku S-Y. A new possibility in fertility preservation: The artificial ovary. Journal of Tissue Engineering and Regenerative Medicine. 2019;13(8):1294–315.

Chapter

15

Ethical Issues in the Use of Assisted Reproductive Technology in Women over Age 40

Nicole Yoder and Gwendolyn P. Quinn

Prevalence of ART over Age 40

Advances in assisted reproductive technology (ART) now allow women to pursue pregnancy at progressively later ages in life. While pregnancy after age 40 was previously considered a rare event, an increasing number of women in their 40s and 50s have been able to achieve pregnancy due to the increased success and availability of ART. In addition to the use of in vitro fertilization (IVF) with autologous eggs in this age group, there has also been a significant increase in the availability, utilization, and acceptability of oocyte donation. This now allows women of advanced maternal ages and even post-menopausal women to achieve and carry a pregnancy. Similarly, with an increase in egg freezing technology and utilization, many women are opting to freeze their eggs early in life and use them at a later time point when pregnancy may not have been previously possible.

These advances in ART have contributed to the current unprecedented number of pregnancies in women 40 and older. In fact, despite an overall decrease in birth rates in the United States as well as globally since the 1960s [1], birth rates for females age 40–44 and 45–49 have been rising over the past three decades [2]. In the United States, birth rates in females age 40–44 increased from 5.5 per 1,000 people in 1990 to 11.8 per 1,000 people in 2018, and in females age 45–49 increased from 0.2 per 1,000 people in 1990 to 0.9 per 1,000 people in 2018. While birth rates in women over age 50 are not as well quantified, fertility clinics have undoubtedly seen more post-menopausal women seeking pregnancy than ever before. Additionally, case reports of women upward of 60 years of age achieving pregnancy have also been on the rise over the last decade. This trend in increasing birth rates in women of 40 years and older has largely been attributed to ART and is a trend likely to continue.

This movement toward increasing maternal age comes with many new challenges. As reproductive physicians now see increasingly older patients, they are also confronted with complex ethical questions regarding the medical, psychological, and psychosocial implications of providing services to this population. It is well established that increased maternal age is associated with many obstetric complications. These complications may have both short- and long-term effects on the mother as well as the fetus and child. In addition to medical complications, many providers are concerned about psychosocial ramifications of pregnancies at the extremes of maternal age. These concerns largely pertain to the well-being of children born to older parents, and are often subject to societal and cultural norms. These factors combined have led many to question the ethics of providing ART to patients in their 40s and beyond; however, most ethical scrutiny has been aimed at post-menopausal mothers and those greater than 50 years of age.

Guidelines for ART over 40

Given that pregnancy and parenting in the older population have only recently become more prevalent, many clinicians have minimal experience providing reproductive technologies to this age group. Many clinicians desire guidance and recommendations regarding medical and ethical concerns related to fertility treatment in older women; however, few guidelines currently exist regarding the acceptability of ART in this group. As a result, guidelines on age limits for ART are largely left up to individual fertility clinics to establish. In the United States, many clinics choose to review the permissibility of the situation on a case-by-case basis. In other clinics, strict age cut-offs are established based on the age of the mother, the father, or the combined age of both intended parents.

In the United States, national organizations such as the American College of Obstetricians and Gynecologists (ACOG) and the American Society of Reproductive Medicine (ASRM) have both made statements regarding the use of ART in special populations such as those of advanced maternal age. The ACOG does not advise on specific guidelines for age limits for ART but does state in a committee opinion that medical conditions should be taken into consideration before providing this service [3]. The ASRM arguably provides the most comprehensive statements regarding provision of fertility services to special groups, including committee opinions regarding oocyte or embryo donation to women of advanced reproductive age (ARA) [4], provision of fertility services for women at increased risk of complications during fertility treatment or pregnancy [5], and child-rearing ability and the provision of fertility services [6]. However, most of these guidelines only identify factors that should be taken into consideration as opposed to providing distinct inclusion or exclusion criteria for providing ART care. For example, the committee opinion on oocyte or embryo donation to women of ARA acknowledges that pregnancy in ARA patients is associated with medical and possible psychosocial risks. It encourages thorough medical screening, counseling regarding medical risks to the mother and fetus, and a psychosocial evaluation before proceeding with treatments. However, it is ultimately left up to the physician to determine whether the medical and social risks are acceptable or not. The ASRM does, however, advise that the use of oocyte donation in patients over the age of 55 is discouraged due to the limited amount of data regarding maternal and fetal pregnancy outcomes in this age group. The committee opinion on provision of fertility services for women at increased risk of complications during fertility treatment or pregnancy similarly identifies points of consideration for the provider but again does not contain distinct medical criteria for inclusion or exclusion. It is suggested that medical risks be thoroughly discussed and that the patient receives extensive counseling on the medical risks to both the mother and fetus, as well as consultation from subspecialists or second opinions when necessary. The committee opinion states that as long as there has been appropriate evaluation and counseling, the patient has the right to make informed decisions regarding their reproductive choices, which

is a reflection of ASRM's value of a patient's reproductive liberty. Conversely, it also acknowledges that providers may have varying ethical opinions regarding ART for ARA patients as well as varying thresholds for the associated medical risks. The committee opinion states that physicians should be free to provide or decline provision of ART services based on their individual ethics, medical assessments, and values.

While these US organizations have provided broad guidelines for ART in US ARA patients, in European and other countries, there are even fewer guidelines available. This is likely due to the fact that age limits for ART access are set by many individual countries, precluding consideration of treatment even when requested. These regulations tend to limit ART to women under the age of 50. Some of the stricter European policies have age cut offs as low as age 45 in Denmark and on the higher end of the spectrum age 51 in Bulgaria [7].

The paucity of guidelines surrounding reproduction in women over 40 is partially due to the lack of data available on ART outcomes in this population. However, it is important to note that the lack of consensus guidelines also stems from the history of arguments for or against ART in older women. Such arguments against allowing ARA women to use ART originated from cultural and religious norms that vary from individual to individual, as well as country to country [7]. The lack of guidelines from governing bodies often leads to ethical dilemmas for clinicians faced with patients seeking ART at advanced ages. Most providers want to respect the reproductive autonomy and procreative rights of the patient but struggle with whether or not it is ethical given the possible negative outcomes [8]. These outcomes include medical risks, psychosocial risks, and adherence to the four basic ethical principles in relation to the patient as well as the future child.

Medical Ethics

One of the most basic questions regarding ART in women over 40 is whether or not it is a medically ethical procedure. It has been well demonstrated that increased maternal age is associated with an increased risk of several obstetric complications that may have both short- and long-term health effects on the mother, the fetus, or both. While this risk begins to increase around age 35, the risk is most pronounced in women who are aged 45–50 or older [4,9]. Women over 50 years of age presumably incur the highest risks; however, the true incidence is not well understood as there are few data available regarding outcomes of pregnancies at extremely advanced ages. The incidence of almost all obstetric complications increases with advanced maternal age; however, this population is particularly prone to complications associated with pregnancy-induced hypertension, gestational diabetes, and increased rates of cesarean sections [4]. Older women are also more likely to experience more serious adverse events such as myocardial infarction, need for mechanical ventilation, pulmonary embolism, heart failure, and death [9]. However, it should be noted that while the risk for serious adverse events is increased, these events are still relatively uncommon and the absolute risk remains low [9].

In addition to age itself as a risk factor for poor outcomes, older women are also more likely to have chronic preexisting conditions such as cardiac disease, obesity, chronic hypertension, or diabetes [10]. Combined with advanced age, these comorbidities further elevate the risks associated with fertility treatments and pregnancy. A nationwide study of pregnant women from the United States demonstrated that older age was associated with an increased prevalence of a multitude of preexisting conditions including cardiac disease, autoimmune disease, asthma, diabetes mellitus, thrombophilias, antiphospholipid syndrome, chronic hypertension, and renal failure when compared to younger women [9]. Many of these conditions can be exacerbated throughout the course of pregnancy and make pregnancy specific complications more likely to occur. While it is clear that preexisting conditions should be optimized prior to initiation of treatment, it is challenging to determine the absolute risks these comorbidities incur in an ARA pregnancy even after medical optimization is achieved.

Increased maternal age and preexisting comorbidities also translate to increased risk for the fetus. Pregnancies complicated by obstetric conditions such as pregnancy-induced hypertension, diabetes, renal disease, or cardiac disease predispose the fetus to complications such as intrauterine fetal demise, prematurity, or low birth weight. Babies born prematurely or with low birth weight have a higher incidence of conditions such as cerebral palsy or other permanent neurodevelopmental sequelae that often require intensive care throughout the life course. The severity and longevity of these negative effects can vary greatly and range from increased need for neonatal intensive care and increased length of hospitalization, to severe and permanent disability or even early death.

Chromosomal and developmental disorders are also a concern with reproduction at advanced ages. It is well established that increasing maternal age is associated with fetal aneuploidy; however, advances in preimplantation genetic testing (PGT) for aneuploidy and early non invasive prenatal testing have significantly increased the ability to detect chromosomal abnormalities either before embryo transfer or within the first trimester of pregnancy. Women who are using ART at ages 45 and older are almost exclusively using either donor eggs or autologous eggs that were previously frozen at a much younger age. Because the age of the egg is what confers risk for aneuploidy, most women using ART aged 45 and beyond will have aneuploidy risks similar to the age of their donor or the age at which they froze their own eggs. Beyond chromosomal abnormalities, there is evidence to suggest that children born to older parents have higher incidence of developmental disorders and autism spectrum disorders [11]. These risks have been noted mostly with increased paternal age; however, it is likely that increased maternal age usually corresponds to older fathers as well, except in the case of donor sperm.

While the connection between increased paternal age and autism is fairly well known, recent data have also demonstrated an increased risk for Asperger's syndrome in children born to mothers over age 35, and increased risk of schizophrenia with both increased maternal and paternal age [11]. In a recent article, Zweifel et al. importantly note that while many psychiatric and developmental disorders have been documented among children with older parents, the exact circumstances surrounding conception and the pregnancy are often lacking. It is unclear whether these pregnancies were a result of autologous gametes as opposed to donor egg and/or donor sperm, and obstetric complications are not always recorded. Without this information, it is difficult to establish if these disorders are due to chromosomal abnormalities, the intrauterine environment, birth trauma or compilations of prematurity, or epigenetic changes.

Because of the increased risk of maternal and fetal complications, existing guidelines universally recommended that women of advanced maternal age undergo comprehensive health screening prior to initiation of fertility treatments [3–5]. Preexisting conditions should be optimized, and consultation as well as medical clearance from the appropriate subspecialists should be obtained when indicated. While it is challenging to provide robust data on pregnancy complications and outcomes in this group, thorough counseling and education on potential risks, discussion of the most up-to-date medical knowledge, and information on alternatives such as gestational carriers or adoption should be provided.

Once medical screening, health optimization, and patient counseling have been completed, the amount of risk that a patient or a provider is willing to accept, or the degree to which they find fertility treatment and pregnancy to be medically ethical, is largely up to the individual patient and provider. Current literature and guidelines predominantly promote patient reproductive freedom and defend the right of patients to make informed decisions regarding if and how they reproduce [5,12]. Many argue that women of ARA should have the same right to make medical decisions regarding their own reproduction as younger women who also have increased health risks. A systematic review of the ethics of reproduction at advanced maternal ages notes that when considering who should receive reproductive services, younger patients with high-risk medical conditions such as systemic lupus erythematosus, type 1 diabetes, or chronic renal failure are routinely offered ART [12]. Similarly, younger patients with cancer diagnoses also have increased risk with fertility treatments but generally face less scrutiny from society regarding the medical ethics of providing ART services. The general consensus in the literature is that it is the provider's duty to ensure that the patient is fully informed of the risks, benefits, and alternatives to treatment, but it is up to the patient to make their own medical and reproductive decisions.

This same general principle applies to providers who are asked to treat ARA women. The ASRM states that providers may ethically treat ARA women with increased risk as long as medical optimization and medical counseling have been provided [5]. However, it is also permissible for clinicians to decline treatment if they believe the risks are too high. It is important that providers make the decisions objectively and free of bias, but providers can exercise the right to decline treatment if they do not deem it medically safe or appropriate.

Psychosocial Ethics

A second ethical debate regarding ART in patients of advanced reproductive age is the psychosocial consequences of reproduction at an older age. One of the predominant concerns is that older parents may be met with unique emotional or social challenges when raising a child. As the age gap widens between parent and child, critics argue that significant social and generational disconnects develop for children of older parents when compared to peers with younger parents. This can lead to poorer communication, a weaker emotional bond, and discrepancies in the values, beliefs, and interests of the parent and child. These differences may become increasingly pronounced as the child ages, especially in the teenage years [13]. There are also concerns about how this may affect the child's relationship with other children, as they may be more prone to embarrassment or teasing from their peers with younger parents [14], as well as social stigma and isolation [13]. Older parents may also have more difficulty physically keeping up with the demands of young children, leading to less active interaction and recreation between parent and child.

The universally largest concern, however, is the risk of early parental death and the consequences that may have on the child [4,13,14]. The death of a parent at any age is a difficult event to endure, but the death of a parent at a young age can have particularly detrimental effects [14]. Children who experience the loss of a parent at a young age are more predisposed to psychiatric disorders such as anxiety, depression, post-traumatic stress disorder, and substance abuse problems, as well as behavioral problems, social withdrawal, and decreased self-esteem. Loss of a parent at a young age may also influence other long-term outcomes for the child, such as education, mental and physical health, and offspring longevity [13,14]. The concern for early parental death is further exacerbated in ARA women who are pursuing single parenthood. In this case, the question arises of what would happen to the child if their only parent figure were to become ill or pass away? Loss of a single parent at an early age could have particularly significant consequences, and it has been argued that this could result in undue societal burden to care for the child in these instances [13].

There is also concern that older parents may develop age-related health problems requiring the child to become a caregiver at a young age [11]. Studies have noted that children of ailing parents have increased anxiety regarding the health of their parents and risk of death. Additionally, children who assume the role of caregiver may have higher rates of anxiety, depression, substance abuse, and other mental and behavioral health issues [11,12]. Caregiving at a young age may also delay offspring from pursuing advanced education, careers, and partnerships.

While many focus on the negative psychosocial aspects of reproduction at advanced ages, there is abundant evidence to support the idea that there are actually many benefits to parenting at an older age. Older parents tend to be more financially secure, have higher incomes, established careers, and more stable family environments [13]. Older parents also tend to have more life experiences, social resources, and emotional maturity that may better prepare them for parenthood. The theory has also been raised that patients who must undergo fertility treatments to achieve pregnancy are particularly well suited for parenthood. This cohort tends to have invested a great amount of time and effort toward having a child, and as a result are deeply committed to parenthood [12,13].

When considering the psychosocial consequences of providing ART to older women, it has also been noted that other groups of people who may present with similar psychosocial situations or limited life expectancies are often not restricted from pursuing fertility treatments [4]. For example, men of advanced reproductive age frequently achieve pregnancies with the assistance of ART without restriction, and patients who may have life limiting illnesses are not restricted from pursuing fertility treatment. This makes it challenging to justify restriction of ART services to women of advanced maternal age based solely on the psychosocial ramifications of their age.

While some fertility programs require psychological evaluation before attempting

pregnancy at advanced ages, the practice is not universal, and may even be seen, in some cases, as discrimination. But similar to medical risks, it is important for both the patient and provider to recognize and discuss any potential psychosocial concerns that may exist prior to initiation of treatment. The ASRM recommends psychosocial counseling on both long- and short-term consequences of parenting at advanced ages [4], as well as in situations where there may be concern for unsafe child-rearing environments [6]. If there are substantial concerns for parental or child outcomes, the provider may ethically decline services based on these concerns. But as with medical risks, providers must take great care to make these decisions objectively and free of bias.

Ethical Principles
When considering the ethical acceptability of medical treatments, it is important to view each scenario in light of the four basic principles of medical ethics: autonomy, beneficence, nonmaleficence, and justice.

Autonomy
Many advocates for the provision of ART in women over 40 argue that reproductive autonomy supports the idea that women can make independent decisions regarding their own reproduction, despite the opinion of the provider or society at large. In the setting of appropriate medical screening and counseling, the ASRM supports the reproductive freedom of women of ARA [4], arguing that women of advanced maternal age should enjoy the same autonomy as other high-risk groups. For example, it has been noted that the reproductive autonomy of younger women with life limiting illnesses is rarely questioned. This group of patients may also bear offspring that are subject to poor obstetric outcomes or early loss of a parent. In these cases, ART is usually supported rather than scrutinized, despite having potentially similar outcomes. Similarly, men of advanced paternal age enjoy reproductive autonomy, despite increased health risks and potential early parental loss.

Opponents of providing ART based solely on the principle of reproductive autonomy argue that patient autonomy should not be prioritized over fetal health, and the desires of the mother should not trump the overall well-being of the future child. The debate between autonomy and medical risk to mother or fetus often dictates a provider's philosophy behind providing ART to women of advanced ages. It is important to note that the degree to which reproductive autonomy is observed can also vary greatly depending on cultural values, religion, and societal norms. In many countries post-menopausal pregnancy is seen as unnatural or a disruption to the traditional family structure. In these cases, the societal values often override autonomy of the individual, and nationwide limits on ART are subject to much lower age limits.

Beneficence and Nonmaleficence

The principles of beneficence and nonmaleficence are very familiar to most physicians, as the core of medical training is to first do no harm. Assisted reproductive technology and pregnancy provide unique challenges when considering these principles because pregnancy itself comes with inherent risks that are exacerbated as age increases. When considering ART at elevated ages it is the physician's responsibility to assess and minimize the risks that exist, but the age at which the harm to benefit ratio becomes excessively dangerous is not always clear. Part of this assessment includes evaluation of absolute contraindications to pregnancy versus relative contraindications to pregnancy. In the case of absolute contraindications, the ethical principles of beneficence and nonmaleficence are easy to apply and interpret. But in cases with relative contraindications, the balance between benefit and harm is less clear. Ultimately, it is up to the physician to decide the balance they are willing to accept in order to honor the promise to first do no harm.

Justice

The issue of justice in the use of ART among women over 40 represents problems of fairness, access, and equality. Typically, these issues are considered in the healthcare setting in relation to *distributive justice* or fairness of allocation of resources, *utility* or restricting scare resources to those who have the highest chance of success, and *social justice* or the distribution of services and creation of guidelines/laws made in accordance with socially acceptable mores. Issues of distributive justice are twofold; the first being that in the

United States, access to ART is often restricted to those with higher incomes. The costs associated with ART range from $10,000 for each IVF cycle to upwards of $30,000 for the use of IVF and PGT. Some of these costs may be covered by a patient's insurance, but many are not. This means patients who are uninsured or underinsured may not be able to use ART. As such, even consultations about ART among women over 40 may be restricted to the wealthy. If one considers access to the use of ART a personal right, then there is potential discrimination against lower-income women of any age. The second half of distributive justice is related to access to care. Accessibility to reproductive specialists (REI) is not only about ability to pay but also the knowledge of where and how to access specialists. Reproductive specialists may be overabundant in cities such as New York City but less available in rural areas such as Wyoming or the Appalachian communities. Issues of utility may also be considered if one believes the use of ART represents "scarce" resources. Principle of utility would dictate that only women (and future children) who have the highest likelihood of success should be able to use ART, notwithstanding ability to pay [15]. If a woman needs to use donated oocytes should those eggs only go to those who have the highest potential for success, thus maximizing utility? If those principles hold true, some women will never have the chance to use ART. As Pennings argues, "If each individual is entitled to an equal opportunity to benefit from the healthcare system, then each woman has the right to receive oocytes, even with a very slim chance of becoming pregnant or having a live, healthy birth" [15]. At times, a threshold principle is used when considering the pros and cons of utility [16]. However, such thresholds imagine there is finite "line" between safe and harmful. Such lines are less clear when applied to ART. Further, the considerations of safety and harm apply in several contexts: the woman, the fetus/future child, and society.

The third aspect of justice, social considerations, is even more difficult to apply as societal and cultural mores differ not only between countries but also within smaller macro and microcosms such as religious affiliations, race, ethnicity, and even neighborhoods and workplaces. Issues of age or ageism are prevalent in multiple social contexts and vary in meaning in each context. For example, the average age of death for a woman in the United States is 78. Thus the likelihood of a woman having a child in her late 40s or early 50s and remaining alive until that child reaches the age of 18 is quite high. Concurrently, women who give birth under the age of 15 have a greater chance of dying during childbirth than any other age group, except those aged over 45. Contributing factors to death during childbirth include socio-economic status, parity, and access to adequate healthcare. Thus, factors of social justice and pregnancy/childbirth affect women of all ages. The odds of a woman dying in childbirth and the odds of a person dying an accidental death or death attributed to morbidities are inversely related to socioeconomic status, that is, the more wealth a person has the less likely they are to die from accident or disease. Thus, it may be likely that women whose wealth affords them the opportunity to seek ART at older ages are also more likely to see their child into adulthood.

References

1. The World Bank. Birth rate, crude (per 1,000 people). https://data.worldbank.org/indicator/SP .DYN.CBRT.IN.

2. Centers for Disease Control and Prevention. NCHS – Birth Rates for Females by Age Group: United States. https://data.cdc.gov/NCHS/NCHS-Birth-Rates-for-Females-by-Age-Group-United-S/ yt7u-eiyg/data.

3. American College of Obstetricians and Gynecologists' Committee on Obstetric Practice, Committee on Genetics, U.S. Food and Drug Administration. Committee Opinion No 671: Perinatal Risks Associated With Assisted Reproductive Technology. *Obstet. Gynecol.* 2016;**128**(3):e61–8.

4. Ethics Committee of the American Society for Reproductive Medicine. Oocyte or embryo donation to women of advanced reproductive age: an Ethics Committee opinion. *Fertil. Steril.* 2016;**106**:e3–e7.

5. Ethics Committee of the American Society for Reproductive Medicine. Provision of fertility services for women at increased risk of complications during fertility treatment or pregnancy: an Ethics Committee opinion. *Fertil. Steril.* 2016;**106**:1319–23.

6. Ethics Committee of the American Society for Reproductive Medicine. Child-rearing ability and the provision of fertility services: an Ethics Committee opinion. *Fertil. Steril.* 2017;**108**:944–7.

7. Calhaz-Jorge, C. *et al.* Survey on ART and IUI: legislation, regulation, funding and registries in European countries: The European IVF-monitoring Consortium (EIM) for the European Society of Human Reproduction and Embryology (ESHRE). *Hum. Reprod. Open* 2020;**2020**:hoz044.

8. Klitzman, R. L. How old is too old? Challenges faced by clinicians concerning age cutoffs for patients undergoing in vitro fertilization. *Fertil. Steril.* 2016;**106**:216–24.

9. Grotegut, C. A. *et al.* Medical and obstetric complications among pregnant women aged 45 and older. *PLoS One* 2014;**9**:e96237.

10. Sauer, M. V. Reproduction at an advanced maternal age and maternal health. *Fertil. Steril.* 2015;**103**:1136–43.

11. Zweifel, J. E., *et al.* Is it time to establish age restrictions in ART? *J. Assist. Reprod. Genet.* 2020;**37**:257–62.

12. Harrison, B. J. *et al.* Advanced maternal age: ethical and medical considerations for assisted reproductive technology. *Int. J. Womens Health* 2017;**9**:561–70.

13. Kocourková, J., *et al.* How old is too old? A contribution to the discussion on age limits for assisted reproduction technique access. *Reprod. Biomed. Online* 2015;**30**:482–92.

14. Zweifel, J. E. Donor conception from the viewpoint of the child: positives, negatives, and promoting the welfare of the child. *Fertil. Steril.* 2015;**104**:513–19.

15. Pennings, G. Distributive justice in the allocation of donor oocytes. *J. Assist. Reprod. Genet.* 2001;**18** (2):56–63.

16. Smajdor, A. How useful is the concept of the "harm threshold" in reproductive ethics and law? *Theor. Med. Bioeth.* 2014;**35**(5):321–36.

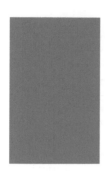

Epilogue

David B. Seifer and Dimitrios S. Nikolaou

Women have healthy babies in their 40s and the number presenting to antenatal services is increasing steadily. The statistics around maternal morbidity in the 40s are troubling. The number of women who are trying to conceive in their 40s and ask for help has also been increasing. What is possible today is significantly better than 15 years ago.

However, for those who practice medicine at the beginning of the third decade of the twenty-first century, reproductive aging represents a contemporary medical Gordian knot. At present, reproductive aging cannot be effectively reversed or stopped. It is controversial whether it can really be slowed. Some of the therapeutic approaches (i.e., stem cells, platelet-rich plasma injections, mitochondrial transplantation, in vitro gametogenesis, etc.) that are reviewed in the last chapter of this book may at some time in the future hold real promise for achieving what currently seems impossible. However, for now we can do our best to do what we can to optimize the fertility of those women with advanced reproductive age.

We believe the comprehensive approach that our team of experts have provided in this book articulate such approaches. The chapter on patient support and patient experience architecture includes the key steps of a comprehensive clinical strategy. The advances in cryobiology and the better understanding of "early ovarian ageing," combined with the wider application of ovarian reserve screening tools, have led to rethinking and redefining "family planning," or perhaps "fertility planning" which is more adaptive to the twenty-first century.

Success can have different meaning to different people. It must include the feeling of having been heard carefully, having tried properly, having achieved what was achievable, and, if not, the peace of mind that one was not dismissed. We hope that this book will contribute to the perspective and knowledge of those practitioners who care for their patients whose main fertility concerns center upon the hurdle of reproductive age.

David B. Seifer, MD
Dimitrios S. Nikolaou, MD

Index

Note: Page numbers followed by *f* indicate a figure on the corresponding page. Page numbers followed by *t* indicate a table on the corresponding page.